P9-ART-759

NSCA's Guide to Program Design

National Strength and Conditioning Association

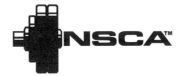

Jay R. Hoffman, PhD

University of Central Florida, Orlando

EDITOR

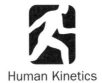

Human Kinetics

Library of Congress Cataloging-in-Publication Data

National Strength & Conditioning Association (U.S.)
 NSCA's guide to program design / National Strength and Conditioning Association ; Jay R. Hoffman, editor.
   p. ; cm. -- (Science of strength and conditioning series)
 Guide to program design
 Includes bibliographical references and index.
 ISBN-13: 978-0-7360-8402-4 (print)
 ISBN-10: 0-7360-8402-9 (print)
 I. Hoffman, Jay, 1961- II. Title. III. Title: Guide to program design. IV. Series: Science of strength and conditioning series.
 [DNLM: 1. Physical Education and Training--methods. 2. Athletic Performance. 3. Muscle Strength. 4. Program Development. QT 255]

 613.7--dc23
                    2011034871

ISBN-10: 0-7360-8402-9 (print)
ISBN-13: 978-0-7360-8402-4 (print)

Copyright © 2012 by the National Strength and Conditioning Association

All rights reserved. Except for use in a review, the reproduction or utilization of this work in any form or by any electronic, mechanical, or other means, now known or hereafter invented, including xerography, photocopying, and recording, and in any information storage and retrieval system, is forbidden without the written permission of the publisher.

The web addresses cited in this text were current as of July, 2011, unless otherwise noted.

Developmental Editor: Katherine Maurer; **Assistant Editors:** Steven Calderwood and Brendan Shea; **Copyeditor:** Joy Wotherspoon; **Indexer:** Betty Frizzell; **Permissions Manager:** Dalene Reeder; **Graphic Designers:** Nancy Rasmus and Fred Starbird; **Graphic Artist:** Denise Lowry; **Cover Designer:** Keith Blomberg; **Photographer (interior):** Neil Bernstein. Photo on p. 7 by Kelly Huff, photos on p. 31 and p. 202 by Tom Roberts. All photos © Human Kinetics; **Photo Asset Manager:** Laura Fitch; **Visual Production Assistant:** Joyce Brumfield; **Photo Production Manager:** Jason Allen; **Art Manager:** Kelly Hendren; **Associate Art Manager:** Alan L. Wilborn; **Art Style Development:** Jennifer Gibas; **Illustrations:** © Human Kinetics; **Printer:** Sheridan Books

We thank the National Strength and Conditioning Association in Colorado Springs, Colorado, for assistance in providing the location for the photo shoot for this book.

Printed in the United States of America   10 9 8 7 6 5 4 3 2 1

The paper in this book is certified under a sustainable forestry program.

Human Kinetics
Website: www.HumanKinetics.com

United States: Human Kinetics, P.O. Box 5076, Champaign, IL 61825-5076
800-747-4457
e-mail: humank@hkusa.com

Canada: Human Kinetics, 475 Devonshire Road Unit 100, Windsor, ON N8Y 2L5
800-465-7301 (in Canada only)
e-mail: info@hkcanada.com

Europe: Human Kinetics, 107 Bradford Road, Stanningley, Leeds LS28 6AT, United Kingdom
+44 (0) 113 255 5665
e-mail: hk@hkeurope.com

Australia: Human Kinetics, 57A Price Avenue, Lower Mitcham, South Australia 5062
08 8372 0999
e-mail: info@hkaustralia.com

New Zealand: Human Kinetics, P.O. Box 80, Torrens Park, South Australia 5062
0800 222 062
e-mail: info@hknewzealand.com

E4868

Science of Strength and Conditioning Series

NSCA's Guide to Sport and Exercise Nutrition

NSCA's Guide to Tests and Assessments

NSCA's Guide to Program Design

National Strength and Conditioning Association

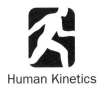

Human Kinetics

Contents

Preface

Jay R. Hoffman, PhD

In my 30 years as an athlete, coach, and scientist I have seen tremendous change in the field of strength and conditioning. Early in my career, strength and conditioning, at least in North America, was a phenomenon primarily associated with the sport of football. In fact, most strength coaches arose from that sport. When the strength and conditioning coach position became a paid one, it generally was limited to the football program. Many other sports shied away from the weight room because it was believed that resistance training would make their athletes muscle-bound and compromise their skill in playing basketball, baseball, or any other sport. It wasn't until the mid-1990s that strength coaches were employed by teams in both Major League Baseball and the National Basketball Association. Today, all professional teams in the major professional sports of the United States and all NCAA Division I athletic programs have full-time strength and conditioning professionals.

The National Strength and Conditioning Association (NSCA) has become an international standard setter in the field, with more than 30,000 members representing 52 countries. Through education, science, and of course the athletes who became the trend setters for strength and conditioning in their sports, the benefits associated with appropriately designed training programs are being realized. Athletes today are bigger, faster, stronger, and quicker due in large part to the training, instruction, and oversight they receive. Technological and dietary improvements have also helped in providing more effective, more specific, and safer training equipment and superior information on nutrition, all readily accessible to coaches and athletes. But even the most knowledgeable experts and best-equipped training centers will produce modest gains at best without sound, progressive, and appropriately challenging strength and conditioning programs to guide athletes' development.

Despite the proliferation of strength coach positions and the resources available to professionals and athletes, it appears that the basic mission of the NSCA is needed more than ever. Every year athletes are injured, or even die, during off-season conditioning. Some coaches are moving away from evidence-based research when developing their strength and conditioning programs; instead they are moving toward conditioning programs that purport to develop mental toughness or are inappropriately designed for the specific athlete at the specific time of year. Programs that are not based on scientific evidence can needlessly increase the risks associated with strength training and conditioning.

Fortunately, we have a wealth of experience and research to consult, which permits us to identify exactly what training regimen will produce the desired results for athletes of all types. This book presents guidance in designing scientifically based training programs. Chapters 1 and 2 provide the basis for a sound sport-specific strength and conditioning program by detailing the process of an athlete's needs analysis and evaluating the effectiveness of a training program. In chapter 3, warm-up recommendations for enhancing performance and preventing injury in all types of training programs are discussed.

Chapters 4 through 10 present a detailed discussion of program design for various types of training, including insights on developing athletes' strength, power, anaerobic conditioning, endurance, agility, speed, and balance. The research evidence for training recommendations is detailed and select drills and exercises are illustrated. Finally, in chapters 11 and 12, *NSCA's Guide to Program Design* brings it all together to show professionals how to design complete and effective training programs. Chapter 11 contains an in-depth discussion of the theory and practice of periodization. Chapter 12 discusses implementing the training program and presents real-world examples and numerous sample workouts. Throughout the rest of the text, cross-reference boxes direct readers to chapter 12, helping to make the connections between in-depth understanding of various training modes and implementation of the total program.

This book will help eliminate the guesswork and missteps that coaches and athletes find so frustrating. It also offers extensive reference lists of supporting research for all readers who wish to explore specific topics more deeply. Using this text, and drawing on the wealth of information on strength and conditioning now available, coaches and other strength and conditioning professionals can continue to design safe and effective programs for the populations and athletes they work with.

Acknowledgments

This book provides a bridge between a love of athletics and the desire to understand the optimal way to maximize human performance. This is precisely the mission that the National Strength and Conditioning Association has set for itself. It has been an honor to have worked with such passionate people whose primary goal is to share knowledge and ensure the dissemination of it so that coaches and athletes can achieve their goals and do so with minimal risk of injury. Thanks to all these outstanding contributors!

To Yaffa, Raquel, Mattan, and Ariel: If a man is judged by the character of his offspring and the love of his wife, then I have truly been blessed!

Athlete Needs Analysis

William J. Kraemer, PhD, CSCS, FNSCA
Brett A. Comstock, MA
James E. Clark, MS
Courtenay Dunn-Lewis, MA

By the early 1980s, research in the field of exercise science had demonstrated that changes in specific variables related to exercise influenced the type of adaptations and performance improvements seen. The concept of *acute program variables* was put forth to better describe all the components of a workout (18). These acute program variables, which have been well established over the past 25 years, consist of the following:

- Choice of exercise
- Order of exercise
- Resistance used
- Number of sets
- Amount of rest between sets and exercises

It had also been established by that time that an effective training program had to be tailored to the demands placed on athletes by their specific sport (19). The many choices within each of the domains of these acute program variables required a preliminary process in order to gain information about the sport and the athlete. The concept of a needs analysis was introduced, allowing the exercise-prescription process to reflect informed choices for each of the acute program variables and to design an appropriate program for an optimally periodized training program (21). This provided a theoretical paradigm for program design for different sports and, more importantly, for individual athletes.

A needs analysis answers three general questions:

1. What are the metabolic demands of the sport?
2. What are the biomechanical demands of the sport?
3. What are the common injuries observed in the sport profile?

The needs analysis, initial testing data, and evaluations of athletes and the sport allow for intelligent program design (9). This process, along with initial testing data, helps strength and conditioning professionals examine athletes' general fitness base, sport-specific fitness, and injury history, as well as the physiological and biomechanical demands of the sport and its potential risk for injury. By gathering this preliminary information, they can make informed choices in regard to program design, tests needed to monitor progress, and other evaluations necessary for athletes in a given sport (2). This allows them to better understand the needs of the strength and conditioning program and to develop a set of appropriate training goals (9). Thus, the ultimate goal of needs analysis is to develop a total conditioning program to improve athletic performance and reduce injuries (21).

Metabolic Demands of the Sport

Not all sports are performed under the same metabolic conditions. The predominant metabolic pathway varies depending on the demands of the sport. It can also be specific to the muscles being used. When a muscle is activated in the recruitment process to produce force, the amount of energy used and the predominant energy system source vary, yet most sports have an inherent, recognizable metabolic profile that ranges in nature from highly aerobic to highly anaerobic. As table 1.1 demonstrates, aerobic endurance and ultraendurance events (e.g., marathons or triathlons) are at one end of the spectrum, and very short-duration or explosive strength/power events (e.g., shot put, maximal clean and jerk) are at the other end. In between these two extremes are sports that use a combination of these metabolic systems during competition. Metabolism changes rapidly based on external demands, allowing dramatic shifts to the anaerobic system when sprinting and then to the aerobic system during recovery (e.g., a soccer player sprinting down the field and then jogging back to position when the ball goes downfield). Table 1.1 presents the general profile of energy dominance for various sports.

Although an emphasis on metabolic training appears to exist in the athletic realm, it is important to carefully evaluate the actual metabolic demands of the sport prior to prescribing exercise. The metabolic demands can be estimated as a total metabolic profile of the sport. One can estimate what the predominant metabolism will be for the primary muscles used, based on a time–motion analysis of the sport. For example, baseball's metabolic demands are predominately related to the ATP–CP system; thus, short rest

TABLE 1.1 Approximate Energy Demands for Various Sports

Sport	ATP–CP system	Lactic acid system	Aerobic system
American football	70	25	5
Archery	100	–	–
Auto racing	30	10	60
Basketball	20	20	60
Baseball	95	5	–
Bicycle racing (road)	10	10	80
Bowling	100	–	–
Boxing	30	45	25
Fencing	85	10	5
Field events	100	–	–
Field hockey	20	25	55
Gymnastics	90	5	5
Ice hockey	30	30	40
Lacrosse	20	25	55
Marathon	–	–	100
Rowing	10	40	50
Rugby	25	25	50
Skiing (downhill)	35	25	40
Soccer	15	25	60
Swimming (sprints)	75	25	–
Swimming (distances)	10	10	80
Skateboarding	80	10	10
Tennis	50	5	45
Track (long distance)	5	5	90
Track (middle distance)	15	50	35
Track (short sprints)	90	5	5
Volleyball	80	15	5
Wrestling	30	45	25

programs that place high demands on the lactic acid system (glycolysis) are really not needed (9, 21, 26).

Many training programs related to developing maximal strength and power require athletes to be rested and recovered when performing the workouts (20). Therefore, a program that places high demands on the lactic acid system and leads to fatigue can compromise other aspects of training. The often-prescribed short rest protocols are only one style of training within the multitude of workouts that can be designed for athletes. Thus, sport-specific conditioning should include attempts to train the same metabolic systems used in the sport. Furthermore, this method allows athletes to express strength and power within the context of metabolism for their sports.

Adenosine triphosphate (ATP) is the body's energy molecule. It is produced by the anaerobic and aerobic energy systems. All muscle fibers use ATP molecules as a source of fuel during exercise to produce chemical and, eventually, mechanical energy. ATP is a crucial requirement in the sliding filament mechanism of muscular contraction that produces force. Primary concerns in sports include the amount of ATP energy required, how rapidly it must be available, and whether the metabolic conditions present can be tolerated. Thus, conditioning programs should place a major emphasis on improving capabilities to produce energy and tolerating the associated metabolic demands of the sports (e.g., compare a 100 m race, an 800 m race, and a marathon).

Generally, the physiology of a sport can be described by the energetic demands of the sport (i.e., aerobic or anaerobic). Although different sports may be classified as aerobic or anaerobic, it is important to remember that no sporting competition will tax a single energetic system alone (see figure 1.1). Additionally, the idea of energetics can be extended further to include sprint, strength, power, and cardiorespiratory (aerobic) endurance sports. As athletes move through this cascade of energy and fuel systems, the level of oxygen required within the system goes from low (none needed to perform a given skill, such as lifting a heavy weight one time) to high, being predominantly dependent on the aerobic system for ATP production in order to sustain the activity (e.g., running a marathon).

The energy systems utilized by the body in training or during a sport are as follows:

- Phosphagens (ATP–CP system)
- Glycolysis (lactic acid system)
- Krebs cycle or citric acid cycle (aerobic system)

The ATP–CP system immediately supports muscular contraction, since it uses energy obtained from intramuscular stores of adenosine triphosphate (ATP) and creatine phosphate (CP). This system is typically utilized during short-duration, high-intensity physical activity. The other anaerobic system, more commonly known as the *lactic acid system*, is called *glycolysis*. Glycolysis results in ATP production from the breakdown of glucose in the sarcoplasm of muscle fibers. The glucose can be obtained from either blood glucose or intramuscular stores of glycogen. Therefore, it is a less rapid source of ATP energy than the ATP–CP system.

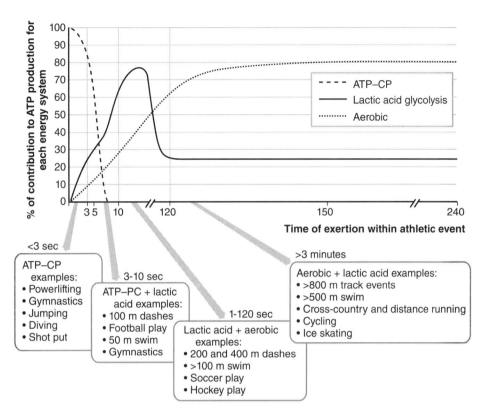

FIGURE 1.1 Contributions of the three energy systems to athletic performance over time. As the duration of a movement increases, the primary energy system at work shifts from the ATP–CP system, to the lactic acid (glycolysis) system, and, finally, to the aerobic system.

Most often referred to as the *Krebs cycle* or the *citric acid cycle*, the aerobic system is the most robust system for producing ATP energy, yet it is the slowest in getting ATP to the active musculature. The aerobic system is obviously very important for performing cardiorespiratory endurance activities, due to its ability to produce large amounts of ATP without generating fatiguing products. It differs from glycolysis in that carbohydrates, fats, and proteins can all enter into the aerobic cycle for breakdown and the eventual production of ATP through the electron transport system in the mitochondria.

Generally, the ATP–CP cycle begins to fatigue and exhaust itself roughly 6 seconds after exercise is begun. Once exercise duration extends beyond this time, the glycolytic pathway begins to take over, providing the energy required for the athlete to continue. However, the glycolytic pathway is a short-lived energy system, lasting only a few minutes. This means that if the exercise intensity allows athletes to sustain activity for longer than a minute or two, then they need to shift predominantly into the final energy system (aerobic metabolism) for support, even when exercising intensely.

Regardless of the sport and the position played, athletes must be able to meet, and preferably exceed, the metabolic demands for the sport. This simply means that athletes need to be able to withstand the stresses (metabolic, biomechanical, and physical) of the sport for the duration of competition. A properly designed training program should have metabolic demands that approximate those of the sport. However, because of the timing of individual movements within the event, custom exercises that increase the ability to tolerate metabolic demands may need to be prescribed. For example, consider the large differences in metabolic demand between a midfielder and a goaltender in soccer or between a forward and a goalie in ice hockey. The conditioning program should be specific to the physiological analysis of each position.

In order to determine the most appropriate training and testing protocols and requirements for individual athletes, the balance between the energy systems and fuels used within a sport must be understood. Some workouts within a periodized training program should mimic the sport metabolism. For example, wrestlers need to develop strength and power, but they also need to perform conditioning activities that utilize short rest periods in order to develop buffering capabilities so that they can express their maximal muscular strength and power under the metabolic conditions of the sport (i.e., high levels of lactic acid and lower blood–pH values) (24). This is why an effective training program must incorporate a variety of workouts and why different athletes require different programs (9).

Biomechanical Demands of the Sport

The next step in the needs analysis is a basic biomechanical assessment, based on the types of generalized body and limb movements that are encountered during an athletic event. This includes the position of the body in space, the timing and coordination of various parts of the body needed to execute the desired movements, the speed of the athlete's body (or parts of the body) during the desired movement, and the length of time of exertion for the athlete (6). Along with an examination of the primary muscle actions used and the planes of motion in which they take place (i.e., sagittal, frontal, transverse), strength and conditioning coaches can examine the pattern of movement, the joints involved during competition, the pattern of muscle actions, and the planes of movement in which actions take place.

By undertaking this very basic biomechanical analysis of the athletic movements required for the sport, a strength and conditioning professional can determine key aspects of the movement, including the type of movements involved, the range of motion (ROM) of joints during activity, the required speed of movement, the pattern of muscle action during movements, and the metabolic demands of the sport or event based on the length of time of each exertion within the athletic event (34). These factors are important when it comes to choosing exercises to be used in a resistance training program. This analysis of the planes of motion and the type of muscle actions used will help strength and conditioning professionals choose resistance exercises that are biomechanically similar to the demands of the sport. From these generalized patterns of movement, they can focus on the specific movements required to perform various sport skills.

Describing Sport Movements

The general pattern of movement will be described as either static or dynamic within a specific plane or planes of movement (34). Within dynamic movement nomenclature, movement can be further described as either *open* or *closed* (34). When the movement is open, the hand or foot will be free to move and the body will remain relatively static (see figure 1.2). In a closed movement, the hand or foot is relatively static and the body moves relatively freely (see figure 1.3).

Three primary types of muscle actions are used in sport skills (isometric, concentric, and eccentric). Isometric action results in no change in the length of the muscle (the muscle produces force that is equal to the force being applied to the bony attachment of the muscle). The concentric movement of the muscle decreases the length of the muscle (the muscle produces more force than is being applied to the bony attachment of the muscle). Eccentric movement

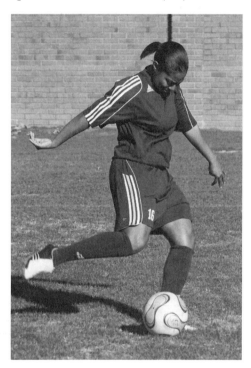

FIGURE 1.2 Kicking a soccer ball is an example of an open-chain sport movement.

results in a lengthening of the muscle (the force applied to the bony attachment of the muscle is greater than the force produced by the muscle). An understanding of these three types of action will ensure that exercises are achieving the desired effect.

Along with the type of movement, another consideration is the speed of movement, or angular velocity of the involved joint. The description for speed of movement is generally given in reference to limb movement or rotational speed of the body around a central (vertebral) axis (34). Although accurately measuring speed of movement requires sophisticated equipment, strength and conditioning professionals can use their best

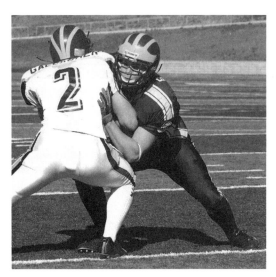

FIGURE 1.3 American football linemen pushing against each other during a block is an example of a closed-chain sport movement.

judgment to estimate the rate of speed that athletes need to utilize in the sport. The important issue with the analysis of speed of movement is to observe joints that are vital to movements within the action. For a majority of athletic movements, this entails observing speed of movement at the hip, knee, or ankle of the leg and at the shoulder, elbow, wrist, or hand of the arm (34). Further, attention should be paid to the positioning of the trunk and the movement of the torso throughout all athletic movements (6, 33, 34).

In addition to the type and speed of movement, there must also be consideration for the speed of muscle force development that is required both for performing athletic movement and stabilizing the torso and body throughout (6, 33) (e.g., holding the torso upright during a spiking motion in volleyball). Through careful analysis of the movement patterns, strength and conditioning coaches can determine and distinguish when the muscle action is causing a movement to occur, stabilizing the body in a static position, or controlling the loading of a limb from an external force (33, 34). It can be generally understood that the acceleration of the body or limb of the body will be done through a concentric contraction, while the deceleration of the body or limb of the body will be done through an eccentric contraction (34). When the body or limb is being stabilized without movement, the contraction type is considered to be isometric (34).

Furthermore, by analyzing movements and muscle actions within the athlete's sport, strength and conditioning professionals can also determine the energy system being utilized (27). They can use motion analysis to determine the length of time for each of the individual points of exertion so that the conditioning program can match the energetic demands of the sport (3, 5, 23). The area of interest for strength and conditioning professionals with this type of analysis is to determine the amount of time that the athlete will be actively engaged in an athletic movement during a sporting event. This analysis gives them a guide to follow for establishing the metabolic demands for the conditioning program as it relates to time of exertion, amount of rest time available within a sporting event, and the type of muscular forces the athlete is required to produce (e.g., a shot put versus a wrestling match versus a 10K race). From this time analysis, strength and conditioning professionals can manipulate various training variables to generate regimens that provide both the neurological and metabolic stresses (3-5, 7, 23) that allow adaptations related to the needs of the sport to be made (19, 32).

Biomechanical Analysis in Practice

For the purpose of understanding the movement being analyzed, strength and conditioning professionals should use the following four questions. First, what are the patterns of movement (i.e., concentric, eccentric, or isometric), and in which planes do they take place? Second, what joints are involved during the activity? Third, what muscles are recruited, and what are the muscle actions? Finally, what is the duration of time that the athlete will be actively engaged in the athletic event? With these key questions, strength and conditioning professionals can determine the demands placed on the body during the sport (6, 33, 34). The ultimate goal of analysis is to manipulate and match the acute variables that govern the program's design to match the metabolism and movements involved in the sport.

Typically, biomechanical evaluations require strength and conditioning professionals to analyze videos of athletes performing their sports. Those without access to advanced video equipment can accomplish this type of analysis by watching simple video of athletes during practices or games. The following are some very basic procedures for video analysis that strength and conditioning professionals can follow (9).

1. View a video of an athletic performance or activity.

2. Select a specific movement in the sport (e.g., a jump shot in basketball or a takedown in wrestling). To completely analyze the sport, several movements or skills may need to be examined. Look at the entire sequence of competition to get a feel for the demands of the sport.

3. Identify the joints around which the most intense muscular actions occur. Running and jumping, for example, involve intense muscle actions at the knee, hip, and ankle. Intense exertion doesn't necessarily involve movement. Considerable isometric force may have to be applied to keep a joint from flexing or extending under external stress.

4. Determine whether the movement is concentric, isometric, or eccentric.

5. For each joint identified above, determine the range of angular motion. Observe how the joint angle changes throughout the movement and which plane it occurs in.

6. Try to determine where the most intense effort occurs within the range of motion around each particular joint. Sometimes facial grimaces or tense muscles seen on video can help identify points of peak intensity.

7. Estimate the velocity of movement in the early, middle, and late phases in the range of motion. If using video, determine the time between frames to examine the movement over the time of the activity.

8. Select exercises to match the limb's ranges of motion and angular velocities, making sure that the exercises are appropriately concentric, isometric, or eccentric.

Through this type of biomechanical analysis, strength and conditioning professionals can make sure that training programs reflect these demands (see table 1.2).

It is important to remember that although analyzing sporting movements and matching the proper exercises in the weight room are vital to the sport-specific nature of resistance training programs, many exercises might be considered universal in that all athletes need them. These exercises include squats, pulling motions (e.g., hang cleans), and presses, such as the bench press. Such exercises provide the core around which a program is built. Integration of whole-body, multijoint exercise movements is vital because single-joint exercises alone cannot improve neurological coordination between joints.

Injury Risks of the Sport

Before discussing injury prevention and how to use a needs analysis to design a program that diminishes the risk of injury, it may be important to step back and review some of the basic concepts of injury and risk for athletes (3, 5, 7, 18, 19, 27). Although it may be defined in many ways, an *injury* is generally any trauma to the body. In athletics, the majority of injuries affect the musculoskeletal system (bones, ligaments, muscles, and tendons), while additional injuries may include the neurological and cardiopulmonary systems (concussions, asthma, and heart attacks). For the most part, an exercise regimen can be designed by analyzing the biomechanical and metabolic demands of the sport and using this information to reduce the risk of injuries that can occur. Although risk of injury can be diminished through needs analysis, proper programming, and periodization of training programs, it must be remembered that sometimes injury is unavoidable.

Musculoskeletal injuries can occur due to either mechanical overload or repetitive overuse of a joint, limb, or muscle group. Mechanical overload injuries can be categorized as *contact* (two athletes hitting each other or an object hitting an athlete) or *noncontact* (athlete is injured without direct contact with another athlete or object). All types of injuries can be addressed within proper exercise program design, but they will be addressed in different fashions based on the exercises utilized to reduce the risk for that particular type of injury.

TABLE 1.2 Patterns of Biomechanical Movement

Type of movement	Descriptive analysis	Type of movement	Descriptive analysis
Flexion	• Movement of the hand or foot toward the torso • Movement of the arm or leg in front of the body	Supination	• Turning the hand so that the palm faces away from the torso (toward the sky) • Turning the foot so that the sole of the foot faces away from the ground (increasing the arch of the foot)
Extension	• Movement of the hand or foot away from the torso • Movement of the arm or leg behind the body	Pronation	• Turning the hand so that the palm faces the torso (toward the ground) • Turning the foot so that the sole of the foot faces the ground (decreasing the arch of the foot)
Abduction	Movement of the arm or leg away from the midline of the body	Inversion	Turning the foot so that the big toe moves inward and toward the nose
Adduction	Movement of the arm or leg toward the midline of the body	Eversion	Turning the foot so that the little toe moves out and toward the nose
Internal (medial) rotation	Inward rotation of the humerus or femur (at the shoulder or hip joint, respectively)	Deviation	Gliding the wrist and hand toward either the thumb side (radial) or pinky-finger side (ulnar)
External (lateral) rotation	Outward rotation of the humerus or femur (at the shoulder or hip joint, respectively)	Circumduction	Movement of the shoulder joint in all directions, making a circular action around the arm
Protraction	Rounding the shoulders (allowing the shoulder blades to move away from each other)	Rotation	• Circular movement of the limb or part of the limb • Movement of the torso around the vertebral column (vertebral rotation)
Retraction	Bringing the shoulder blades in close proximity to each other	Horizontal abduction/ adduction	Movement of the arm or leg: • Toward the midline (adduction) • Away from midline (abduction) while holding it in a flexed position
Elevation	Raising the joint	Depression	Lowering the joint

Regardless of the type of injury, most injuries seem to coincide with two factors. First, injury occurrence increases when an athlete becomes fatigued. Second, the rate of injury increases when the athlete experiences tissue fatigue (where the joint, bone, ligament, tendon, or muscle cannot respond to the forces placed on it). This phenomenon can be thought of as a fatigue-induced cascade of events, which begins with fatigue of either the central or local tissue and results in injury (1, 2).

In terms of biomechanical demands, injury prevention should be based on how accidents typically occur in the sport. Two primary means exist for athletic injury in sports: contact injuries and noncontact injuries. The difference between the two is not the type of injury that the athlete may suffer; it lies in the mechanism of injury. All contact injuries come from a limb or joint being exposed to an excessive load that is caused by an external force (e.g., a tackle in American football hits a knee). From this excessive load, the tissue around the limb or joint fails to meet the demand and becomes injured (most notable are fractures to bones or ligament ruptures). Most noncontact injuries occur during an acceleration of movement (either speeding up or slowing down). They are more readily seen in the change-of-direction movements that occur at various points within a competition (e.g., a running back in American football who is changing direction plants his leg while moving at full speed). Outside of acceleration, noncontact injuries also occur through overuse of certain muscles, muscle groups, tendons, or ligament structures of the body, based on the demand of the sport.

Needs Analysis for Injury Prevention

Regardless of the sport, a cascade of events often eventually leads to injuries (see figure 1.4). For example, for wrestlers, reducing fatigue or learning to better tolerate the fatigue processes during practice and competition is the easiest way to prevent injury (29, 36, 37). By understanding the means by which athletes encounter risk, strength and conditioning professionals can integrate exercise programs that may offset one of the steps toward injuries (e.g., short rest circuits for wrestlers help them develop buffering capacities to offset the decreases in pH that are related to fatigue).

When determining how injury prevention fits within the needs analysis of a sport, strength and conditioning professionals must ask the following questions. First, how likely is an injury to occur in the sport? Second, what

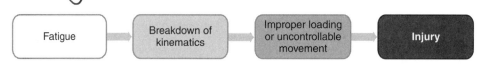

FIGURE 1.4 Sport injuries are often the result of several interconnected factors. Fatigue can lead to poor technique or body positioning, which, combined with an overload resulting from contact or poor positioning, leads to injury.

are the common injury sites and how are these injuries most likely to occur? Third, which athletes are most prone to these risks for injury? Fourth, how can an exercise program be developed that will diminish these risks? This is where strength and conditioning professionals can work with athletic trainers and team physicians to get a handle on each athlete's injury or medical status and to integrate a training program for injury prevention.

The role of prevention within athletics is to design programs that address the need for reducing the risk of injury during competition. This is truly a team approach. It needs to combine the skills and knowledge of the team physician, the sports medical staff (i.e., athletic trainer and physical therapists), the strength and conditioning professional, and the sport coaching staff. Within this team approach, the overall needs analysis should focus on the general concept of what an injury is and how it occurs for a particular athlete, all the while addressing the following questions as they relate to that specific person:

- How is the athlete predisposed to injury within the sport?
- Is this athlete at greater risk based on a predisposition to injury?
- When will injuries most likely occur during the athletic event?
- Is the athlete recovering from an acute or chronic injury that can affect athletic performance?

Biomechanical observations show where the athlete is most at risk for injury, based on the demands of the sport. They will also demonstrate how to counteract the risk of injury through strength training. Strength and conditioning professionals must keep in mind that although different sports may have similar injury profiles, each sport has different demands that change the required training stimuli athletes need to encounter during training to decrease the risk for injury. Table 1.3 shows some common injuries by sport and position.

This part of the analysis should include a careful examination of the individual athlete's injury and training history. Does the athlete reflect or deviate from the expectations of the sport in terms of past injuries? Some athletes are more or less prone to injury than others. In addition, evidence-based predictions of injury that use testing or profile parameters (e.g., body fat, exercise performances, core strength) are an emerging trend in athletic training that should be discussed with the athletic trainer and included in a needs analysis.

The strength and conditioning professional and athlete should also use the injury-prevention portion of the needs analysis to develop testing methods for aspects of sports performance that are not normally addressed in other phases. This additional portion should examine passive, static, and dynamic ranges of motion that the athlete is able to attain in many positions. Such analysis can be done by having the athlete perform various exercise-related

TABLE 1.3 Common Injuries by Sport and Position

Sport	Position	Type of injury[1]
Baseball and softball	Pitcher	Rotator cuff tendinitis Medial elbow strain/sprain Trunk rotator strain Knee sprain (ACL/MCL)
	Infielder/outfielder	Knee sprain (ACL/MCL) Ankle inversion sprain Trunk rotator strain Medial elbow strain/sprain
	Catcher	Knee sprain, patella-femoral pain Knee meniscus injury Rotator cuff tendinitis Muscle strain (especially lower body)
Basketball	All	Knee sprain (ACL/MCL) Patella tendinitis Ankle inversion sprain Muscle strain (especially lower body)
American football and rugby	Quarterback (American football)	Rotator cuff tendinitis Medial elbow sprain/strain Knee sprain (ACL/MCL) Shoulder dislocation/separation Ankle inversion injury
	All other positions*	Knee sprain (PCL) Vertebrae compression Shoulder dislocation/separation Hand and wrist sprain/strain
Football (soccer)	All	Ankle inversion sprain Knee sprain (ACL/MCL) Patella-femoral injury
Gymnastics	N/A	Muscle strain Knee sprain Shoulder tendinitis Ankle inversion Vertebrae compression Hip strain Shoulder separation Elbow sprain/strain

Sport	Position	Type of injury[1]
Hockey (field or ice) and lacrosse	Goalie	Groin strain Knee sprain (ACL/MCL, PCL/LCL) Trunk rotator strain Hip flexor strain Hand and wrist sprain
	All other positions*	Vertebrae compression Foot and ankle sprains/strains Shoulder dislocation/separation
Running (cross-country and distance)	N/A	Plantar fasciitis Iliotibal band tendinitis Patella tendinitis Knee bursitis
Swimming	N/A	Shoulder tendinitis
Tennis	N/A	Ankle sprain Muscle strain Knee sprain Hip bursitis Elbow tendinitis Inflammation of elbow ligaments
Track (sprinting or mid-distance)	N/A	Ankle sprain Muscle strain Knee sprain Hip bursitis
Water polo	All	Shoulder tendinitis Muscle strain
Wrestling	N/A	Muscle strain Shoulder sprain Shoulder dislocation Vertebrae compression Hand and wrist sprain Knee sprain

*Denotes that injuries are in addition to those listed for a single position within the sport for all other positions.

[1]These are examples of injury types that can occur within the sport. They are not an indication of specific diagnoses that can occur. This list is only a sample. It does not include all injuries that may occur in the sport. *Type of injury* denotes the major categories of injuries that can be seen by athletes within a position for a given sport. This list is given as an indication for direction of training as it relates to injury prevention.

ACL = anterior cruciate ligament; MCL = medial collateral ligament; PCL = posterior cruciate ligament; LCL = lateral collateral ligament.

movements while the strength and conditioning professional notes a deficit in the athlete's ability to attain the desired range of motion. Additionally, the strength and conditioning professional should take time to analyze the athlete's movements during training in the weight room. This will provide insight on the athlete's movement patterns, both statically and dynamically. The strength and conditioning professional will then be able to prescribe the exercises that will best address deficits in the desired muscle action, posture, or ROM (2).

When the risk of injury within a sport is combined with its biomechanical analysis, this information allows strength and conditioning professionals to set definable risks of injury based on the athletic position within a sport (2). For example, baseball pitchers are typically at a greater risk for elbow and shoulder injuries (primarily due to overuse) than first basemen. The relationship between gender and the risk of injury has left room for debate (4, 5, 28). However, trends for gender difference in injury rates within a sport do exist. Using the type of injuries that occur based on gender, sport, and position played, exercise protocols can be implemented to minimize the risk of properly periodized training programs.

With the advent of pretesting and training preparation for athletes, many strength and conditioning professionals have been pushed outside of their realm of expertise. They may need to work with members of a sports medicine team (e.g., team physician, athletic trainers, and physical therapists) to integrate measures that might allow them to better manage the chance of injury for each athlete by using evidence-based medical practices for identifying risk. As previously noted, this is an emerging science within athletic medicine. Strength and conditioning professionals should use this information to enhance the adaptations of each athlete at risk by incorporating exercises into the program to achieve higher adaptations (e.g., improved core strength, improved upper back strength, improved body composition, and so on) (10). This will provide the *prehabilitation effect* often referred to in the sports medicine community (30).

By using this information, any strength and conditioning professional can use a needs analysis to establish an injury-prevention program that will ultimately improve the strength and endurance of athletes' musculoskeletal and cardiorespiratory systems. This approach will also prevent fatigue and injury within the body.

Athletes Recovering From Injury

Athletes recovering from an existing injury may require the manipulation of training stimuli in multiple directions within a single program (21, 23). For example, the program may be able to make athletes bigger, faster, and stronger, despite their inability to perform full squats due to a prior knee or ankle injury. Recovery from injury requires making adjustments in the training regimen that will allow healing from the tissue trauma. As previously stated, in this situation, sport coaches need to use the sports medicine team (team physician, athletic trainers, physical therapists, and the strength and conditioning professional) to appropriately recognize and apply the training stimulus that the athlete will need to both recover from the injury and to improve performance (21, 23, 35).

Strength and conditioning professionals must examine both the training history and the injury profile of each athlete. This examination should involve input from all members of the sports medicine team who are involved with the injury-prevention portion of the program. Furthermore, by knowing the training history and injury profile, the strength and conditioning professional can adjust exercises, as previously mentioned with the squatting example, so that the athlete can still participate in training without causing further stress to the body (25).

Integrating the Needs Analysis

Before designing a training program, strength and conditioning professionals must consider the needs of the athlete based on the demands of the sport, position played on the team, genetic and morphological differences, and any previous injuries or medical conditions (13, 15-17). One key aspect to remember when developing the training program is the athlete's training history. The first aspect of this assessment is to catalogue previous training and the point in the training calendar when the athlete begins training. In completing this assessment, the strength and conditioning professional should talk with athletes to determine what they have been doing in their previous strength training, their athletic history, their injury history, and any other questions that may seem pertinent to forming a comprehensive background profile. Testing is also important to assess sport-fitness status, develop injury-prediction models, motivate athletes to improve or maintain a given fitness parameter, examine the effectiveness of a conditioning program, and to motivate athletes to take responsibility for their physical development in order to prevent injuries and improve their physical potential and performance. The maturity of the athlete and the amount of prior training and competition will affect the comprehensive approach.

The strength and conditioning professional is faced with the realities of the length of time allotted to train, the facilities available, and the training goals of each athlete (9). These goals should always be based in facts and scientific data, not simply in philosophy. The best indicator of how well programming goals have been met is to evaluate how closely the training program matched the demands of the sport. Training variables must be manipulated so that training is specific to the

For more information on constructing an integrated and periodized annual training plan, see chapter 12.

muscle actions, muscle groups, movement group, velocity, and energy system required for the sport. It sounds intuitive to say that a training program should focus on the areas the athlete wants to improve. This concept is generally accepted, and yet it is sometimes ignored. The needs analysis will help determine the needed areas of emphasis.

With a full understanding of the physiological demands of the sport, the strength and conditioning professional can develop a program that will enhance the athletes' physiological capacity for the sport, yet not push them into a pattern of overuse that can set them up for injury. Again, knowledge of the athletes' personal and competitive schedules and the use of periodized training are vital in this process. This is especially important when sport governing organizations (e.g., National Collegiate Athletic Association) limit practice time. Thus, sport coaches may be forced to compete with the strength and conditioning professional for valuable training time.

Too often, sport coaches do not allow appropriate time for rest and recovery, consequently overloading athletes with too much practice (e.g., often soccer [football] coaches scrimmage too much and spend too much time with running conditioning drills, sacrificing time for strength and power training). This behavior may predispose athletes to overuse or noncontact injuries by reducing the body's time to repair and recover from the stresses of exercise and activity. By analyzing the exertion-to-rest intervals, the strength and conditioning professional can determine which types of exercises can help develop both athletic prowess within a competition model and methods for recovery within and between competitions. Identifying the potential recovery problems is part of the process. From that point, solutions must be devised to ensure the athlete can meet the demands of practice, competition, and recovery.

Now that the foundational information concerning metabolic demands of the sport, biomechanics, and injury prevention has been reviewed, this information must be used in each athlete's workouts and conditioning program. Strength and conditioning professionals have a multitude of information to gather and consider. It is their duty to spend time understanding the fundamentals, putting them into practice, and re-evaluating and changing the program to meet the demands of various sports.

Functional and Nonfunctional Overreaching and Overtraining

Strength and conditioning professionals must manipulate exercise selection and tailor training stimuli to attain the desired adaptations for a particular sport (9, 23). When training variables and exercise selection are manipulated, a stimulus is created that varies based on the goal of training (i.e., hypertrophy, power, strength, local muscular endurance, or capacity for cardiorespiratory endurance of the musculoskeletal system). This forces the athlete to adapt in response to the training program through neurological, structural, and hormonal changes. These changes are only achieved by stressing the athlete beyond comfort levels (typically called *overload*).

By providing overload in the training program, strength and conditioning professionals ensure that the athlete will functionally overreach within the training program and progress as expected (11, 12, 14). Thus, a staircase effect results. The athlete experiences acute fatigue and a temporary reduction in performance, but quickly returns to normal or even slightly increased function (9). With long-term overreaching, the body's functional capabilities may be suppressed for several days. However, they rebound (i.e., increase beyond pretraining values) dramatically when the overreaching stimulus is removed (31). Here, the strength and conditioning professional is in control of this positive adaptation, or the structural and functional differences that occur with training (37).

 The manipulation of training variables is a delicate balancing act. Close monitoring of both workout logs and testing is required. If manipulation of the training variables is not tailored correctly to the desired adaptations and specific training goals, the athlete will experience symptoms of nonfunctional overreach. In this scenario, the athlete's body will have the same neurological, structural, and hormonal responses to exercise as with functional overreach, but he will be unable to positively adapt without rest. Performance will begin to suffer and some training adaptations may be lost. This means that the total conditioning program is flawed and that the athlete is not successfully adapting or maintaining functional capabilities or body composition (22). If this process continues, the athlete can enter into an overtraining syndrome, and may need months to recover performance capabilities (11) (see figure 1.5).

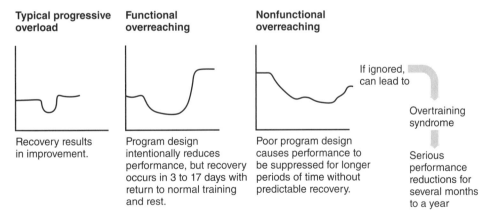

FIGURE 1.5 Functional overreaching results in a temporary drop in performance, followed by adaptation and performance gains. If this pattern does not occur, though, it could be a sign of nonfunctional overreaching. Over time, this could result in overtraining syndrome and a prolonged drop in performance.

Compatibility of Concurrent Training Programs

Once the design of a program is complete, strength and conditioning professionals must consider how to integrate various training goals into the total conditioning program, especially when both resistance training and a high element of cardiorespiratory endurance training are involved.

It has been shown that when athletes perform resistance and cardiorespiratory training simultaneously at high intensity, increases in adaptations to muscle size and power are compromised (8, 25). In addition, some sport coaches use too much aerobic conditioning or think it is necessary to develop an aerobic base. In fact, short-distance sprint-interval programs can be used to accomplish the same goals (9). Soccer (football), basketball, hockey, field hockey, lacrosse, and rugby all have important speed-endurance requirements. However, professionals should not diminish the speed and power components required for many sports by using too much aerobic conditioning training. In contrast, athletes in aerobic endurance sports benefit from heavy resistance training because of the need to strengthen tissues and prevent injury. When done appropriately, it has been shown to positively affect aerobic endurance performance (8, 25).

Another factor that might influence the compatibility of exercise selection is the need to incorporate speed and agility training (5) and sport-specific activities into the training program. Therefore, the judgment on compatibility of training should focus on two issues. First, strength and conditioning professionals should review their analysis on the physiological and biomechanical demands of the sport and the position of the athlete to evaluate the power, strength, and cardiorespiratory endurance demands that must be met. Second, they should determine and monitor with testing what level of detriment, if any, to performance will occur if cardiorespiratory endurance and resistance training are combined within the program. Proper periodization and rest periods are important to recovery and reduce overtraining.

SUMMARY POINTS

- Strength and conditioning professionals must carefully evaluate the individual athlete and the sport in order to understand the needs within a resistance training program and the demands of a total conditioning program.

- The essential aspects of a needs analysis for any athlete include the metabolic demands, biomechanical demands, and potential injury risks of the sport.

- Integrating the resistance training program with other conditioning activities is an important aspect for total conditioning. Training goals must be prioritized, training must be periodized, and nonfunctional overreaching and overtraining must be addressed.

- Professionals must be dedicated to improving the physical development of athletes within the construct of their age, psychological development, physical toleration of training, and proper progression of the program. As such, a needs analysis is a vital part of the design of any conditioning program, especially the resistance training program (9).

2

Athlete Testing and Program Evaluation

Jay R. Hoffman, PhD, CSCS*D, FNSCA

The development of strength and conditioning programs is based on scientific evidence gathered through quantitative assessment. In part, the science of coaching involves appropriately interpreting results from assessment programs and filtering this information to the end user (either the athlete or sport coach). A number of justifications for program evaluation exist. It can help strength and conditioning professionals develop athletic performance profiles for specific sports, evaluate the effectiveness of specific training paradigms and athletes' potential for success in a specific sport or position, and set training goals for both teams and individual athletes. This chapter focuses on developing an assessment program, including selecting and administering tests, properly interpreting assessments, and understanding popular laboratory and field tests used to evaluate athletes.

The development of an evidence-based training program is connected to the needs analysis of a sport (see chapter 1). However, to understand the basic physical requirements of a sport, an athletic profile must be developed. The development of this profile requires a detailed battery of testing that provide a thorough analysis of all components comprising athletic performance (i.e., strength, anaerobic power, speed, agility, maximal aerobic capacity and endurance, and body composition). Results from this assessment can determine the relevance and importance of each fitness component for a particular sport. It can also allow appropriate emphasis to be placed on that specific variable in the athlete's training program. A sport-specific athletic profile establishes standards that can be used to predict future success in that sport and to assist in player selection. As discussed previously, both athletes and strength and conditioning professionals can use the sport-specific profile as a motivational tool and to establish training goals by comparing the results with normative data from similar athletic populations. Performance testing can also be used to provide baseline data for individual exercise prescription, to evaluate the efficacy of specific training programs, and to assist in issues relating to recovery from injury and return to play.

Factors That Affect Performance Testing

Athlete evaluation needs to be interpreted in relation to a number of factors. When comparing athletes to one another or when comparing the performance results of a single athlete, the strength and conditioning professional must understand that test results are influenced by several factors. These include body size, muscle-fiber type, the training status of the athlete, and the specificity, relevance, validity, and reliability of the test.

Body Size

In general, strength is positively related to body size. That is, larger athletes are stronger than smaller athletes. For sports that do not have a weight class, absolute strength is an appropriate way to compare athletes. However, sometimes reporting strength relative to body mass may be more appropriate, especially when comparing athletes of varying mass on strength and power performance.

The issue of body size is also seen in other performance measures. The importance of this can be easily understood when examining vertical jump height and power performance. Two athletes, one weighing 198 pounds (90 kg) and the other 242 pounds (110 kg), are evaluated for lower body power with a vertical jump test. Both athletes jumped 27 inches (68.6 cm). However, which athlete is more powerful? Based on jump height alone, one may assume that both athletes have similar lower body power. However, if power relative to the person's body mass is examined, then the heavier athlete was much more powerful. The heavier athlete jumped the same distance but with a heavier load. If you recall that power is equal to force $\times$ velocity, the greater weight (force) resulted in greater power development. The way the data are examined can result in two substantially different outcomes!

Fiber Type Composition

The contractile properties of muscles play a significant role in their ability to generate power, sustain performance, and delay fatigue. Athletes with a higher percentage of fast-twitch fibers have the inherent ability to produce greater force and faster contraction velocity (23). In contrast, athletes whose muscles are composed primarily of slow-twitch fibers have a slower rate of fatigue but do not perform as well on strength and power assessments. These athletes will find more success in aerobic endurance sports. Athletes have very little ability to significantly alter their fiber-type composition through training. Therefore, in evaluating athletic speed or agility, it needs to be recognized that athlete's physiological limitations will influence the extent of their improvement. Although it may be possible to make a slow athlete faster, it is highly unlikely that a strength and conditioning professional can make a slow athlete fast.

Training Status

The training experience of the athlete determines to a great extent the magnitude of potential performance improvements. The greater the training experience, the smaller the potential for achieving performance gains (see figure 2.1). For athletes with limited training experience, the capacity for improvement will be quite high. However, as the duration of training increases, the rate of improvement in performance declines. As training continues further, changes in performance are difficult to achieve. Athletes will appear to have reached a plateau. This plateau may be considered a genetic ceiling, suggesting that performance improvements at this level are limited to the athletes' physiological makeup. Strength and conditioning professionals should also be aware that athletes with a high ability level, regardless of training status, may also be limited in terms of attaining significant performance improvements, even when participating in training programs for the first time (25, 27). Thus, strength and conditioning professionals must understand where their athletes sit on the training curve, and set training goals based on realistic expectations.

Recognizing the athlete's experience level is also essential for interpreting performance results. For instance, in a one-year investigation of elite

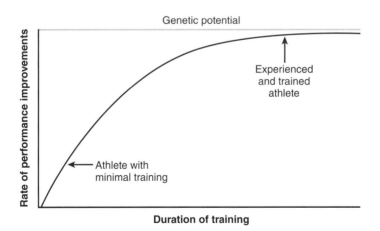

FIGURE 2.1 Theoretical training curve. Note that as athletes become more and more trained, the speed and degree of improvement in response to training is slower. However, for elite athletes, these small gains may still be significant.

Adapted, by permission, from J.R. Hoffman, 2002, *Physiological aspects of sport training and performance* (Champaign, IL: Human Kinetics), 74.

weightlifters, small increases in strength were observed. However, these increases did not reach statistical significance (18). Although they could not see statistical change, practically speaking, the athletes and the strength and conditioning professionals could rate the training program a success. In a group of elite athletes, training improvements are so difficult to achieve that even small improvements can mean the difference between winning and losing. When interpreting test results, especially in an elite athletic population, practical significance should take precedence over statistical significance (24).

Test Selection

The selection of a testing battery is generally based on the relevance of each particular fitness component within a particular sport. A typical testing battery may include strength tests for the upper and lower body, power tests, and assessments for speed and agility, cardiorespiratory endurance, body composition, and flexibility.

When developing athletic assessments, the appropriate testing battery is initially determined by the needs analysis of the sport. Once the type of assessments are determined (e.g., strength, power, aerobic endurance, speed, and so on), the next step is to ensure that the tests selected are reliable, valid, specific, and relevant to the sport being assessed. If any of these concerns are not met, the testing battery would be flawed and would yield very little information.

Specificity and Relevance of the Test

For a performance test to be of significant value, it is imperative that each test used is specific to the athlete's training program. For instance, when strength training and testing are performed using a similar mode of exercise (i.e., squats), testing results can accurately reflect the magnitude of strength improvements. However, if training and testing are performed on different training modes (e.g., machines versus free weights) or exercises (e.g.. squats versus leg press), the actual magnitude of strength improvement will not be seen.

A 10-week training study examined two groups of subjects (40). The first group trained on a variable resistance machine (performing leg presses), while the other group trained using free weights (doing squats). The group of subjects that trained with the leg press increased their leg-press strength by 27%. However, when tested on the squatting exercise, the magnitude of their strength improvements was only 7.5%. In contrast, the group that trained with the squatting exercise realized a strength gain of 28.9%, yet their improvement in leg-press strength was only 7.5%. It appears from this study that strength testing in a mode of exercise that is different from (but uses similar muscle groups to) the one used in training may only reflect 25% of the magnitude of strength gains.

When testing athletes, it is also necessary to select assessments that have relevance to the specific sport. Tests should be selected that provide the athlete and strength and conditioning professional with information concerning the athlete's ability to succeed in a specific sport. For example, the Wingate anaerobic power test is considered to be the gold standard in laboratory-based power measurements. However, because it is performed on a cycle ergometer, its relevance for sports that do not involve cycling is questionable. As a result, efforts have been made to develop anaerobic power tests that are more specific and have a greater relevance to sports consisting primarily of running or jumping movements (43). An example of a sport-specific anaerobic power test is the vertical jump test. The athlete can perform it on a force plate or while attached to an accelerometer for the sports of basketball and volleyball.

Validity and Reliability of the Test

One of the most important characteristics of a test is its validity and reliability. *Validity* refers to the degree that each test measures what it is intended to or claims to measure. For example, the 1RM squat exercise is considered a valid measure of lower body strength, primarily because it recruits the greatest muscle mass in the lower body. *Reliability* refers to the ability of each test to produce consistent and repeatable results. Tests selected that have proven reliability can reflect even slight changes in performance when evaluating a conditioning program. If a test is unreliable, then differences in testing may reflect only the variation of the test, not the effectiveness of the training program.

Practical Considerations for Test Administration

To attain accurate assessments, tests need to be administered safely and in an organized fashion. Assessment timing should be carefully planned, and the tests should be administered in a proper sequence. In addition, all athletes being tested should have a clear understanding of the purpose of each test.

Safety Considerations

All athletes, regardless of level of competition, should be medically cleared before participating in any health or performance assessment. The goal of attaining medical clearance is to determine whether athletes have any contraindication to participation in either an exercise program or a fitness assessment. It is the responsibility of each strength and conditioning professional to ensure that medical clearance has been obtained. It is highly recommended that the issue of medical clearance be included in the manual for standard operating procedures. The procedure manual should be completed with the assistance of the team physician or sports medicine team associated with the facility.

Timing of Assessment

To maximize the information provided by assessment programs, it is imperative that evaluation periods are conducted throughout the training year. The goal of each evaluation period may be different, focusing on determining training goals, assessing the effectiveness of the training program, or evaluating the readiness of athletes to compete.

To evaluate the effectiveness of a training program, assessments should be performed at its onset and conclusion. To assess the physical readiness of the athletes to participate in a competitive season, testing should occur at the onset of training camp. Novice athletes who are being evaluated prior to beginning a fitness program should be allowed sufficient time to learn how to perform each of the tests. This will allow the athletes to perform each of the tests safely, resulting in more accurate assessments and more effective exercise prescription.

Figure 2.2 shows examples of specific testing periods throughout a training year. This testing schedule is for collegiate American football players, with a competitive season lasting from September to November. The first testing session should be held before off-season (winter) workouts begin in order to guide exercise prescription, establish training goals, and serve as a motivational tool for the athletes. The second round of testing should occur at the end of winter workouts and before summer workouts begin, about three months before the start of the competitive season. This testing session helps strength and conditioning professionals evaluate the winter conditioning program, check the athletes' progress, and continue to motivate them. The final testing session, at the very start of training camp, serves as a final evaluation of the effectiveness of the summer training program.

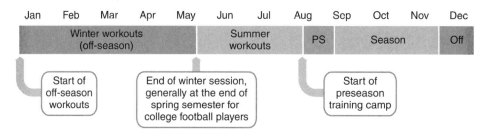

FIGURE 2.2   Timing of athlete assessments for a collegiate American football team.

Adapted, by permission, from J.R. Hoffman, 2006, *Norms for fitness, performance, and health* (Champaign, IL: Human Kinetics), 9.

Testing Sequence

One of the most important administrative concerns is the order in which the testing battery is performed. In general, the least fatiguing tests should be performed first. Tests that require high-skill movements, such as agility measurements, should be performed prior to any fatiguing tests. Any performance test that fatigues the athlete will confound the results of any subsequent tests. For example, aerobic endurance exercise preceding strength training appears to cause a significant decrease in strength expression (33). However, no detrimental effects on aerobic endurance performance have been noted when strength testing is performed first. Thus, it would be prudent for athletes to perform the more fatiguing tests (e.g., 300-yard shuttle runs, line drills, 1.5-mile run) last during a testing battery.

Many factors influence testing sequence, including the number of athletes being tested, the length of the testing period (e.g., 2 hours, one day), and the number of strength and conditioning professionals available to assist. In an ideal testing scenario, all athletes would perform the testing in the same sequence. If testing is performed over an extended time period (e.g., over two days), the most fatiguing tests should be performed last. However, due to time constraints, the ideal testing sequence may not always be realistic.

Testing a team or other large group of athletes may require simultaneous use of several different testing stations. Athletes often rotate through various stations within a set time period. Some athletes may perform a 40-yard sprint, followed by strength measures. Other athletes perform their strength tests before sprint and agility tests.

A testing scenario likely to yield accurate results includes the performance of endurance and shuttle runs (the most fatiguing tests) at the end of the testing battery and the provision of proper rest, which involves at least 5 minutes between stations for the phosphagen energy system to be restored (20). Strength and conditioning professionals should also consider how muscle potentiation may be affected by test sequence. Performing maximal squat testing first may significantly enhance vertical jump height (28).

Interpretation of Test Results

Once testing is completed, the information obtained must be communicated to both the athlete, and when appropriate, to the sports coach. Individual results can be compared to previous results to evaluate progress in the team's conditioning program. Performance results can also be compared with those of other athletes playing in the same sport and position to assess the athlete's potential. Results can also be used to prescribe exercises, develop training goals, and motivate athletes.

Tests for Needs Assessment and Program Evaluation

The remainder of this chapter discusses tests that are common to each of the performance variables. It is not meant to be an all-inclusive list of potential tests. However, the discussion focuses on tests that are widely accepted and used.

 For more on the use of tests in the context of an annual training plan, see chapter 12.

Strength

When assessing strength, strength and conditioning professionals must decide which type of exercise to use and whether to test maximal strength or predict it from submaximal assessment. In regard to test selection, they must remember the importance of specificity. The test should be part of the athlete's resistance training program. As mentioned previously, this allows a clear understanding of the effectiveness of the conditioning program and provides a true measure of the athlete's ability. If initial testing occurs prior to the onset of a conditioning program (for example, freshman athletes being tested on the first day of practice), the exercises used to assess strength may be novel to the athletes. These tests would be appropriate as long as the exercises are part of the resistance training program that follows, the same tests are used to reassess the athletes at the conclusion of the training program, and the tests are not too technically demanding (e.g., 1RM cleans). Another benefit of using an exercise that is part of the athlete's conditioning program is to ensure proper technique, thereby reducing the potential for injury during testing and to provide appropriate selection of the resistance attempted during the strength test.

Strength testing can be performed with either dynamic, constant-resistance exercises (i.e., free weights), isokinetic testing, or an isometric dynamometer. The mode of exercise used to assess strength depends on the goals of the testing program. If strength tests are part of an evaluation to predict potential sports performance, they should incorporate similar movement patterns and involve the same muscle mass that is routinely recruited during actual sport performance. Strength testing should involve exercises that engage multiple joints and large muscle mass.

Generally, strength tests are used to provide a measure of strength for a certain area of the body (e.g., upper body or lower body). Thus, tests should be selected that are common to the athlete's training program and that recruit the largest amount of muscle mass for a particular body area. In general, the bench press exercise is commonly used to assess strength in the upper body and the squat exercise is commonly used to assess strength in the lower body. Both of these tests recruit a great amount of muscle mass.

Isokinetic Testing

In some cases, an exercise that recruits a smaller muscle mass or an isolated joint action may provide additional information. For example, comparing muscle groups from bilateral limbs (i.e., right-knee flexors with left-knee flexors) or agonist versus antagonist muscle groups (i.e., knee flexors versus knee extensors) may indicate a potential weakness that can predispose the athlete to injury. Isokinetic testing isolates these muscle groups in order to make these important comparisons. Isokinetic testing devices (see figure 2.3) measure joint movements at a constant velocity. The force exerted by a moving body segment is met with an equal and opposite resistance that is constantly altered as the body segment moves through its full range of motion. The force exerted by the body segment to produce rotation around its axis is referred to as *torque*, and is expressed in newton-meters (N · m).

Since isokinetic devices only permit the evaluation of a single-joint, unilateral movement, their role in strength evaluation is primarily limited to determining the athlete's potential for muscle injury as a result of either a bilateral deficit or a muscle–joint imbalance (24). This mode of testing is also time consuming. Therefore, it is typically used by athletic trainers who work individually with rehabilitating athletes.

Research that evaluates antagonistic-to-agonist strength ratios and their ability to predict injury is equivocal (23). The primary issue is the large variability seen among athletes of different sports, the effect of resistance training on strength improvements in specific muscle groups, and the

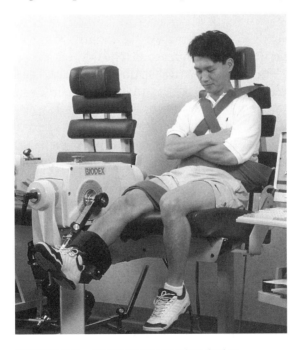

FIGURE 2.3   An isokinetic testing device.

differences seen in antagonistic–agonistic ratios between different joints. The examination of bilateral strength differences appears to be a bit more promising in regard to predicting risk for injury. Bilateral strength deficits of 15% or greater may indicate a significant risk for injury (32). For athletes with strength imbalances greater than 15%, an incidence of muscle injury has been reported that is 2.6 times greater (32). However, much debate still exists about the effectiveness of the use of bilateral deficits.

In some athletes in sports that rely predominantly on unilateral arm action (e.g., tennis, baseball pitching), bilateral deficits are often noticed in the muscle groups of the shoulder, elbow, and wrist (9, 13). Strength differences approaching 20% in the upper limb have been seen in tennis athletes and baseball pitchers. These large bilateral-strength differences may be compounded by the non-weight-bearing requirements of the upper body musculature. It is still not fully understood whether this large bilateral strength difference negatively affects performance or increases the risk for injury in these athletes.

Dynamic Constant Resistance Testing

The use of dynamic constant resistance exercises, performed with free weights, is the most popular mode of strength testing. This is related to several factors, including the likelihood that the exercises used for testing are also part of the athlete's training program, the exercises selected can better simulate actual sport movement, and the large muscle mass that these exercises generally recruit. The issue that is frequently encountered in testing maximal strength is whether to directly measure one-repetition maximum (1RM) or to predict maximal strength from the number of repetitions performed with a submaximal load. Often, the decision is based on practicality. When testing large groups of athletes (as is often the case when strength testing a team), time is an important and valid consideration.

Another issue that has been raised with maximal strength testing is the potential risk for injury. It is important to note that absolutely no research supports this contention. As long as the athlete is using appropriate loads, a qualified strength and conditioning professional is present, spotters are used properly, and the equipment and testing area is safe, the use of 1RM testing does not increase the risk for injury. The bench press, squat, and the power clean are widely used measures to assess upper body strength, lower body strength, and explosive power, respectively. These tests have been demonstrated to have strong test–retest reliability ($r > 0.90$) (24). A protocol for assessing a 1RM is presented in the sidebar on the next page.

The validity of submaximal tests to predict maximal strength has previously been demonstrated (correlation coefficients >0.90) (33, 36, 37). It should be noted that the number of repetitions performed at selected percentages of the 1RM is quite variable among exercises, and that the variance within an exercise is also quite large (22). Table 2.1 provides examples of published formulas that can be used to predict a 1RM.

Protocol for Testing Maximal Strength (1RM)

The athlete should do the following:

1. Perform a warm-up set of 10 repetitions at a resistance that is approximately 50% of the expected 1RM
2. Perform another warm-up set of 5 repetitions at a resistance that is approximately 75% of the expected 1 RM
3. Rest 3 to 5 minutes
4. Perform one repetition with a resistance that is approximately 90% to 95% of the expected 1RM
5. Rest 3 to 5 minutes
6. Attempt 1RM lift
7. Rest 3 to 5 minutes
8. If the attempt is successful, increase the resistance and attempt a new 1RM
9. Continue this protocol until failure

TABLE 2.1 Equations for Predicting the 1RM Strength Test

Equation	Reference
Repetition weight / (1.0278 – 0.0278 × reps)	(8)
(0.033 × reps × repetition weight) + repetition weight	(14)
(100 × repetition weight)/(101.3 – 2.67123 × reps)	(33)

Another concern is the number of repetitions that are performed to predict maximal strength. When a submaximal bench-press test is used to assess maximal upper body strength, the validation of the prediction model is maintained as long as the number of repetitions performed is 10 or fewer. If more than 10 repetitions are performed, the equations lose their validity and tend to underestimate actual strength levels (37). Thus, if a strength and conditioning professional decides to use a submaximal test to predict maximal strength, it is recommended that the loading be relative to the strength level of the athlete. For example, some American football teams use loads specific to the player's position. For instance, linemen perform as many bench press repetitions as possible with 330 pounds (150 kg), linebackers perform as many repetitions with 300 pounds (136 kg), and so on. This time-efficient method gives athletes a better opportunity to produce a valid test.

Anaerobic Power and Anaerobic Fitness

Anaerobic power can be assessed in both laboratory and field settings. For most strength and conditioning professionals, the ability to work with a human performance laboratory is limited. However, if the opportunity presents itself, a human performance laboratory allows for greater sophistication and sensitivity in athletic assessment. This section discusses tests for both the laboratory and the field that can be used to assess anaerobic power and fitness. Anaerobic power provides information about an athlete's potential, whereas anaerobic fitness describes the athlete's ability to perform high-intensity exercise for a prolonged duration of time (e.g., a game). For example, seeing how high a basketball player can jump provides information to help determine his potential. However, it does not provide any information as to whether the athlete's physical condition is good enough for playing basketball.

Laboratory Tests

A variety of laboratory tests can be used to assess anaerobic power. These tests differ in the mode of exercise, sensitivity of the assessment, and the extent of information provided. Anaerobic power can be evaluated through sprints on a nonmotorized treadmill (14, 43), repeated jumps on a force plate or contact mat (7), and maximal-effort cycling tests (3, 31, 44). These tests assess peak power (highest power output attained during the test), mean power (average power output of entire test), or both. Additionally, fatigue rate (the athlete's ability to maintain power output throughout the duration of the test) may be reported.

The gold standard for laboratory-based anaerobic power tests is the Wingate anaerobic power test (WAnT) (5). This 30-second maximal-effort cycling test is performed against a resistance relative to the subject's body weight. The WAnT was first developed at the Wingate Institute in Israel. Of all the laboratory-based anaerobic power tests available, the WAnT has the most extensive research base to date. Test–retest reliability has consistently been shown to exceed $r > 0.90$ (5).

The WAnT provides assessments of an athlete's peak power and mean power, as well as a fatigue index. However, as the sophistication of computer programs evolved, many human performance laboratories have begun to vary the duration of the test. Some have used repeated trials of shorter duration (10-20 s), or have performed a longer, 60-second test (26, 29). Although it is not clear whether the fatigue index is a good indicator of anaerobic fitness, the index does appear to correlate highly with the percent of fast-twitch fibers (6). Typically, a greater fatigue index is seen in athletes with a greater percentage of fast-twitch fibers. Athletes who are trained for aerobic endurance generally have a lower fatigue index. Figure 2.4 depicts a sample performance diagram produced from a 30-second WAnT.

The primary drawback of WAnT, and the reason that it has not achieved widespread acceptance among strength and conditioning professionals, is related to questions concerning specificity of muscle and activity patterns. Few sports are performed using motions similar to those on a cycle ergometer. Anaerobic power assessment of a basketball player, for instance, may

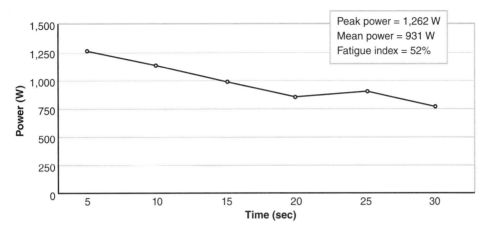

FIGURE 2.4　Example of power output over the course of 30 seconds in a Wingate anaerobic power test (WAnT).

Reprinted, by permission, from J.R. Hoffman, 2006, *Norms for fitness, performance, and health* (Champaign, IL: Human Kinetics), 54.

be more specific if performed with a vertical-jump power test. This test requires the athlete to perform repeated countermovement jumps on a force plate or contact mat. The flight time of each jump is recorded (from the moment subject breaks contact with the mat until he or she makes contact when landing). The time in flight is used to calculate the change in the body's center of gravity (7). Using body weight and the calculated jump height, mechanical work is calculated. Anaerobic power can be determined by using both mechanical work and the length of contact time between jumps. A vertical jump anaerobic power test does have greater sport specificity, especially for basketball and volleyball (24).

Field Tests

When testing large groups of athletes, several administrative concerns (equipment availability and the fact that only a single subject can be tested at any one time) may preclude use of any of the previously mentioned tests. As a result, most strength and conditioning professionals use a field-based test to provide similar assessments to those obtained from laboratory-based measures. The vertical jump is a popular field test for anaerobic power. A few field tests can be used to evaluate anaerobic fitness. Two of the most popular are discussed in the following section.

Vertical Jump　The vertical jump is perhaps the most popular field test for assessing anaerobic power. It is relatively easy to perform and provides a specific measure of power for athletes participating in sports that involve jumping. The primary drawback of the vertical jump test is that it can only measure jumping height. To provide a more accurate assessment of power, a formula can be used to estimate power output from the vertical jump test (19). Keep in mind that power outputs are recorded in watts (W). The equations to calculate peak and mean power are as follows:

Peak power (W) = 61.9 × jump height (cm) + 36 × body mass (kg) + 1,822

Mean power (W) = 21.2 × jump height (cm) + 23 × body mass (kg) − 1,393

300-Yard Shuttle Run   The shuttle run is a field test often used to assess anaerobic capacity. Following an adequate warm-up, the athlete lines up at the starting point. At the signal, the athlete sprints to a point 25 yards (23 m) away and then returns to the starting line. A total of six round trips are performed (12 × 25 yards = 300 yards, or 273 m). As the athlete crosses the line on the final sprint, the time is recorded to the nearest 0.1 second, and a 5-minute rest interval is begun. Following the 5-minute rest interval, the athlete repeats the 300-yard shuttle. The average of the two times is recorded.

Line Drill   The line drill is a field test used to measure anaerobic fitness in athletes. The line drill can be performed on a regulation-size basketball court or in any outdoor or indoor facility with similar space dimensions (see figure 2.5). The athlete begins from a standing position and sprints from the baseline to four separate cones placed at the near foul line (5.8 m), half-court line (14.3 m), far foul line (22.9 m), and far baseline (28.7 m). As athlete arrives at each cone, he sprints back to the original starting point and proceeds as rapidly as possible to next cone.

When performing this test in an outdoor facility such as a football field, yard line markers can be used. For instance, when testing football players, the goal line would be the starting point and cones would be placed at the 10-, 20-, 30-, and 40-yard lines (9, 18, 27, 36 m). The procedure would then be the same as if performed indoors. When testing a large group of subjects, athletes should touch the lines instead of touching the cones. In order to accurately assess each athlete, a strength and conditioning professional with a stopwatch must be present for

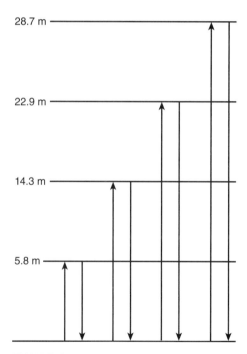

FIGURE 2.5   Sprinting pattern for a line drill performed on a regulation-size basketball court.

Reprinted, by permission, from J.R. Hoffman, 2006, *Norms for fitness, performance, and health* (Champaign, IL: Human Kinetics), 200.

each athlete who is running. A total of three trials are often used, with a 2-minute rest period between each trial. All sprint times are recorded and the fastest time is reported. A fatigue index is generated by dividing the fastest score by the slowest score.

Aerobic Capacity and Aerobic Endurance

Success for athletes in aerobic endurance sports, such as cross-country skiing, running, swimming, and cycling, often depends on a large aerobic capacity. Although many factors determine aerobic performance (i.e., capillary density, mitochondrial number, muscle-fiber type), the $\dot{V}O_2$max of the athlete provides important information concerning the capacity of the aerobic energy system. Maximal aerobic capacity can be either determined by directly measuring oxygen consumption ($\dot{V}O_2$) while exercising to exhaustion or predicted through submaximal exercise tests.

Direct Laboratory Measurement

The most common laboratory method for assessing aerobic capacity is directly measuring oxygen consumption while an athlete performs a graded exercise test on a treadmill to exhaustion. Maximal aerobic capacity can also be determined while an athlete performs on a cycle ergometer, during tethered swimming, or while swimming in a swimming flume. The choice of exercise should be determined by the athlete's sport.

Aerobic capacity measured on a treadmill will produce the greatest results. In a study of triathletes, the $\dot{V}O_2$max from tethered swimming and cycle ergometry were 13% to 18% and 3% to 6% lower, respectively, than values obtained from treadmill running (38).

Figures 2.6a and 2.6b describe popular treadmill-testing protocols for assessing maximal aerobic capacity for the general population. Many protocols have been developed, and some are population specific. For instance, some exercise protocols are designed primarily for cardiac rehabilitation, while others are primarily designed for athletes. The primary differences between the two are the initial starting points (elevation and speed of the treadmill) and the increments for each stage of exercise (increases in elevation and speed). For an athletic population, the exercise protocol for may require the subject to begin exercising at a self-selected speed between 134 and 188 m/min. The athlete should maintain the self-selected speed for the duration of the test, while the treadmill elevation will increase by 2% every 2 minutes until the athlete reaches exhaustion.

Prior to the onset of a maximal exercise test, the subject should be allowed to warm up for at least 5 minutes or until he or she feels ready to proceed. Generally, the warm-up is performed at 0% grade on a treadmill, at a speed that the subject considers comfortable. Following the warm-up, the subject is attached to the breathing apparatus, and the testing protocol begins. The test ends when the subject indicates that he or she has reached

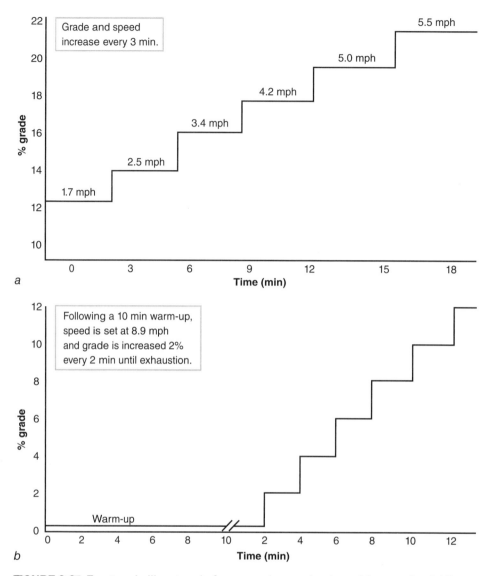

FIGURE 2.6 Two treadmill protocols for assessing maximal aerobic capacity: (*a*) Bruce Treadmill Protocol for Assessing Maximal Oxygen Consumption, (*b*) Costill and Fox Treadmill Protocol for Assessing Maximal Oxygen.

Figure 2.6a Reprinted, by permission, from J. Hoffman, 2006, *Norms for fitness, performance, and health* (Champaign, IL: Human Kinetics), 68.

Figure 2.6b Adapted, by permission, from D. Costill and E.L. Fox, 1969, "Energetics of marathon running," *Medicine and Science in Sport Exercise* 1: 81-86.

exhaustion or when subject has met three of these four criteria to ascertain that $\dot{V}O_2$max has been reached:

1. The increase in oxygen uptake is no greater than 150 ml/min, despite an increase in exercise intensity (plateau criterion)
2. Attainment of age-predicted maximal heart rate (HRmax)

3. A respiratory exchange ratio ($\dot{V}CO_2/\dot{V}O_2$) greater than 1.10
4. A plasma-lactate concentration of at least 8 mmol/L within 4 minutes of ending exercise

Indirect Laboratory Measures

Considering the costs that are associated with the equipment, space, and personnel needed to directly measure oxygen consumption, this methodology of testing is generally reserved for research or clinical settings. When direct measurement of $\dot{V}O_2$max is not possible, a variety of submaximal tests are available to predict aerobic capacity. The validity of these tests has been well established. They are based on several assumptions, including that a steady-state heart rate is obtained for each stage of exercise, a linear relationship exists between heart rate and the intensity of exercise, the maximal heart rate for a given age is consistent, and the efficiency of exercise (i.e., $\dot{V}O_2$ for the intensity of exercise) is the same for everyone. If any of these assumptions are not met, the validity of the test may be reduced. These tests are generally performed in a controlled environment. They are administered on an individual basis.

Submaximal aerobic testing can be performed on either a cycle ergometer or a treadmill. Generally, a submaximal test uses an endpoint of 85% of age-predicted maximal heart rate. A treadmill protocol for submaximal aerobic testing is shown in figure 2.7. If using a treadmill, the speed and grade of the final stage can be used to estimate $\dot{V}O_2$max. The following formula may be appropriate to use (11):

$$\dot{V}O_2\text{max } (ml \cdot kg^{-1} \cdot min^{-1}) = 15.1 + (21.8 \times \text{speed in mph})$$
$$- (0.327 \times \text{heart rate}) - (0.263 \times \text{speed in mph} \times \text{age})$$
$$+ (0.00504 \times \text{heart rate} \times \text{age}) + (5.98 \times \text{gender})$$

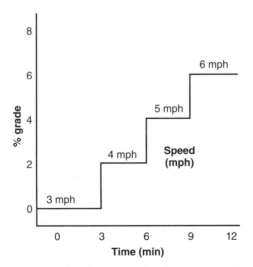

FIGURE 2.7   A testing progression for submaximal aerobic testing on a treadmill. Each stage should be maintained for 3 minutes to allow a steady-state heart rate to be achieved.

Reprinted, by permission, from J.R. Hoffman, 2006, *Norms for fitness, performance, and health* (Champaign, IL: Human Kinetics), 70. Based on data from Ebeling et al. 1991 (12).

For gender, insert *0* for females and *1* for males. This formula is reported to predict $\dot{V}O_2$max within 4.85 ml · kg^{-1} · min^{-1} of actual $\dot{V}O_2$max.

The benefit of using a treadmill is primarily related to the fact that most people are more familiar with either walking or running as compared to riding a cycle ergometer. However, cycle ergometers may still be a more popular mode of testing because they make it easy to perform other measures (i.e., blood pressure and ECG readings) during the test. The test is also non-weight-bearing in nature. In addition, cycle ergometers are relatively inexpensive compared with treadmills. They are also safer (e.g., the chance of a subject tripping or falling while cycling is lower than that of running on a treadmill). All these reasons may contribute to a greater use of submaximal cycle-ergometer testing.

For the YMCA submaximal cycle-ergometer test, the initial workload is set at 150 kg · m · min^{-1} (0.5 kp). Each stage is 3 minutes in duration. The work load at each subsequent stage varies depending on the heart rate in the last minute of the previous stage (see figure 2.8*a*). The heart rate measured during the last minute in each stage is then plotted against work rate. The line generated from the plotted points is extrapolated to the athlete's age-predicted maximal heart rate. A perpendicular line is dropped to the *x* axis to determine the work rate that would have been achieved if the athlete had worked to maximum (figure 2.8*b*). $\dot{V}O_2$max can then be calculated with the following formula:

$$\dot{V}O_2\text{max (ml/min)} = \text{workload (kg · m · min}^{-1}) \times (2 \text{ ml · kg}^{-1} \cdot \text{m}^{-1})$$
$$+ (3.5 \text{ ml · kg}^{-1} \cdot \text{min}^{-1}) \times \text{body mass (kg)}$$

Field Tests

When testing large groups of athletes, it may be more feasible to administer a field test to estimate aerobic capacity. These tests include measuring the time to run a given distance or the distance that can be run in 12 minutes. The most popular tests are the Cooper 12-minute run and the 1.5-mile test for time (1). The goal of the Cooper test is for the athlete to run as far as possible in the 12-minute time period. To estimate the athletes' $\dot{V}O_2$max for the 12-minute run, the following formula can be used:

$$\dot{V}O_2\text{max (ml · kg}^{-1} \cdot \text{min}^{-1}) = (0.0268 \times \text{distance covered in meters}) - 11.3$$

The distance for a single lap for most oval tracks is 400 m. For instance, if an athlete ran six laps, he has run 2,400 m. Using the formula, the estimated $\dot{V}O_2$max for that athlete would be 53.0 ml · kg^{-1} · min^{-1} [(0.0268 × 2,400) − 11.3]. The primary drawback for this test is that it may be quite difficult to estimate distance run, especially if the athlete did not complete a set fraction of a lap. Administratively, it may be easier to have athletes run a given distance. This allows a single administrator to call out the times of

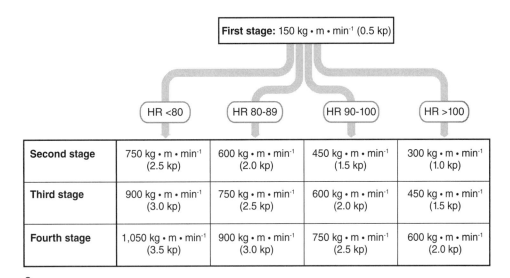

	HR <80	HR 80-89	HR 90-100	HR >100
Second stage	750 kg • m • min⁻¹ (2.5 kp)	600 kg • m • min⁻¹ (2.0 kp)	450 kg • m • min⁻¹ (1.5 kp)	300 kg • m • min⁻¹ (1.0 kp)
Third stage	900 kg • m • min⁻¹ (3.0 kp)	750 kg • m • min⁻¹ (2.5 kp)	600 kg • m • min⁻¹ (2.0 kp)	450 kg • m • min⁻¹ (1.5 kp)
Fourth stage	1,050 kg • m • min⁻¹ (3.5 kp)	900 kg • m • min⁻¹ (3.0 kp)	750 kg • m • min⁻¹ (2.5 kp)	600 kg • m • min⁻¹ (2.0 kp)

a

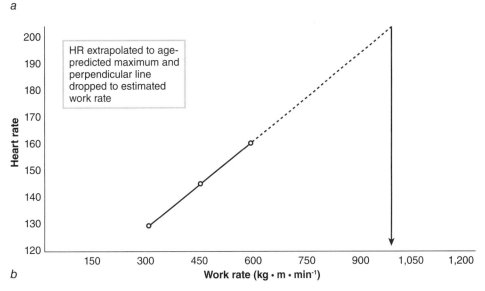

b

FIGURE 2.8 (*a*) Work loads, based on heart rate, for stages 2 through 4 of the YMCA submaximal cycle-ergometer test. (*b*) The line graphed from the heart rates measured in the last minute of each stage can be extended to the age-predicted maximal heart rate to estimate maximal work rate.

Reprinted, by permission, from J.R. Hoffman, 2006, *Norms for fitness, performance, and health* (Champaign, IL: Human Kinetics), 200-201.

each runner as he completes the six laps. Aerobic capacity can be estimated for the 1.5-mile run by the following formula:

$$\dot{V}O_2max \ (ml \cdot kg^{-1} \cdot min^{-1}) = 3.5 + (483 \div time \ in \ minutes \ to \ run \ 1.5 \ miles)$$

If an athlete ran 1.5 miles in 11.0 minutes, the $\dot{V}O_2max$ would be calculated as 47.4 ml · kg⁻¹ · min⁻¹ [3.5 + (483/11.0)].

Speed

Speed is the ability to perform a movement in as little time as possible. It is relatively easy to measure, requiring only the use of a stopwatch and track or field area. For programs with larger training budgets, electronic timers are becoming more popular. The major issue with using a stopwatch is the potential for measurement error. Even under ideal conditions with an experienced tester, stopwatch times may be 0.2 seconds faster than electronically measured times because of the tester's reaction-time delay in pressing the stopwatch's start and stop buttons as the athlete begins and ends the sprint (24).

The 40-yard sprint is the most popular distance used in most speed assessments. This is probably due to the familiarity that most strength and conditioning professionals have with sprint times associated with this distance. The 40-yard sprint has achieved tremendous popularity among American football coaches. It is a staple of most football testing programs. Considering the large player rosters and the number of strength and conditioning professionals who have a football background, the 40-yard sprint has become a staple for most athletic testing programs in the United States. However, the justification for the 40-yard distance is not entirely clear. It may have originated as an arbitrary distance that has become well accepted over time.

Other sports have used either shorter or longer distances, depending on the specific needs of the sport. Some strength and conditioning professionals for basketball use a 30-yard sprint (the approximate length of a basketball court) to assess speed. Baseball, on the other hand, often uses the 60-yard sprint (the distance between three bases, such as home to second or first to third).

Agility

Agility refers to the ability to change direction rapidly. It is a common variable measured during most athletic performance testing. Like speed, it is relatively easy to measure. All that is needed is a stopwatch and cones. A variety of different agility tests can be selected. However, the most relevant agility performance test is one that incorporates movements that are similar to those performed by the athlete during competition. The test used should also be part of the athlete's training program.

For example, movement patterns in basketball involve sprints, side shuffles and backward runs. The T test is an agility measure that utilizes those specific movement patterns. It is very appropriate for assessing agility in basketball players. Popular agility tests include the T test, Edgren side-step test, the pro-agility (5-10-5) test, and the Illinois test.

T Test

For the T test, arrange four cones as seen in figure 2.9. Cones A and B are 10 yards (9 m) apart. Cones C and D are placed 5 yards (4.5 m) from either side of cone B. Following a warm-up, the athlete begins by standing at cone

A. At the *go* command, the athlete does the following:

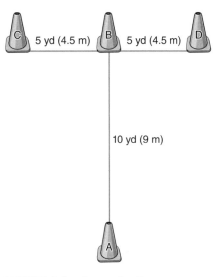

1. Sprints to cone B and touches the base of the cone with the hand

2. Sidesteps either to the left to cone C or to the right toward cone D and touches the base with the closest hand

3. Sidesteps to the other far cone (C or D) and touches the base of the cone with the closest hand (The athlete does not touch cone B as he crosses to the other cone.)

4. Sidesteps back to cone B and touches the base of the cone

FIGURE 2.9   Set-up for T test.

Reprinted, by permission, from J.R. Hoffman, 2006, *Norms for fitness, performance, and health* (Champaign, IL: Human Kinetics), 202. Adapted, by permission, from D. Semencik, 1990, "Tests and measurements: The T-test," *NSCA Journal* 2(1): 36-37.

5. Runs backward to cone A (The time is stopped when the athlete crosses the cone.)

The athlete should face forward at all times and should not cross the feet. Crossing the feet or failing to touch a cone results in disqualification.

Edgren Side-Step Test

For the Edgren side-step test, a 12-foot-wide (4 m) gymnasium floor is divided into four 3-foot (1 m) sections using five lines (see figure 2.10). After a warm-up, the athlete straddles the center line. On the *go* command, the athlete does the following:

1. Sidesteps to the right until the right foot has touched or crossed the right outside line

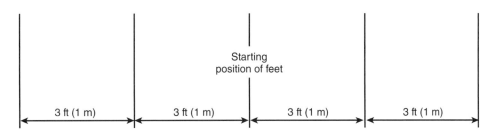

FIGURE 2.10   Setup for the Edgren side-step test.

Reprinted, by permission, from J.R. Hoffman, 2006, *Norms for fitness, performance, and health* (Champaign, IL: Human Kinetics), 202. Adapted, by permission, from NSCA, 2000, Administration, scoring, and interpretation of selected tests, by E. Harman J. Garhammer, and C. Pandorf. In *Essentials of strength training and conditioning*, 2nd ed., edited by T.R. Baechle, and R.W. Earle (Champaign, IL: Human Kinetics), 300.

2. Sidesteps to the left until the left foot has touched or crossed the left outside line

3. Continues to sidestep back and forth to the outside lines as rapidly as possible for 10 seconds

The total number of lines crossed, including the outermost lines, for the 10 seconds are recorded. A point will be deducted from the total score any time that the athlete crosses the feet.

Pro-Agility Test

The pro-agility test is also known as the *20-yard shuttle run*. The test is often performed on a football field, but it may be performed on any marked field or any place where three lines can be drawn 5 yards apart. On a football field, the athlete straddles the 15-yard line, then sprints to the 20-yard line. He then changes direction and sprints to the 10-yard line, then changes direction again and returns to the 15-yard line (figure 2.11). The stopwatch begins on the athlete's initial movement and stops when he crosses the 15-yard line.

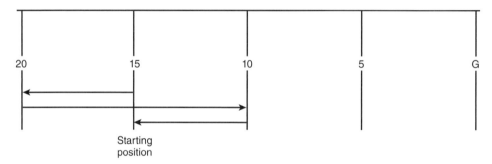

FIGURE 2.11   Set-up for the pro-agility test.

Reprinted, by permission, from J.R. Hoffman, 2006, *Norms for fitness, performance, and health* (Champaign, IL: Human Kinetics), 204.

Illinois Test

Eight markers are required to set up this test. Four of the markers are used to form a rectangle 10 m long by 5 m wide. The other four are placed in a straight line in the center of the rectangle at 3.3 m intervals. This test requires the athlete to begin by lying facedown at marker A. When given the *go* command, the athlete sprints forward 10 m to marker B, performs a U-turn, and sprints back in the opposite direction. When approaching the starting position, the athlete veers diagonally to the left, and enters an agility course consisting of four markers in the center of the rectangle. The athlete runs in a zigzag, weaving around the obstacles. When he reaches the end of the course, the athlete turns around and performs the same pattern back to the starting position. After weaving through the last marker, the athlete makes a U-turn to the left and sprints toward marker C, then makes a final U-turn and sprints straight ahead to marker D (see figure 2.12).

Body Composition

Body composition generally reports the percentage of body weight that is fat. The range in body-fat percentages varies among different athletes. This is related primarily to the specific demands of each sport. Aerobic endurance athletes or gymnasts are generally on the very lean side, but some American football players (primarily linemen) may be borderline obese. A number

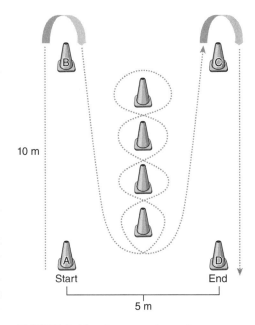

FIGURE 2.12 Setup and running pattern for the Illinois test.

of methods can be used to assess body composition. These methods vary in terms of complexity, cost, and accuracy. The following sections briefly describe their methods.

Dual-Energy X-Ray Absorptiometry

Dual-energy X-ray absorptiometry (DEXA) has become the new gold standard of body-composition assessment. It is a noninvasive procedure that provides regional and total body measurements of lean and fat tissue, bone density, and bone mineral content. The reliability and validity of DEXA for body-composition assessment has been established at low, moderate, and high levels of body fat and with athletic and nonathletic populations (16, 45). One of the major advantages of DEXA measurements is that it uses a three-compartment model (fat mass, lean tissue mass, and bone density) to determine body composition. Such a method is superior to the more common two-compartment model (fat and lean tissue mass). It appears to result in a more accurate measurement of body composition, eliminating additional sources of error seen during estimation of body density (e.g., residual volume). The major drawback to DEXA measurements is the cost of purchasing and operating the machine. In addition, because the DEXA is an X-ray device, the radiological boards in some states require physician prescription and operation by a licensed X-ray technician. These requirements make body-composition testing through this technique unrealistic for most assessment facilities.

Hydrostatic Weighing

For years, hydrostatic weighing was considered to be the gold standard of body-composition analysis. Hydrostatic weighing measures body composition based on the amount of water that is displaced when an athlete is submerged. As the body is immersed under water, it is buoyed by a counterforce equal to the weight of the water displaced. The loss of weight in water, corrected by the density of water, allows body density to be calculated. Once body density is calculated, then the body-fat percentage can be calculated through various equations that depend on age, growth and maturation, gender, and ethnicity.

In addition, calculation of lung residual volume is needed to accurately assess body density. This can be either measured directly or predicted through various formulas. Although this method of body composition is highly reproducible, several factors that may reduce the accuracy of measurement still remain. For instance, the accurate measure of residual volume is important to reduce error. It may not account for possible air in the intestines. Calculation of body density also makes several assumptions that may increase the error in atypical populations. It is generally assumed that body-composition analysis using the hydrostatic method provides an estimation of body fat within 2.5% of the true value (17).

Plethysmography

Plethysmography is a viable method of assessing body composition, especially for athletes who are uncomfortable being fully immersed in the hydrostatic tank. The use of an air-displacement plethysmography (closed chamber that measures body volume by changes in pressure) has been found to be highly reliable in a number of subject populations (2, 10). Air-displacement plethysmography has been shown to be a valid measure of body composition (4, 38, 41). However, it may overestimate body-fat percentage in comparison to DEXA (37, 40). Although the use of air displacement provides an accurate assessment of body-fat percentage, the calculation may be higher than that seen from DEXA measures. Thus, comparisons between these modalities may be difficult to perform.

Skinfold Measurements

Skinfold measurements are the most popular method used to assess body composition. They take significantly less time to complete than the other modalities discussed. The principle behind skinfold measurements is that the amount of subcutaneous fat is proportional to the amount of body fat. By measuring skinfold thickness at various sites on the body, body-fat percentage can be calculated through a regression equation. Commonly used skinfold sites include the following:

- Abdomen: Horizontal fold, 2 cm to the right of the umbilicus
- Biceps: Vertical fold on the anterior aspect of the arm over the belly of the biceps muscle

- Chest: Diagonal fold, one-half of the distance between the anterior axillary line and the nipple (men), or one-third of the distance between the anterior axillary line and the nipple (women)
- Midaxillary: Horizontal fold on the midaxillary line at the level of the xiphoid process of the sternum
- Subscapular: Diagonal fold at a 45° angle, 1 to 2 cm below the inferior angle of the scapula
- Suprailiac: Diagonal fold in line with the natural angle of the iliac crest taken in the anterior axillary line
- Thigh: Vertical fold on the anterior midline of the thigh midway between the proximal border of the patella and the inguinal crease
- Triceps: Vertical fold on the posterior midline of the upper arm midway between the acromion process of the scapula and the inferior part of the olecranon process of the elbow

However, because the ratio between subcutaneous fat and total body fat varies according to age, gender, and ethnicity (35), the appropriate regression equation must be selected. In addition, regression equations also vary in the needed number of skinfold sites. Even when the appropriate regression equation is used, a 3% to 4% error may be associated with the body-fat percentage attained from skinfold measurements (35). Thus, care must be taken in selecting the correct regression equation. Table 2.2 provides several examples of commonly used regression equations. Table 2.3 provides population-specific equations for converting body density to body-fat percentage.

Bioelectrical Impedance

Bioelectrical impedance is another popular modality used to estimate body composition. It is similar to skinfold measures in regard to accuracy, and it may be easier to use because it eliminates potential error among testers. The basic principle behind bioelectrical impedance is the relationship between total body water and lean body mass. Since lean tissue contains a large concentration of water, and water is an excellent conductor of electricity, the resistance to an electrical current passing through the body provides a potential indicator of body-fat percentage. Lean athletes would have minimal resistance, indicating that a higher percentage of lean tissue is present. A higher resistance to the electrical current would suggest a greater amount of body fat.

Because body water content is critical to these measures, any change in body fluid can have a significant effect on body-fat calculation. If bioelectrical impedance is to be used, it is highly recommended that subjects refrain from drinking or eating within four hours of the measurement, void completely prior to the measurement, and refrain from ingesting any

TABLE 2.2 Commonly Used Regression Equations for Computing % Body Fat From Skinfold Measurements and Description of Skinfold Sites

Sites	Sex and age	Formula
DURNIN AND WOMERSLEY 1974 (10)		
Biceps, triceps, subscapular, and suprailiac	**Males (age in years)**	
	17-19	$D = 1.1620 - 0.0630 \times (\log \Sigma \text{ skinfolds})$
	20-29	$D = 1.1631 - 0.0632 \times (\log \Sigma \text{ skinfolds})$
	30-39	$D = 1.1422 - 0.0544 \times (\log \Sigma \text{ skinfolds})$
	Females (age in years)	
	17-19	$D = 1.1549 - 0.0678 \times (\log \Sigma \text{ skinfolds})$
	20-29	$D = 1.1599 - 0.0717 \times (\log \Sigma \text{ skinfolds})$
	30-39	$D = 1.1423 - 0.0632 \times (\log \Sigma \text{ skinfolds})$
JACKSON AND POLLOCK 1985 (28)		
7-site		
Chest: midaxillary, triceps, subscapular, abdomen, suprailiac, and thigh	Males	$D = 1.112 - 0.00043499 \, (\Sigma \, 7 \text{ skinfolds}) + 0.00000055 \, (\Sigma \, 7 \text{ skinfolds})^2 - 0.00028826 \, (\text{age})$
	Females	$D = 1.097 - 0.00046971 \, (\Sigma \, 7 \text{ skinfolds}) + 0.00000056 \, (\Sigma \, 7 \text{ skinfolds})^2 - 0.00012828 \, (\text{age})$
3-site		
Chest, abdomen, and thigh	Males	$D = 1.10938 - 0.0008267 \, (\Sigma \, 3 \text{ skinfolds}) + 0.0000016 \, (\Sigma \, 3 \text{ skinfolds})^2 - 0.0002574 \, (\text{age})$
Triceps, suprailiac, thigh	Females	$D = 1.1099421 - 0.0009929 \, (\Sigma \, 3 \text{ skinfolds}) + 0.0000023 \, (\Sigma \text{ skinfolds})^2 - 0.0001392 \, (\text{age})$

D = body density

TABLE 2.3 Population-Specific Formulas for Conversion of Body Density to % Body Fat

Population	Age	Sex	% body fat (%BF) formula
White	17-19	Males	$\%BF = 4.99 \div (D - 4.55)$
		Females	$\%BF = 5.05 \div (D - 4.62)$
	20-80	Males	$\%BF = 4.95 \div (D - 4.50)$
		Females	$\%BF = 5.01 \div (D - 4.57)$
Black	18-32	Males	$\%BF = 4.37 \div (D - 3.93)$
	24-79	Females	$\%BF = 4.85 \div (D - 4.39)$

Data from Heyward and Stolarczyk 1996 (19).

alcohol, caffeine, or any diuretic agent prior to assessment (23). Failure to comply will increase measurement error. Performing this measurement when dehydrated may overestimate the body-fat percentage (less body water leads to less conductance).

SUMMARY POINTS

- An assessment program can be used to examine the effectiveness of training programs, evaluate athlete potential, develop training programs, and set training goals.

- To maximize the effectiveness of the assessment program, the tests must be reliable and valid, and must provide relevant information to both the strength and conditioning professional and the athlete.

- A testing battery for an athlete should be developed based on the needs assessment in order to reflect the metabolic, biomechanical, and other demands of the sport.

- Concerns for test administration include the ordering of tests and the timing of testing. These variables must be adjusted to allow athletes to perform their best on the tests and to provide information at important points in the competitive cycle.

- It is highly recommended that readers refer to the following textbook for a thorough and in-depth discussion of normative values for all assessments discussed in this chapter:

  Hoffman JR. *Norms for Fitness, Performance, and Health.* Champaign, IL: Human Kinetics; 2006.

3

Dynamic Warm-Up

Avery D. Faigenbaum, EdD, CSCS*D, FNSCA, FACSM

It is important for all athletes to warm up before practice and competition. A well-designed warm-up can mentally and physically prepare athletes for the demands of sports training and athletic events by increasing blood flow to active muscles, raising core body temperature, enhancing metabolic reactions, and improving joint range of motion (26). These effects can boost athletic performance by enhancing oxygen delivery, increasing the speed of nerve-impulse transmissions, improving rate of force development, and maximizing strength and power (2, 5, 45). Moreover, a well-designed warm-up can set the tone for upcoming activities and establish a desired tempo for practice or competition. Indeed, warm-up procedures that are consistent with the needs, goals, and abilities of each athlete should be considered an integral component of every sport practice and competition.

Although well-designed warm-up procedures can enhance athletic performance, reduce the risk of injury, and lessen the potential for muscle soreness after exercise (1, 21, 26), it is important to realize that warming up and stretching are two different activities. A warm-up consists of preparatory activities and functionally based movements that are specifically designed to prepare the body for exercise or sport. In contrast, the primary goal of stretching is to enhance flexibility. These distinctions are important because long-held beliefs about traditional warm-up procedures have recently been questioned. Some scientists and practitioners now propose that it may be advantageous to exclude static stretching from warm-up routines prior to sport training and athletic competitions (32, 49, 52, 59).

Interest is growing in warm-up procedures that involve dynamic activities and sport-specific movements that maximize active ranges of motion at different movement-specific speeds while preparing the body for the demands of sport training and competition (10, 13, 15, 29, 55). This chapter reviews the components of a traditional warm-up and examines the potential benefits of a dynamic warm-up. Although it discusses different types of warm-ups, this chapter focuses on the influence of dynamic warm-up protocols on athletic performance. It also discusses the proposed physiological mechanisms that may enhance the preparedness of athletes for sport practice and competition and outlines program design considerations for developing warm-up protocols that emphasize the movement requirements of the sport or activity.

A traditional warm-up usually consists of two components. The first is a general warm-up of 5 to 10 minutes of low- to moderate-intensity cardiorespiratory exercise, such as jogging or stationary cycling, followed by several minutes of static stretching. The second is a specific warm-up that involves less intense movements similar to the sport or activity about to be performed. The purpose of this type of warm-up is to allow the body to gradually adjust to the changing physiological demands of the exercise session without undue fatigue. A general warm-up of basic exercises for the major muscle groups increases heart rate, blood flow, muscle temperature, and core body temperature, as evidenced by the onset of sweating. Static stretching exercises, in which a body position is held stationary for a predetermined period of time (typically 10-30 seconds), are habitually recommended by some sport coaches to improve range of motion within joints, enhance performance, and reduce the risk of injury prior to activity (30, 36, 46). However, conventional beliefs regarding the routine practice of pre-event static stretching have recently been questioned (48, 50, 53).

Static Stretching and Performance

Although static stretching enhances flexibility, which is a well-recognized component of health-related fitness (1), there is little scientific evidence to suggest that pre-event static stretching prevents activity-related injury or enhances athletic performance (32, 47, 50, 53). Even athletes who compete in sports that require high levels of flexibility, such as gymnastics or diving, must consider both the potential benefits and the related concerns when deciding whether or not to include static stretching exercises in the warm-up routine.

A growing body of research evidence indicates that pre-event static stretching of the prime movers may actually have a negative effect on force production, power performance, strength endurance, reaction time, and running speed (4, 10, 11, 19, 34, 40, 41). In one research study that examined the effects of static stretching on sprint performance in collegiate track-and-field athletes, researchers reported a 3% decrease in sprinting performance at 40 m following pre-event static stretching (57). It has also been shown that pre-event ballistic stretching (i.e., bouncing movements) and stretching techniques for proprioceptive neuromuscular facilitation (PNF), which involve both passive movements and active muscle actions, can also inhibit strength and reduce explosive power (6, 39). Although some data suggest that pre-event static stretching has no short-term effect on performance measures (23, 33), a majority of the available evidence indicates that it can have detrimental effects on subsequent performance.

This stretching-induced effect is thought to be related to a decrease in neural activation, reduced musculotendinous stiffness, or a combination of neural and muscular factors (3, 20, 24). Since static stretching can result in muscle damage (as evidenced by elevated levels of creatine kinase in the blood), it is also possible that tissue damage could explain, at least in part, stretching-induced decrements in performance (51). While the undesirable effects of an acute bout of static stretching on performance are increasingly apparent, additional research is needed to determine the precise mechanisms underlying the performance decrements, as well as the particular stretching protocols and performance conditions that produce this adverse effect.

Of note, the observed reductions in performance following static stretching may, in some cases, last up to one hour (20). Since even a 1% change in performance can have a noticeable influence on the outcome of an athletic event in both individual and team sports, the small but significant changes in performance following an acute bout of static stretching should be considered by sport coaches and strength and conditioning professionals. Indeed, several fitness and medical organizations, including the American College of Sports Medicine (1), the National Strength and Conditioning Association (28), and the President's Council on Physical Fitness and Sports (32) contend that pre-event static stretching may adversely affect athletic performance, particularly in sports that involve strength and power.

This is not to say that static stretching should be eliminated from an athlete's program, but it should be sensibly incorporated into the daily training regimen, since chronic stretching can enhance the range of motion around a joint and potentially improve strength and power performance (35, 52). Consequently, most athletes should perform static stretching during the cool-down or as part of a separate training session. In some cases, however, athletes who participate in sports that require high levels of flexibility may benefit from pre-event static stretching. For example, gymnasts who need to improve flexibility may perform pre-event stretching exercises after a general warm-up, provided that they perform a series of dynamic movements prior to training or competition.

Because static stretching has traditionally been a part of many warm-up routines, strength and conditioning professionals need to genuinely appreciate each athlete's prior beliefs about pre-event static stretching when prescribing flexibility training protocols for sport teams. In some instances, athletes who routinely perform static stretching (and have strong beliefs about its value) may need to be educated about the undesirable consequences of an acute bout of static stretching on athletic performance. They should be gradually introduced to pre-event protocols that include dynamic activities.

Dynamic Warm-Up and Performance

Since the current practice of pre-event static stretching has been based more on intuition and tradition than on scientific evidence, dynamic warm-up protocols that simulate movements that occur in daily activities and sport have become more popular as we continue to better understand methods of training that enhance performance. This type of training typically includes movements of low, moderate, and high intensity that increase body temperature, enhance motor-unit excitability, develop kinesthetic awareness, and maximize active ranges of motion (10, 24, 28, 55). Instead of focusing on individual muscles, dynamic exercises emphasize the movement requirements of an exercise or sport. The term *movement preparation* is also used to describe this type of training because it actually prepares athletes to move (55).

Again, it is important to note that dynamic exercises do not involve the bouncing type movement that is characteristic of a ballistic stretch, but rather a controlled elongation of specific muscle groups. During this type of continuous movement, the muscles are stretched to a new range of motion. They then contract to perform the desired action. As such, the muscles do not relax during the dynamic movement, remaining active throughout the entire range of motion. For example, during the lunge walk (figure 3.1), the athlete exaggerates the length of each stride as the lunge movement is performed for the prescribed number of repetitions, keeping the lead knee over or slightly behind the toe and the back knee just off the floor.

Ideally, a seamless progression from dynamic movements that are less intense to more intense activities that resemble sport movements should occur during a dynamic warm-up routine. Higher intensity movements are needed to optimize performance; therefore, they should be recognized as an important component of the pre-event protocol (54). For example, track-and-field athletes, such as long jumpers, could begin their warm-up with side shuffles and then progress to power skips. Sprinters could begin with high steps and then perform

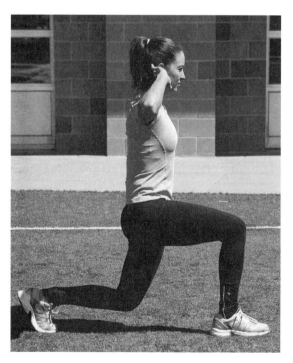

FIGURE 3.1 The lunge walk is an example of a dynamic warm-up exercise.

a series of sprint drills to better prepare to perform at maximal levels during sport practice and competition. Prior to a weightlifting workout, plyometric jumps and explosive exercises with medicine balls could be used to prepare athletes for the upcoming training session (37, 56). Regardless of the movement, strength and conditioning professionals must emphasize proper technique and highlight important mechanics in order to reinforce key skill factors that are required to perform the movement correctly. This type of pre-event warm-up can contribute to an acutely enhanced muscular performance effect. If dynamic warm-up protocols are well conceived and consistent with the needs and abilities of the athletes, some observers suggest that subsequent explosive performance may improve between 2% and 10% (54).

Postactivation Potentiation

In preparation for explosive sporting events, such as the long jump, pole vault, or high jump, a technique known as postactivation potentiation (PAP) may be used as part of the athlete's dynamic warm-up (44). Postactivation potentiation may create an optimal environment for athletic performance by increasing phosphorylation of the regulatory myosin light chains, enhancing neuromuscular function, or possibly changing pennation angle (54). Although the exact mechanisms of PAP are not totally understood, evidence exists that the response of skeletal muscle to the demands placed on it is influenced by its contractile history (43). A brief time of repetitive stimulation can result in an enhanced contractile response (potentiation), while continued stimulation can impair the contractile response (fatigue) (43).

Given that potentiation and fatigue can coexist in skeletal muscle during repetitive stimulation and for some time afterward (43), strength and conditioning professionals must consider the interaction between these two phenomena when designing and implementing warm-up procedures for athletes. In short, the net difference between potentiation and fatigue will determine the outcome of the pre-event protocol.

A number of studies involving youths and adults have examined the short-term effects of various warm-up procedures (static stretching versus dynamic) with respect to their effect on muscle force and power performance (7, 14, 18, 38, 42, 58, 60, 61). A majority of the existing literature suggests that a well-designed dynamic warm-up protocol can enhance acute muscle performance in athletic populations due, at least in part, to the effects of activity-related PAP. However, many factors need to be considered when applying the principles of PAP to athletic performance. Namely, training experience, individual power-strength ratio, intensity and volume of the pre-event activity, and the recovery period can influence the efficacy of any performance-enhancing stimulus. Additionally, individual variability should be considered when examining the application of PAP to activities that require dynamic muscle contractions.

An important issue regarding the practical application of PAP is the time between the cessation of the PAP activity and the start of training or competition. Although an optimal time probably exists when the muscle has recovered but is still potentiated, it is likely that this potential window of opportunity depends on a complex interaction of factors, including the fiber type of the athlete, training experience, and the design of the preload activity. Preliminary evidence suggests that the optimal time to maximize the PAP effect on power performance (such as during a high jump) is within 4 to 12 minutes after the preload stimulus (8, 17, 22, 31). Of note, fatigue tends to be more dominant in the early phase of recovery, but it subsides at a faster rate than PAP, so potentiation can be realized during subsequent sport activities (54). Limited data suggest that the effects of pre-event muscle activation may linger for several hours, possibly extending into the second half of a team game (12).

Mental Preparation

Although a well-designed warm-up increases body temperature and enhances flexibility, the incorporation of dynamic movement activities can also establish a desired tempo for upcoming events and set the tone for strength and conditioning activities. If the warm-up protocol is slow and monotonous (e.g., low-intensity jog around the field and static stretching), performance during the practice session or game that follows may be less than expected. On the other hand, if the pre-event protocol is dynamic, engaging, and diverse, performance during the practice session or game that follows may be enhanced. In short, a warm-up that includes dynamic flexibility exercises may help to better focus the athletes' attention on listening, learning, and noting task-relevant cues.

Developing a Dynamic Warm-Up Protocol

Unlike a traditional warm-up protocol, a dynamic warm-up can result in noticeable improvements in fundamental movement skills. It also prepares the body for the vigorous, random movements that can occur during sports training and competition. As such, this phase of training can provide an opportunity for younger athletes to gain confidence in their abilities to perform movement skills. Additionally, warm-up activities that are active, engaging, and somewhat challenging are far more enjoyable than traditional stretch-and-hold activities.

A well-designed dynamic warm-up should turn on the neuromuscular system to prepare athletes for the demands of sports training and competition. The general idea is to (1) warm up, (2) activate, and (3) motivate. *Warm up* highlights the importance of increasing body temperature, *activate* refers to exciting or potentiating the neuromuscular system, and *motivate* draws attention to the need to psychologically prepare athletes for the demands of sports practice and competition. Instead of jogging around the playing field, a general warm-up of jumping rope, body-weight calisthenics, medicine ball exercises, footwork patterns with an agility ladder, or sport-specific actions, such as dribbling a soccer ball around cones, can contribute to movement skill development and make a valuable contribution to the overall conditioning process. In one study, the incorporation of a four-week dynamic warm-up into the daily preseason training regimen of college wrestlers positively influenced measures of strength, power, agility, muscular endurance, and flexibility as compared to an active control condition (25).

For a sample dynamic warm-up protocol, see chapter 12.

A fundamental principle of a dynamic warm-up is to perform large muscle group exercises that are similar to the movement patterns that will be performed during training or competition. Dynamic warm-up routines do not require equipment or a lot of space. Athletes typically perform each functionally based movement in place for a prescribed number of repetitions (e.g., 8 to 12) or cover a predetermined distance (e.g., 10 to 20 m). Normally, athletes complete 8 to 12 different exercises that progress from relatively simple movements to more challenging exercises, involving more complex movement patterns that require greater ranges of motion. To this end, a well-designed warm-up can enhance the physical fitness of athletes and contribute to the overall conditioning program in a time-efficient manner. However, it is important to keep in mind that the goal is to warm up, activate, and motivate without undue fatigue. Performance may deteriorate if the warm-up is too intense or if the muscles do not have an opportunity to recover from the fatigue induced during the pre-event dynamic warm-up protocol.

If appropriate, dynamic exercises can be combined to add variety to the warm-up routine in a time-efficient manner. For example, knee lifts can be added to the lunge walk to stretch more muscles in a shorter period of time. In any case, athletes should perform each movement while receiving instruction on correct exercise technique (e.g., vertical torso, up on toes, knee toward chest) in order to reinforce proper movement mechanics. Since literally hundreds of exercises can be incorporated into a dynamic warm-up, the sample exercises described in this chapter should be considered a general guide or starting point to help strength and conditioning professionals develop a 10- to 15-minute routine that is consistent with the fitness and skill level of their athletes.

Ideally, different dynamic warm-up protocols that are specific to the unique demands of strength and conditioning workouts, practice sessions, or games should be developed. Athletes who have limited or no experience performing dynamic exercises should be exposed to this type of training during the preseason (or earlier) to limit any potential muscle soreness that can result from performing novel dynamic movements that maximize active ranges of motion. Additional ideas for incorporating dynamic flexibility exercises into warm-up protocols are available elsewhere (9, 16, 27, 55).

Dynamic Warm-Up Exercises

ARM HUGS

The athlete should do the following:

1. Stand erect and raise both arms out to the side to shoulder height
2. Cross the arms in front of the body and grab the opposite shoulder
3. Hold briefly, then spread arms open as wide as possible, stretching the pectoral muscles
4. Repeat the pattern

HEEL-TO-TOE WALK

The athlete should do the following:

1. Stand erect with both feet approximately shoulder-width apart
2. Step forward, placing the heel of the right foot on the ground (*a*)
3. Immediately roll forward and rise onto the ball of the right foot (*b*)
4. Repeat with left leg, moving forward with each step (*c*)

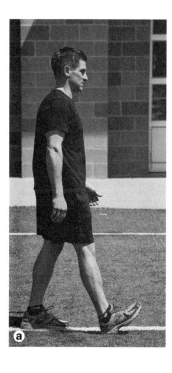 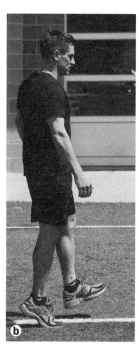 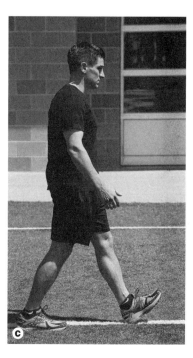

HIGH-KNEE WALK

The athlete should do the following:

1. Step forward with the left leg
2. Lift the right thigh up toward the chest while maintaining an upright posture
3. Grasp the front of the right knee with both hands
4. Pull the right thigh toward the chest
5. Lower the right leg and repeat on opposite side, moving forward with each step

WOODCHOPPERS

The athlete should do the following:

1. Stand erect with feet shoulder-width apart, arms overhead, and hands clasped together (*a*)
2. Lower the body to a full squat position, keeping the arms straight and moving the hands down between the knees (*b*)
3. Return to the starting position, extending the arms overhead as high as possible

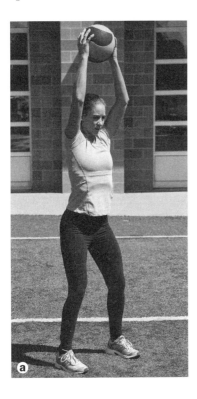
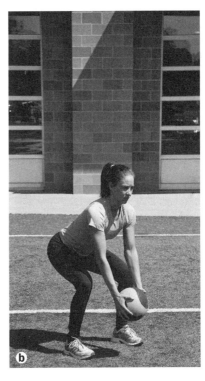

TRUNK TWISTS

The athlete should do the following:

1. Stand erect with the feet approximately shoulder-width apart, knees slightly relaxed, arms slightly bent in front of body, and hands clasped together
2. Bend forward at the waist (about 45°) (*a*)
3. Twist the whole upper body to the right and then to the left, keeping the hips and lower body facing forward (*b*)

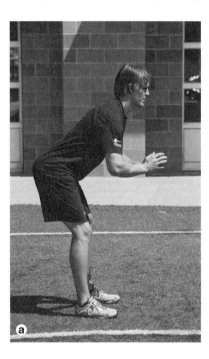
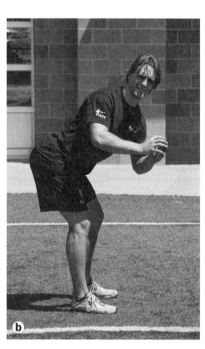

STEPPING TRUNK TWIST

The athlete should do the following:

1. Stand erect with the hands clasped behind the head (*a*)
2. March in place (*b, d*)
3. Rotate the hips to the right 90° and then to the left 90°, keeping the upper body forward and upright (*c, e*)

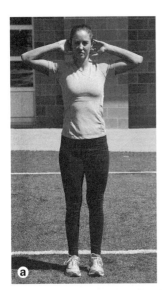
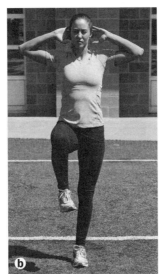
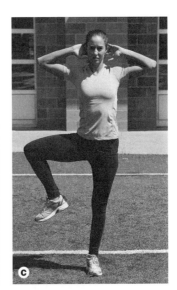

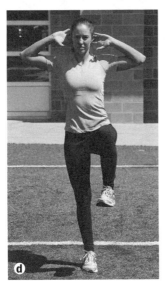
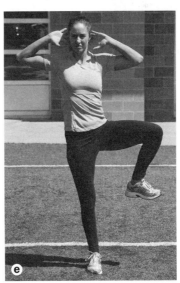

TRAIL-LEG WALKING

The athlete should do the following:

1. Stand erect with the hands on the hips
2. Walk forward, lifting the left knee out to the side (abduction) and up to waist height (*a*)
3. Adduct the leg back to the midline of the body (*b*) before lowering it to the ground
4. Repeat on the opposite side (*c*), moving forward with each step

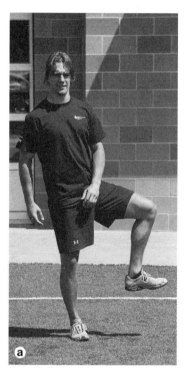
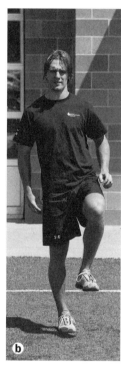
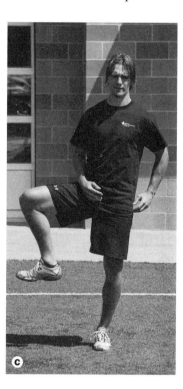

LEG CRADLE

The athlete should do the following:

1. Step forward with the left foot
2. Lift the right knee as high as possible, turning the knee outward (*a*)
3. Place the right hand on the right knee and the left hand on the right ankle (avoid grasping the foot)
4. Pull the lower leg toward the chest (*b*)
5. Maintain an erect body position during the movement
6. Release the right leg and repeat on the other side while walking forward

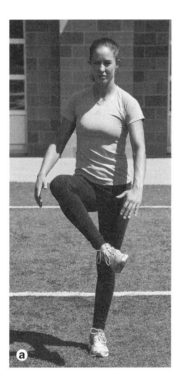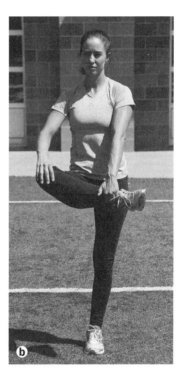

QUAD WALK

The athlete should do the following:

1. Step forward with the left foot
2. Lift the right foot behind the body, maintaining an erect body position
3. Grasp the right ankle with the right hand and pull the foot toward the buttocks
4. Lower the right leg and repeat on the other side while walking forward

HAND WALK (OR INCHWORM)

The athlete should do the following:

1. Stand with the feet shoulder-width apart and the knees slightly flexed
2. Bend forward at the waist and place both hands on the floor, keeping the buttocks in the air and maintaining only a slight bend in the knees
3. Walk hands alternately forward until the body is in the push-up or plank position
4. Walk the feet to the hands using small steps and maintaining straight arms and a slight bend in the knees
5. Repeat the motion

STRAIGHT-LEG KICK

The athlete should do the following:

1. Stand with both arms extended overhead and the feet approximately shoulder-width apart
2. Step forward with the left leg
3. Kick the right leg upward, keeping the torso erect and the leg straight
4. Move both hands toward the toes of the right foot
5. Lower the right leg and return the arms to the starting position
6. Repeat on the opposite side, moving forward with each step

INVERTED HAMSTRING

The athlete should do the following:

1. Stand erect and balance on the right foot
2. Bend forward at the waist, simultaneously extending the left leg back and moving both arms out to the sides
3. Keep the body parallel with the ground while maintaining a neutral spine (the line between the shoulders and the left foot should be straight)
4. Return to the starting position with a small backward step
5. Repeat on the opposite side

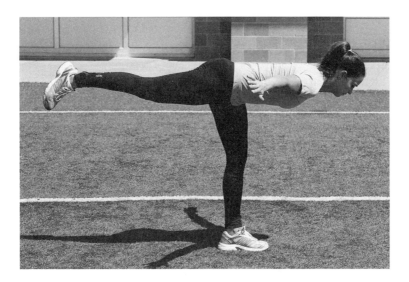

LUNGE WALK WITH REACH

The athlete should do the following:

1. Stand erect with the feet approximately shoulder-width apart and the hands in front of the body

2. Take an exaggerated step forward with the left leg, keeping the left knee directly over the left foot

3. Lower the right knee until it is about 1 to 2 inches (3 to 5 cm) above the floor

4. At the same time, reach both arms in different directions (i.e., forward, overhead, to the left, or to the right) while maintaining proper body position

5. Push off the floor by extending the left knee and hip

6. Return the arms to the starting position

7. Place the right foot next to the left foot

8. Step forward with the right leg and move the arms into a different position

LUNGE WALK WITH ELBOW TO INSTEP

The athlete should do the following:

1. Stand erect with feet shoulder-width apart and the arms at the side of the body
2. Take an exaggerated step forward with the left leg, keeping the left knee directly over the left foot
3. Lower the right knee until it is about 1 or 2 inches (3 to 5 cm) above the floor (*a*)
4. Lean forward and bring the left elbow toward the instep of the left foot (*b*)
5. Lean back and return to an erect torso position
6. Push off the floor by extending the left knee and hip
7. Bring the right foot forward and place it next to the left foot
8. Step forward and repeat the motion on the other side

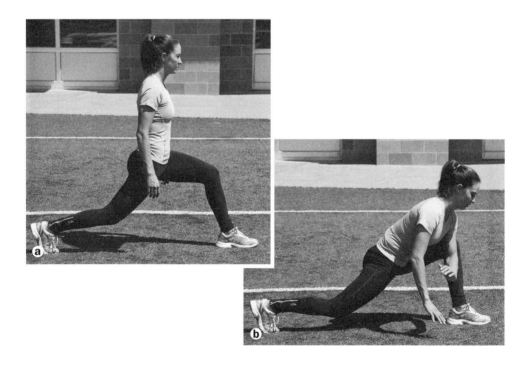

BACKWARD LUNGE

The athlete should do the following:

1. Stand erect with the feet shoulder-width apart and the hands clasped behind the head
2. Keeping the torso perpendicular to the floor, take an exaggerated step backward with the left leg
3. Lower the body until the left knee is about 1 to 2 inches (3 to 5 cm) above the floor
4. Push off the floor by extending the right knee and hip
5. Bring the left leg back to the starting position
6. Lunge backward with the right foot

LATERAL LUNGE

The athlete should do the following:

1. Stand erect with the feet shoulder-width apart and the arms extended in front of the body
2. Take an exaggerated step with the left leg to the side
3. Lower the hips toward the floor
4. Keep the right leg extended and both feet pointed forward
5. Return to the standing position
6. Repeat for the desired number of repetitions, performing the motion in both directions

HIGH HURDLE STEP

The athlete should do the following:

1. Stand erect with the feet shoulder-width apart
2. Mimic the motion of stepping laterally over a high hurdle with the left foot (*a*)
3. Repeat this motion with the right foot
4. Raise each knee as high as possible (*b*)
5. Perform the desired number of repetitions and then repeat in opposite direction

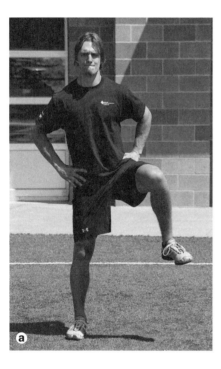 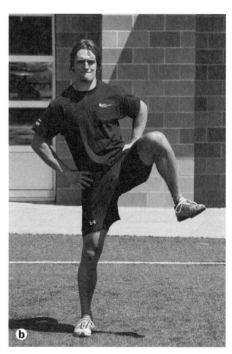

CARIOCA

The athlete should do the following:

1. Stand erect with the feet shoulder-width apart
2. Move laterally to the left by crossing the right foot in front of the left
3. Step laterally with the left foot
4. Cross the right foot behind the left and repeat
5. Perform the motion rapidly with as much hip rotation as possible
6. Perform the motion in both directions

GLUTE KICKS

The athlete should do the following:

1. Move forward using short steps and vigorous arm action, keeping the torso erect
2. At the same time, rapidly kick the right heel toward the buttocks, followed by the left heel

SKIP TAPS

The athlete should do the following:

1. Skip forward, emphasizing a high knee lift
2. At the same time, touch the inside of the foot of the raised leg with the opposite hand (*a*)
3. Alternate taps to each foot for the desired distance (*b*)

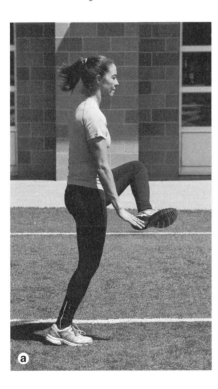
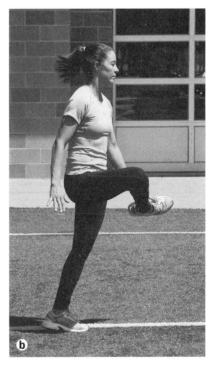

SUMMARY POINTS

- Active participation in a well-designed dynamic warm-up can prepare athletes both physically and mentally for the demands of sport training and competition.

- Despite the conventional wisdom that favors pre-event static stretching, a growing body of evidence indicates that dynamic movements that are sensibly incorporated into a warm-up protocol may improve performance during sports training and competition by increasing body temperature, enhancing ranges of motion, and improving neuromuscular function.

- Although additional research is needed to optimize warm-up procedures for athletes and to better understand the influence of dynamic warm-up protocols on sport-related injury risk, the available data indicate that well-conceived dynamic warm-up activities can have a favorable influence on athletic performance.

- A warm-up should be carefully planned and thought out to the same degree as the main exercise session or event.

4

Resistance Training

Nicholas A. Ratamess, PhD, CSCS*D, FNSCA

Resistance training is a modality of exercise that is well known for its role in improving performance by increasing muscular strength, power and speed, hypertrophy, muscular endurance, motor performance, balance, and coordination. Athletes in essentially every sport have benefited greatly from resistance training. However, the critical element that dictates acute exercise response and chronic adaptation is the design of the resistance training program. A resistance training program is a composite of several variables interacting with each other to provide a stimulus for adaptation. The intricate manipulation of these variables by the strength and conditioning professional or the athlete makes the training program successful. Because infinite ways to design programs exist, many resistance training programs can be successful if they adhere to the training guidelines discussed in this chapter. The training programs of elite athletes demonstrate this point.

Guidelines have been established by the National Strength and Conditioning Association and the American College of Sports Medicine for proper prescription of each variable of acute training programs. If the training stimulus consistently surpasses the athlete's threshold of adaptation for a specific component of fitness, performance can increase, leading to positive physiological adaptations. Thus, only progressive resistance training programs lead to long-term performance enhancement. This chapter discusses the finer points of program design in a way that provides strength and conditioning professionals with a framework for building a template.

Adaptations to Resistance Training

A general understanding of the human body's acute physiological responses to training and subsequent adaptations is essential for optimally designing resistance training programs. Although it is beyond the scope of this

TABLE 4.1 Physiological Adaptations to Resistance Training

Variable	Adaptation
Neural	
Reflex potentiation	Increases
Muscle fiber recruitment and firing rate	Increase
Recruitment timing and efficiency	Increase
Neurotransmitter release	Increases
Tension inhibition	Decreases
Nerve–muscle interface	Expands
Skeletal muscle	
Size	Increases
Protein content	Increases
Fiber number	May not change or slightly increases
Fiber-type transitions (fast to slow)	Increases
Growth-factor expression	Increases
Resting energy substrate levels	Increase
Metabolic anaerobic enzyme activity	May increase, decrease, or not change
Architectural changes (fiber angle, length)	Increase
Buffer capacity	Increases
Capillary number	Increases (but density decreases with fiber growth)
Mitochondrial number	Increases (but density decreases with fiber growth)
Connective tissue	
Ligament size and strength	Increases
Tendon size and strength	Increases
Bone mineral density	Increases
Collagen content	Increases
Cartilage size and strength	May increase or maintain matrix
Endocrine	
Resting hormones: testosterone, growth hormone (GH), IGF-1, cortisol	No change (unless significant change in RT program takes place)
Acute testosterone and GH response	May be augmented or may not change
Androgen receptors	Up-regulated transiently

Variable	Adaptation
Cardiorespiratory	
Resting blood pressure and heart rate	May not change or may decrease
Resting stroke volume	May increase with body size increases
Acute heart rate response	May be less per absolute workload
Acute blood pressure response	May be less per absolute workload
Acute cardiac output and stroke volume	Increase
Ventricular and septal mass or thickness	Increase
Ventricular chamber size	No change or slight increase

chapter to provide a detailed description of training adaptations, table 4.1 briefly presents several of the critical adaptations that lead to performance enhancement.

Resistance training elicits numerous beneficial adaptations to the nervous, muscular, connective tissue, cardiorespiratory, and endocrine systems that enable increases in muscle size, strength, power, and endurance (12, 29). Adaptations to the nervous system enable athletes to recruit more muscle fibers and to preferentially use the muscle fibers most beneficial for strength and power activities. In addition, some neural defense mechanisms (which stimulate inhibition or the onset of fatigue, such as the reflex of the Golgi tendon organ) may be desensitized, thereby allowing athletes to progressively train at a higher tolerance level. Muscular adaptations entail increases in size, substrate concentrations and enzyme activity, fiber transitions (e.g., type IIx to IIa), architectural changes, and enhanced oxidative capacity (increased capillary and mitochondrial density are characteristic of resistance training programs with strong aerobic components). Connective tissue hypertrophy and ultrastructural changes are needed to support strength increases and muscle hypertrophy.

The endocrine system is of great significance during an acute bout of resistance exercise, since some hormones (i.e., catecholamines, testosterone) augment performance, but are especially critical in mediating the post-exercise tissue-remodeling process. Cardiorespiratory changes occur mostly in enhancing the heart's capacity to tolerate stress. Although aerobic exercise produces more comprehensive changes in cardiorespiratory function, resistance training is a potent stimulus for increasing the heart's musculature and contractile characteristics. Collectively, these adaptations can enhance sport performance. They are also highly dependent on the resistance training program used (i.e., the magnitude of progressive overload, variation, and specificity).

Customizing Resistance Training Programs

The most effective resistance training programs meet individual needs or the goals that result from performing a needs analysis (see chapter 1). Individualized resistance training programs are most effective because they ensure that the design is goal oriented and that the principle of training specificity is realized. When all relevant information is gathered and the athlete is deemed healthy enough to perform resistance training, the process of program design is initiated. Some common concerns and questions that need to be addressed are as follows (9, 21):

- *Are health concerns or injuries present that may limit the exercises performed or the exercise intensity?* A pre-existing condition may limit the exercises an athlete can perform at that time. This could potentially limit training intensity until the athlete has sufficiently recovered.

- *What type of equipment (e.g., free weights, machines, bands, tubing, medicine and stability balls, balances, and so on) is available?* The type of equipment available is paramount to exercise selection. Although outstanding programs can be developed with minimal equipment, knowledge of what is available allows strength and conditioning professionals to select appropriate exercises.

- *What is the targeted frequency? Are there any time constraints that may affect workout duration?* The total number of training sessions per week needs to be determined, since it will affect all other training variables (e.g., the exercises selected for each workout, volume, and intensity). Some training sessions may be scheduled for specific periods of time. For example, if the training session is scheduled to last 1 hour, then the program needs to be developed within that time frame. This will affect the type and number of exercises selected, the total sets performed, and the rest intervals used between sets and exercises.

- *What muscle groups need to be trained?* All major muscle groups need to be trained, but some may require prioritization based on the athlete's strengths and weaknesses or the demands of the sport. It is critically important to maintain muscle balance between opposing muscle groups when designing training programs. Thus, exercises must be selected that stress all muscle groups. Appropriate training is essential for muscles with agonist–antagonist relationships (i.e., hamstrings-to-quadriceps ratio) and primary stabilizer roles for large muscle mass exercises. Small muscles are also often weak in comparison to larger muscle groups. For example, attention should be paid to rotator cuffs and scapula stabilizers, as well as deep spinal, core, and trunk muscles. Periodic assessment of athletic performance is needed in order to determine strengths and weaknesses and to monitor progression.

- *What are the targeted energy systems (e.g., aerobic or anaerobic)?* There are three major metabolic systems in the human body: the ATP–CP, glycolytic, and oxidative (aerobic) systems. Resistance training programs mostly target the ATP–CP and glycolytic systems. Few repetitions of high-intensity exercises with long rest intervals stress the ATP–CP system. In contrast, moderate to high repetitions of moderate- to high-intensity exercises, with short to moderate rest intervals, typically target the glycolytic system (i.e., to improve acid–base balance and muscle endurance). Specific attention can be given to either of these energy systems if they match the metabolic demands of the sport. Although the oxidative (aerobic) system is very active during resistance exercise, it tends to be trained more specifically through aerobic training. However, certain programs, such as *circuit training* or high-repetition programs with small rest intervals, can effectively target the aerobic system through resistance training.

- *What types of muscle actions (e.g., concentric [CON], eccentric [ECC], isometric [ISOM]) are needed?* Some athletes may benefit from periodically targeting a specific type of muscular action to elicit a specific adaptive response. For example, a wrestler frequently encounters situations in a match where maximal ISOM strength is necessary. Thus, including more ISOM muscle actions in the program may be a beneficial tool for conditioning.

- *If training for a sport or activity, what are the most common sites of injury?* Special attention can be given to susceptible areas. For example, female athletes are four to eight times more likely to sustain a tear of their anterior cruciate ligament (ACL) than their male counterparts. Thus, special attention should be given to female athletes to strengthen the kinetic chain from the core to the feet. Including exercises that strengthen the knee musculature, the ankle, and the hip in all three planes of motion (and reduce *valgus* stresses) may be beneficial for reducing knee injuries. Resistance training for the core musculature may help as well.

Goals must be determined in order to guide program design. Common goals of resistance training include injury rehabilitation and improvements in muscle size, strength, power, speed, local muscular endurance, balance, coordination, flexibility, percent body fat, general health (e.g., lowered blood pressure, stronger connective tissue, reduced stress). Most programs improve several of these components instead of focusing on a single component. For example, gymnasts require great levels of strength and power, but may experience decreases in performance as a result of excessive hypertrophy. Since these athletes require a high *strength-to-mass ratio*, training programs should be targeted at maximizing neuromuscular components without stressing excessive muscle growth. However, football linemen may benefit from additional lean body mass in addition to strength and power increases. These athletes may be trained to specifically target muscle hypertrophy as well. Thus, the training program must reflect these needs and incorporate sufficient means of overload and variation to attain these goals.

For examples of resistance training programs based on athletes' needs and goals for different parts of the training year, see chapter 12.

Although program goals often include improvement, sometimes athletes need maintenance training. Here, resistance training is used to maintain the current level of fitness rather than for further progression. These programs are used commonly by athletes during the competitive season. Maintenance training could result in *detraining* (cessation of training or substantial reduction in frequency, volume, or intensity that results in decrements in performance) if the training threshold is not met over time. Therefore, cyclical maintenance programs should be designed for progression.

Resistance Training Program Variables

The resistance training program is a composite of several variables. These variables include (1) exercise selection, (2) exercise order and workout structure, (3) intensity, (4) training volume (total number of sets and repetitions), (5) rest intervals, (6) repetition velocity, and (7) training frequency. Altering one or several of these variables affects the training stimuli. Therefore, proper prescription of resistance exercises involves manipulation of each variable to the specificity of the targeted goals.

Exercise Selection

The exercises selected during resistance training play a critical role in performance enhancement and subsequent physiological adaptations. From a biomechanical perspective, exercises can be defined by the type of muscle contraction, type of joint motion, and whether they involve an open or closed kinetic chain. When selecting exercises, strength and conditioning professionals also need to address practical concerns, such as what type of equipment will be used and whether exercises will be performed unilaterally or bilaterally.

Type of Contraction

All exercises consist of concentric (CON), eccentric (ECC), and isometric (ISOM) muscle actions. Each dynamic repetition consists of an ECC (lowering phase or muscle lengthening), a CON (lifting phase or muscle shortening), and an ISOM (static or no change in muscle length) muscle action. Physiologically, ECC actions provide greater force per unit of muscle cross-sectional area, involve less muscle-fiber activation per level of tension, require less energy expenditure per level of tension, and result in greater muscle damage. They are also more conducive to muscle growth than CON or ISOM muscle actions (21, 31). In addition, dynamic strength improvements are greatest when ECC actions are emphasized. Because of these, accentuated ECC training has been used by some advanced lifters.

Most resistance exercise sets may be viewed in a way where the CON action, primarily the *sticking region* (the weak point of the exercise range of motion that is evident during heavy sets or when significant fatigue is present), is the limiting factor of the set. That is, the sticking region is the make-or-break point of the exercise. Because the CON sticking region is the limiting factor in full range-of-motion repetitions (as is most common during resistance training), weight selection ultimately depends on what weight can be lifted through the CON sticking region. For example, during the squat, the lifter encounters the most difficult point of the exercise just above the parallel position. The weight becomes easier to move concentrically throughout the rest of the range of motion once the sticking region has been surpassed. Consequently, other areas of the range of motion, including the ECC phase, may not receive the optimal training stimulus.

Heavy negatives and forced negatives from a partner are a couple of ways in which the ECC muscle action can be emphasized (see the section on supramaximal intensities on page 87). These provide great neuromuscular overload and a novel stimulus for enhancing strength and muscle size. However, heavy ECC training should be used with caution (e.g., short four- to six-week training cycles for only a few sets per workout) to reduce excessive muscle damage and the risk of overtraining and injury. Another form of heavy ECC training involves performing a bilateral exercise with low to moderate weight and then lowering it with only one limb. For example, the athlete can perform a two-leg knee extension, but then lower the weight with only one leg, alternating the negative leg with each repetition or set. These ECC training variations provide significant overload to skeletal muscle.

ISOM muscle actions exist in many forms during resistance exercise: (1) from stabilizer muscles that provide reactive forces to maintain posture during an exercise, (2) in between ECC and CON actions for the agonist muscles in an exercise, (3) while gripping the weights, and (4) as the primary action of the exercise in a specific area of the range of motion. For example, the plank exercise is predominantly ISOM in nature (see figure 4.1). Strong contraction of the core musculature is needed to offset the effects of gravity. In the performance of an overhead squat (see figure 4.2), the upper body

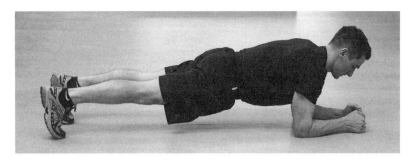

FIGURE 4.1   In the plank exercise, the primary muscle action is isometric.

and trunk isometrically stabilize to maintain the overhead bar position during the descent and ascent phases. ISOM actions of the finger, thumb, and wrist muscles are paramount for gripping the weights (especially during pulling exercises). Grip-strength training is predicated upon ISOM muscle actions to a large extent. ISOM muscle actions included during a set can serve as the primary goal of the exercise. For example, during a pull-up, holding the top position for a specific length of time involves ISOM contraction of back and arm musculature. This action may be used as a specific exercise to enhance strength and muscular endurance specific to range of motion.

Some advanced resistance training programs may include a form of ISOM training known as *functional isometrics*. Functional isometrics involve lifting a barbell in a power rack a few inches until it is up against the rack's pins. The lifter then continues to maximally ISOM push or pull, maintaining for approximately 2 to 6 seconds. Functional isometrics can be performed in any area of the range of motion, but they are effective when performed near the sticking region of the exercise. This is an effective strength

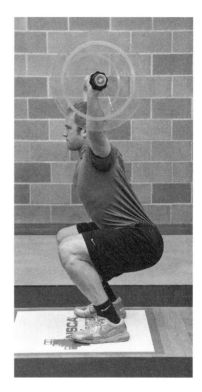

FIGURE 4.2   The overhead squat. Although the squat movement is not isometric, the upper body and trunk muscles must contract isometrically to stabilize and maintain the bar position.

training technique (targeting the exercise's weak point) that has been used for a number of years. Some exercises commonly targeted with functional isometrics are the bench press, deadlift, squat, and clean pull.

Joint Involvement

Two general types of resistance exercises may be selected: exercises for a single joint and exercises for multiple joints. *Single-joint exercises* stress one joint or major muscle group, whereas *multiple-joint exercises* stress more than one joint or major muscle group. Both single- and multiple-joint exercises are effective for increasing muscular strength. Either can be considered sport-specific depending on the athlete. Single-joint exercises (e.g., knee extension, biceps curl) have been used to target specific muscle groups. They may pose a lesser risk of injury due to the reduced level of skill and technique involved. Multiple-joint exercises (e.g., bench press, shoulder press, and squat) are more technically complex in terms of neural activation. They have been regarded as most effective for increasing muscular strength because they enable the athlete to lift a larger amount of weight (21).

Multiple-joint exercises may be subclassified as basic strength or total body lifts. *Basic strength* exercises involve at least two or three major muscle groups, whereas *total body lifts* (e.g., Olympic lifts and variations) involve most major muscle groups. They are the most complex exercises to perform. These lifts are regarded as the most effective exercise for increasing muscle power because they require explosive force production and fast bodily movements. Exercises that work large or multiple muscle groups produce a substantial acute metabolic and hormonal (testosterone and growth hormone) response. In fact, performing large muscle group exercises before small muscle group exercises has been shown to significantly enhance ISOM strength gains of the small muscle group to a larger degree than performing small muscle mass exercises alone does (11). It is thought that exercises that stress large muscle groups produce a greater anabolic hormone environment for the small muscle group exercises (11). Thus, muscle mass involvement is an important consideration when selecting exercises.

Type of Equipment

Alterations in body posture, grip, hand width, foot stance, and position change muscle activation to some degree, thus altering the exercise. Many variations or progressions of single- and multiple-joint exercises can be performed. One facet is the use of either free weights or machines. Both have been recommended for inclusion in resistance training programs. *Free weights* consist of barbells, dumbbells, and associated equipment (i.e., plates, collars, benches). *Machines* encompass a variety of specifically designed pieces of equipment that provide resistance within some prescribed range of motion and movement pattern.

Both free weights and machines are very effective for increasing muscle strength and performance, and both have advantages and disadvantages depending on the needs of the athlete. Machines provide greater stability and control the path of movement. Free weights require the lifter to control all aspects of the exercise. Stabilizer muscles are stressed to a higher degree when free-weight exercises are performed. This has led to the suggestion that machine exercises are safer and easier to learn initially, while free weights stress total muscular development to a larger degree. Due to specificity of training, free-weight training leads to greater improvements in free-weight tests and machine training results in greater performance on machine tests (6). When a neutral testing device is used, strength improvement from free weights and machines appear to produce similar results (38). Free weight training appears more applicable to improving athletic performance.

However, some machines enable the performance of exercises that would be very difficult to perform with free weights (e.g., leg curls, lat pulldowns, tricep pushdowns). These machines may be considered essential. They can provide a benefit to the individual athlete (12). However, the decision to include free-weight or machine exercises may depend on other factors, such as equipment availability and cost.

In addition to free weights and machines, performance of exercises in unstable environments (e.g., with stability balls, wobble boards, and BOSU balls) has become a popular modality of training. These exercises can increase the activity of trunk muscles and other stabilizer muscles (compared to stable environments). However, since lighter weights must be lifted, the stimulus for maximal strength enhancement and force production is limited. In addition, recent research has indicated that structural movements, such as the squat and power clean exercise, are more effective than exercise on unstable surfaces in activating core muscle groups such as the trunk (23). There still may be some usefulness of exercises performed on unstable surfaces (i.e., rehabilitation). Chapter 10 discusses this in further detail. Strongman competition exercises have also become a popular method of training for many diverse populations. Exercises such as stone or barrel lifting, farmer's walk, log press, tire lifting, and truck towing (to name a few) stress all major muscle groups and produce a high level of neuromuscular and metabolic challenge, creating a beneficial stimulus for total body strength and conditioning. Lastly, exercises can be performed with alternative equipment, such as sandbags, kegs, kettle bells, bands and chains (which provide variable resistance to full exercise range of motion), and thick bars. A multitude of exercises can be performed in a variety of conditions that provide many options for the strength and conditioning professional and athlete.

Unilateral and Bilateral Exercises

Another way to vary exercise performance is to alternate between unilateral (one-limb) and bilateral (two-limb) exercises for the same prime movers. The level of muscle activation differs when an exercise is performed bilaterally versus unilaterally. Unilateral training may increase bilateral strength (in addition to unilateral strength), and bilateral training may increase unilateral strength (24), as well as reduce the *bilateral deficit*. This term describes the fact that the maximal force produced by both limbs together is smaller than the sum of the limbs contracting unilaterally. The bilateral deficit may be minimal in well-trained individuals. Thus, unilateral and bilateral exercises are both recommended (31).

Kinetic Chain

From a performance perspective, closed chain kinetic exercises have higher transfer of training effects to specific sporting movements and activities of daily living. A *closed chain kinetic exercise* is one where the distal segments are fixed (squat, deadlift; see figure 4.3), whereas an *open chain kinetic exercise* (leg curl; see figure 4.4) enables the distal segment to freely move against a resistance (25). High correlations between closed chain exercises and performance in vertical and standing long jumps have been shown (4). In addition, Augustsson and colleagues found that training with a closed

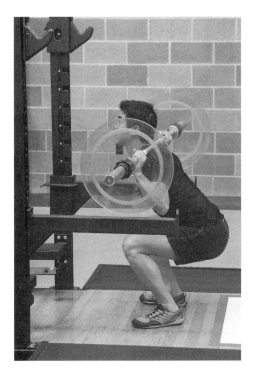

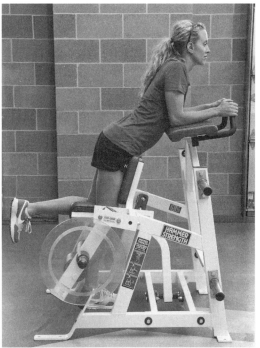

FIGURE 4.3 The squat is an example of a closed chain kinetic exercise, where the distal portion of the body (the legs) is fixed in place, here, by contact with the floor.

FIGURE 4.4 The leg curl is an example of an open chain kinetic exercise, where the distal portion of the body (the legs) moves freely against resistance.

chain kinetic exercise (squat) produced a 10% increase in vertical jump performance, whereas open chain exercises produced no improvement (1). Therefore, closed chain kinetic exercises should form the core foundation of athletic resistance training programs.

Workout Structure and Exercise Order

The number of muscle groups trained per workout needs to be considered when designing the resistance training program. There are three basic workout structures to choose from: (1) total body workouts, (2) upper and lower body split workouts, and (3) muscle group split routines. *Total body workouts* involve exercises that work all major muscle groups (i.e., 1 or 2 exercises for each major muscle group). They are very common among athletes and Olympic weightlifters. In Olympic weightlifting, the primary lifts and variations are total body exercises. Usually, the first few exercises in the workout sequence are the Olympic lifts (plus variations). The remainder of the workout may be dedicated to basic strength exercises. *Upper and lower body split workouts* involve performance of only upper body exercises during one workout and only lower body exercises during the next workout.

These types of workouts are common among athletes, power lifters, and bodybuilders. *Muscle group split routines* involve performance of exercises for specific muscle groups during a workout (e.g., a back and biceps workout in which all exercises for the back are performed, then all exercises for the biceps are performed). These are characteristic of bodybuilding programs.

All of these program designs can be effective for improving athletic performance. Individual goals, time and frequency, and personal preferences determine which structures are selected by the strength and conditioning professional or athlete. The major differences among these structures are the magnitude of specialization present during each workout (related to the number of exercises performed per muscle group) and the amount of recovery time between workouts. Individual needs determine which structure will be used (in addition to the exercises performed) prior to exercise sequencing.

The order of exercises within a workout significantly affects acute lifting performance and subsequent changes in strength during resistance training. The primary training goals should dictate the exercise order. Exercises performed early in the workout are completed with less fatigue, yielding greater rates of force development, higher repetition number, and greater amount of weights lifted. Studies show that performance of multiple-joint exercises (bench press, squat, leg press, shoulder press) declines significantly when done later in a workout (following several exercises that stress similar muscle groups) (35, 36). Considering that these multiple-joint exercises are effective for increasing strength and power, prioritization is typically given to these core structural exercises (i.e., those extremely important to targeting program goals) early in a workout.

For example, Olympic lifts require explosive force production, and creating fatigue reduces the desired effects. These exercises need to be performed early in the workout, especially since they are technically demanding. Sequencing strategies for strength and power training have been recommended (21, 25, 31). It is important to note these can also apply to muscular endurance and hypertrophy training. These recommendations and guidelines are listed in the sidebar.

For hypertrophy and muscular endurance training, some exceptions may exist to these guidelines. Although training to maximize muscle size should include strength training, muscle growth is predicated on factors related to mechanics (force) and blood flow. In contrast, strength training maximizes the mechanical factors. When the goal of training is hypertrophy, training in a fatigued state does have a potent effect on the metabolic factors that induce muscle growth. In this case, the exercise order may vary to stress the metabolic factors involved in muscle hypertrophy.

For example, some bodybuilders have used a technique known as *preexhaustion*. Here, a single-joint exercise is performed first (to fatigue a specific muscle group), followed by a multiple-joint exercise. One example is to

General Guidelines for Exercise Order

When training all major muscle groups in a workout:

- Large muscle group exercises (i.e., squat) should be performed before smaller muscle group exercises (i.e., shoulder press).

- Multiple-joint exercises should be performed before single-joint exercises.

- For power training: Total body exercises (from most to least complex) should be performed before basic strength exercises. For example, the most complex exercises are the snatch (because the bar must be moved the greatest distance) and related lifts, followed by cleans and presses. These take precedence over exercises such as the bench press and squat.

- Alternating between upper and lower body exercises or opposing (agonist–antagonist relationship) exercises can allow some muscles to rest while the opposite muscle groups are trained. This sequencing strategy is beneficial for maintaining high training intensities and targeting repetition numbers.

- Some exercises that target different muscle groups can be staggered between sets of other exercises to increase workout efficiency. For example, a trunk exercise can be performed between sets of the bench press. Because different muscle groups are stressed, no additional fatigue would be induced prior to performing the bench press. This is especially effective when long rest intervals are used.

When training upper body muscles on one day and lower body muscles on a separate day, athletes should do the following:

- Perform large muscle group, multiple-joint exercises before small muscle group, single-joint exercises

- Alternate opposing exercises (agonist–antagonist relationship)

When training individual muscle groups, athletes should do the following:

- Perform multiple-joint exercises before single-joint exercises

- Perform higher-intensity exercises before lower-intensity exercises (The sequence can proceed from the heaviest exercises to those of lower intensity.)

perform the dumbbell fly exercise first to fatigue the pectoral and deltoid muscles, and then perform the bench press. When the bench press is examined, many times the triceps brachii muscle group is the site of failure. This theoretically suggests that the pectorals may not be optimally stimulated. With pre-exhaustion, the pectoral group is prefatigued. As a result, when the lifter performs the bench press after the dumbbell fly, it is likely that the pectoral muscles (i.e., the targeted muscles) will fatigue first. Because a higher number of repetitions are performed when training for hypertrophy, less weight is used. This technique improves hypertrophy and muscle endurance to a greater extent than maximal strength.

For muscle endurance training, fatigue needs to be present for adaptations to take place. Thus, the order can vary in infinite ways. For example, during a preseason conditioning phase, a basketball coach may choose to place the squat exercise later in the workout. This will force the athlete to perform the exercise in a fatigued state, which could replicate a scenario encountered during the sport (e.g., being able to perform a squatting movement similar to jumping in the second half of a game).

Exercise selection can also vary when warm-up exercises are used. For example, some athletes choose to perform a single-joint exercise (leg extension) before the squat exercise as a warm-up. The key distinction here is that the leg extension is performed with light weights and does not fatigue the lifter. Thus, warm-up exceptions can be used effectively to prepare for higher-intensity training.

Intensity

Intensity is the term often used to describe the amount of weight lifted during resistance training. It is highly dependent on other variables, such as exercise order, volume, frequency, repetition speed, and length of rest intervals. Intensity prescription depends on the athlete's training status and goals. Low intensities of 45% to 50% of 1RM or less may increase muscle strength in untrained athletes. However, higher intensities (at least 80% to 85% of 1RM) are needed to increase maximal strength as the athlete progresses to advanced levels of training. Heavy lifting produces a pattern of muscle-fiber recruitment that is distinct from light to moderate loading. Strength, power, muscular endurance, and hypertrophy may only be maximized when the maximal numbers of muscle fibers are recruited.

Repetition Maximum Continuum

An inverse relationship exists between the amount of weight lifted and the number of repetitions performed. Figure 4.5 depicts the relationship between intensity and repetition number. On this continuum, high intensity and low repetitions are most conducive to strength development. As repetitions increase and intensity decreases, a shift to the right occurs and muscle endurance becomes the predominant fitness component stressed. Loads

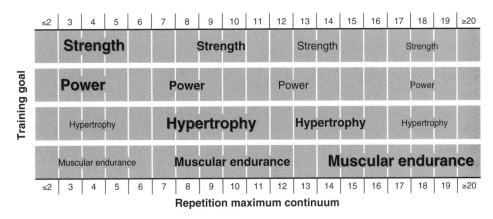

FIGURE 4.5 Theoretical repetition maximum (RM) continuum.

Reprinted, by permission, from NSCA, 2008, Resistance training, by T. Baechle, R. Earle, and D. Wathen. In *Essentials of strength training and conditioning*, 3rd ed., edited by T. Baechle and R. Earle (Champaign, IL: Human Kinetics), 401.

corresponding to 1- to 6RM (repetition maximum), or >85% of 1RM, are most effective for increasing maximal strength (21, 25). Although significant strength increases occur when loads correspond to 6- to 12RM (67% to 85% of 1RM), this range may not be specific to increasing maximal strength in advanced athletes as compared to higher intensities. This range is characteristic of programs that target muscle growth in all trainees and strength training for novice- to intermediate-trained athletes. It has been suggested that this range may provide the best combination of intensity and volume (21, 31). That is, a repetition range between 6- and 12RM may maximize the interaction between mechanical and metabolic growth factors. Intensities lighter than this (12RM and lighter) have only a small effect on maximal strength, but they are very effective for increasing muscular endurance.

Although each training zone on this continuum has its advantages, athletes should not devote 100% of their training time to one general zone as a way to avoid encountering training plateaus or overtraining (21). It is recommended that novice to intermediate lifters resistance train with loads corresponding to 67% to 85% of 1RM for 6 to 12 repetitions. Advanced athletes should alternate this range with training loads of 80% to 100% of 1RM to maximize muscular strength (31). It is also important to note that intensity prescription is exercise dependent. Some exercises, such as multiple-joint structural exercises like power cleans, benefit greatly from periodic high-intensity strength cycles within the training plan. However, other exercises may have different goals associated with them. The intensity may not be as high for every exercise in a workout. For example, an athlete might perform squats with a heavy load (4- to 6RM), followed by the leg curls at a lower intensity (8- to 10RM). The commitment to strength training entails heavy weight lifting. However, this does not mean that every exercise must be high in intensity. Rather, it is the core structural exercises that are typically targeted to be performed at higher intensities.

Power Training

Power training requires two loading strategies. Remember that power is the product of force and velocity. Therefore, both force and velocity components must be emphasized to maximize power. Moderate to heavy loads are required to recruit the fast-twitch muscle fibers needed for maximal strength increases. However, as depicted by the force–velocity relationship when maximal effort and loads are used, concentric force increases as velocity decreases. Thus, greater loading results in such a decrease in velocity that performing heavy resistance training increases force production, but does not optimize the velocity (or time) component (33). A second vital training strategy when training for power is to incorporate low to moderate intensities performed at an explosive lifting velocity (i.e., based on the impulse–momentum relationship). The intensity may vary depending on the exercise in question and the athlete's training status.

Most studies have shown that peak power is attained in a range from 15% to 60% of 1RM for ballistic exercises, such as the jump squat and bench press throw (2, 3, 31, 39). Recent research indicates that perhaps even less resistance (e.g., body weight) can maximize power output during jumps (7, 8). One study has shown that jump-squat training with 30% of 1RM is more effective for increasing peak power than jump-squat training with 80% of 1RM (23). With ballistic resistance exercises, the load is maximally accelerated either by jumping or by releasing the weight. However, repetition of traditional resistance exercises results in a substantial deceleration phase, which limits power development throughout the complete range of motion. The intensities at which peak power is attained during traditional repetitions are generally higher than those for ballistic exercises due to the variance in deceleration (e.g., 40% to 60% of 1RM for the bench press, 50% to 70% for the squat) (34). Peak power for Olympic lifts typically occurs at the 70% to 80% range of 1RM (16).

Although any intensity may enhance muscle power, specificity is needed to ensure that training encompasses a range of intensities, with emphasis placed on those that match the demands of the sport or activity. For example, an American football player (lineman) benefits greatly from power training of moderate to high intensity because this may more closely simulate actions encountered on the field. However, high jumpers in track and field may benefit from lower intensities in this spectrum, since they are essentially competing against only their own body mass. Therefore, lighter training loads may more closely match the sporting demands. Thus, training for maximal power requires a spectrum of resistance exercise intensities performed at high velocity, based on the demands of the sport and or position.

It is recommended that power training include various loading strategies in a periodized manner. Heavy loading (85% to 100% of 1RM) is necessary for increasing strength, and light to moderate loading (30% to 60% of 1RM for upper body exercises, 0% to 60% of 1RM for lower body exercises) performed at an explosive velocity is necessary for increasing fast force production. A multiple-set (3-6 sets) power program that is integrated in periodized manner into a strength training program consisting of one to six repetitions is recommended.

Increasing Intensity

Three basic methods exist for increasing loading during progressive resistance training: (1) increasing relative percents of 1RM, (2) training within a repetition maximum (RM) zone, and (3) increasing absolute amounts. Increasing relative percents is common in periodized programs, especially for Olympic lifts and variations, squats, deadlifts, and bench presses. Athletes may train with 70% of their predetermined 1RM for one set and at 80% during the next set. Percents can be used to vary intensity from set to set or to quantify a training cycle (e.g., hypertrophy cycle may be characteristic of intensities of 67% to 75% of 1RM, versus a strength cycle, which may be characteristic of intensities greater than 85% of 1RM). Over a long training cycle, a relative percent can exceed 100% of the originally calculated 1RM if the strength and conditioning professional is factoring in the athlete's potential strength gains during training. Relative percents are especially useful during unloading weeks. They may vary as a result of strength testing, since the percent will be based on the new 1RM strength value.

Training within a RM zone requires an increase in repetitions with a current workload until a target number is reached. In a zone of 8- to 12RM, the athlete selects an 8RM load and performs 8 repetitions. During the next few workouts, the athlete performs additional repetitions with that load until 12 repetitions are completed on consecutive workouts. The training load is then increased, and the athlete subsequently performs 8 repetitions.

Increasing intensity in absolute amounts is most common, especially among assistance exercises and core structural exercises. For example, the athlete completes six repetitions with 100 kg in the bench press. As strength increases, the athlete continues to perform six repetitions; however, he uses a greater load (e.g., 105 kg). When the athlete feels (or appears) stronger, an absolute amount of weight can be added to the exercise. The absolute increase depends on the exercise, since a large muscle mass exercise (i.e., leg press) can tolerate an increase of 4 to 7 kg, while a small muscle mass exercise (i.e., biceps curl) may only tolerate an increase of 1 to 2 kg. All of these methods have been studied and shown to be very effective for resistance training. Ultimately, which method or combination of methods will be used is up to the preference of the athlete or strength and conditioning professional.

Supramaximal Intensities

In some cases, supramaximal (>100% of the athlete's concentric 1RM) intensities may be used. These provide a high degree of overload. They are used sparingly, mostly at the end of training cycles where peak strength needs to be attained. Remember that a concentric 1RM can alternatively be defined as the maximal amount of weight lifted through the sticking region. Consequently, other muscle actions and segments of the range of motion allow athletes to lift more than their respective 1RM for a given exercise. Techniques such as *forced repetitions* and *heavy negatives, partial range-of-motion training* (in the strongest area of the range of motion), and *overloads* may be used to stimulate the nervous system and to perhaps enhance maximal strength (25). Heavy negatives involve loading the bar with >100% of 1RM (usually by 20% to 40%). The ECC phase should only be performed in the presence of capable spotters or a power rack with the pins set appropriately. This is also the case with forced repetitions, where a spotter assists with the CON phase, but the athlete primarily controls the ECC phase.

Partial range-of-motion lifts may be used to emphasize the natural strength curves that occur during the selected exercises. For example, multiple-joint pushing exercises typically follow an ascending curve (where strength is increased as the exercise progresses through the range of motion), while pulling exercises follow a descending curve (force output decreases as the exercise progresses through the range of motion). Bypassing the weak point and overloading the strongest area of the range of motion can be used to stimulate the nervous system for strength gains.

Overloads involve holding a supramaximal weight without actually performing the exercise. The theory with this method of training is to trick the nervous system by supporting >100% of 1RM. It is thought that this may enhance 1RM strength by making the 1RM feel lighter. Power lifters have often been known to use overloads. For example, an exercise called the walk-out is used to assist in supporting a higher 1RM squat. The lifter supports the supramaximal weight from the lift-off-the-rack phase to the starting position without actually performing the squat. Since all of these techniques are very high in intensity, they must be used with caution. They tend to be reserved primarily for advanced lifters.

Volume

Training volume is a summation of the total number of sets and repetitions performed during a workout. Training volume can be manipulated by changing the number of exercises performed per session, the number of repetitions performed per set, or the number of sets per exercise. Typically, an inverse relationship exists between the number of sets per exercise and the number of exercises performed in a workout. There is also an inverse relationship between volume and intensity. That is, volume should be reduced if significant increases in intensity are prescribed. Strength training is associated with low to moderate training volume, since a low to moderate number of repetitions are performed per set for core structural exercises. Hypertrophy and muscular endurance training are associated with moderate to high intensity and volume. These programs, which are high in total work, tend to stimulate a potent endocrine and metabolic response.

Training volumes of athletes vary considerably and depend on other factors besides intensity (e.g., training status, number of muscle groups trained per workout, nutrition practices, practice and competition schedule). Current volume recommendations for strength training include one to three sets per exercise for novice lifters and two to six sets for intermediate and advanced lifters. Multiple sets should be used with systematic variation of volume and intensity for progression into intermediate and advanced training. Dramatic increases in volume are not recommended, since they may lead to overtraining. Further, not all exercises need to be performed with the same number of sets. The volume of each exercise is related to the program priorities (31).

The number of sets performed per exercise, muscle group worked, and overall structure of the workout is also of primary interest when designing a resistance training program. Few studies directly compare resistance training programs of varying total sets. Most volume studies compare single- and multiple-set training programs. One set of an exercise performed for 8 to 12 repetitions at an intentionally slow lifting velocity has been compared to both periodized and nonperiodized multiple-set programs. These studies have shown similar results in novice athletes regardless of program design (37), but some studies have shown multiple sets to be superior (5). Periodized, multiple-set programs were shown to be superior during progression to intermediate and advanced stages of training (20, 22, 32). One study showed strength reduction in trained women who switched to a single-set program (18). Regarding total sets per workout, one study that examined the current literature suggested that eight sets per muscle group yielded the most substantial effects (28). Most studies used two to six sets per exercise and found substantial strength increases in trained and untrained athletes (21). Typically, two to six sets per exercise are most common during resistance training, but both greater and lesser amounts have also been used successfully.

Set Structures for Multiple-Set Programs

When multiple sets are used, the next decision concerns the way they are structured. The intensity or volume during each exercise can increase, decrease, or stay the same. Three basic structures (as well as integrated systems) are commonly used. The first is a *constant load/repetition* system. The intensity and volume remain the same across all sets. This is very effective for increasing strength, power, hypertrophy, and muscular endurance. It can be easily incorporated into a periodized training program.

A second system is to work from light to heavy. Weight is increased in each set, while repetitions remain the same or decrease. One popular example is the *ascending pyramid*. Ascending pyramids can be used to target any fitness component by manipulating the intensity and volume. This may be advantageous in the sense that there is progression prior to lifting the heaviest weight (i.e., the lifter may be more prepared for the first exercise in sequence due to a more specific warm-up). However, overuse of the ascending pyramid increases the risk of overtraining.

The third system is to work from heavy to light. One popular example of this is the *descending pyramid*. Here, the weight is decreased with each subsequent set, while repetitions remain the same or increase. The advantage is that the heaviest set is performed first when fatigue may be minimal. However, critics of this system typically voice concerns about athletes being inadequately warmed-up when performing the heaviest set. Advantages and disadvantages for each method exist. Because all are effective, use of these may be up to the personal preference of the athlete, coach, or strength and conditioning professional.

Rest Intervals

Rest interval length depends on training intensity, goals, fitness level, and use of the targeted energy system. The amount of rest between sets and exercises significantly affects the metabolic, hormonal, and cardiorespiratory responses to an acute bout during resistance exercise, as well as performance of subsequent sets and training adaptations (21, 30). Acute force and power production are compromised with short rest intervals (30), although these short rest intervals are beneficial for hypertrophy and muscle endurance training. Figure 4.6 depicts acute lifting performance with various rest intervals. A continuum is shown where the greatest reductions in performance are seen with 30-second rest intervals. The performance was best maintained with 5-minute rest intervals (30). Thus, short rest intervals compromise performance, whereas long rest intervals help maintain intensity and volume.

Long-term resistance training studies have shown greater strength increases with long (i.e., 2-3 min) versus short (i.e., 30-40 s) rest periods between sets (25, 31). It is important to note that rest interval length will vary based on the goals of the training program and the demands of individual exercises within that program (not every exercise must use the same rest interval). For novice, intermediate, and advanced strength training, it is recommended that rest periods of at least 2 to 5 minutes be used for strength training (31). These recommendations also apply to training for hypertrophy, although shorter rest intervals can also be effectively used at various points of training. Strength and power performance is highly dependent on the ATP–CP system. It generally takes at least 3 minutes for the majority of repletion to take place. High-intensity lifting performance requires the availability of maximal energy substrate in order to perform the set with minimal or no fatigue. Muscle strength may increase when using short rest intervals, but at a slower rate.

Rest interval selection has a great effect when training for muscular endurance. Training to increase muscular endurance implies the athlete (1)

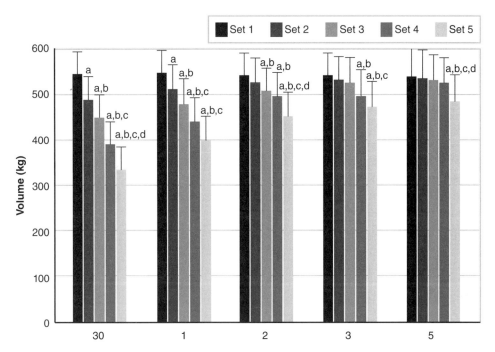

FIGURE 4.6 Lifting performance during 10-repetition sets of the bench press with 30-second, 1-, 2-, 3-, and 5-minute rest intervals. (*a*) Significantly less ($P < 0.05$) than set 1, (*b*) less than set 2, (*c*) less than set 3, (*d*) less than set 4.

With kind permission from Springer Science+Business Media: *European Journal of Applied Physiology,* "The effect of rest interval length on metabolic responses to the bench press exercise," 100: 1-17, N.A. Ratamess et al. Copyright 2007.

performs high repetitions to enhance submaximal muscular endurance or (2) minimizes recovery between sets to enhance high-intensity (or strength) endurance. Thus, it is recommended that short rest intervals be used for muscular endurance training (e.g., ≤30 s).

Repetition Velocity

Lifting velocity affects the neural, hypertrophic, and metabolic responses to training. It is highly dependent on loading and fatigue. For nonmaximal lifts, the velocity that the athlete intends during the movement is critical. Since force = mass × acceleration, significant reductions in force production are seen when the intent is to perform the repetition slowly (33). However, there are two types of slow-velocity contractions: unintentional and intentional. *Unintentional* slow velocities are used during high-intensity repetitions in which either the loading or fatigue level are responsible for the velocity. That is, the athlete exerts maximal force (intending to move the weight fast) but, due to the heavy loading or onset of fatigue, the resulting velocity is slow. These are seen during heavy sets and pose a potent stimulus for strength increases. In addition, repetition velocity may decrease during the last few repetitions of a set during the onset of fatigue (26).

Intentional slow-velocity repetitions are used with submaximal weights where the athlete has direct control of the velocity. Force production is much lower for an intentionally slow velocity than for a traditional (moderate) or explosive velocity with a corresponding (lower) level of muscle-fiber activation (19). Intentionally lifting a weight slower forces the athlete to reduce the weight greatly. One study found that weight needed to be reduced by approximately 30% and that this did not provide an optimal stimulus for improving 1RM strength (17). Thus, intentionally slow velocities may be useful for muscular endurance training, but they appear counterproductive for strength and power training.

Moderate to high velocities (1-2 s CON or less; 1-2 s ECC) are most effective for enhanced muscular performance (e.g., number of repetitions performed, work and power output, and volume) (27). For strength training, the intent to move the weight as quickly as possible (to optimize the neural response) appears to be the critical training attribute. That is, the velocity seen during lifting may viewed as the outcome, but the maximal intent to move the bar quickly is a key stimulus. This technique, which has been termed *compensatory acceleration*, requires the athlete to accelerate the load maximally throughout the range of motion during the CON phase to maximize bar velocity. A major advantage is that this technique can be used with heavy loads. It is quite effective for multiple-joint exercises and is more beneficial for strength training than slower velocities (15). In addition, fast or explosive lifting velocities are recommended for maximizing increases in power (31).

Training for muscle endurance or hypertrophy requires a spectrum of velocities with various loading strategies. The critical component to muscle endurance training is to prolong the duration of the set. Two recommended strategies for prolonging set duration are (1) moderate number of repetitions using an intentionally slow velocity and (2) high number of repetitions using moderate to fast velocities. Intentionally slow velocity training with light loads (5 s CON: 5 s or slower ECC) places continued tension on the muscles for an extended period of time. This is more metabolically demanding than moderate and fast velocities. However, it is difficult to perform a large number of repetitions using intentionally slow velocities. When high repetition numbers are desired, moderate to fast velocities are preferred. Both training strategies of moderate repetitions at slow velocity and high repetitions at moderate to fast velocity increase the glycolytic and oxidative demands of the stimulus, thereby serving as a very effective means of increasing muscular endurance.

Frequency

The number of training sessions performed during a specific period of time may affect training adaptations. *Frequency* indicates the number of times certain exercises are done or muscle groups are trained per week. It depends on several factors, such as volume, intensity, exercise selection, level of conditioning or training status, recovery ability, nutritional intake, and training goals. Numerous resistance training studies used frequencies of two or three alternating days per week for untrained athletes. This has been shown to be an effective initial frequency. It is recommended for beginning lifters (31). An increase in training experience does not necessitate a change in frequency for training each muscle group, but it may be more dependent on alterations in other acute variables, such as exercise selection, volume, and intensity. Increasing training frequency may enable greater specialization (e.g., greater exercise selection and volume per muscle group). In other studies, four or five days per week were superior to three, three days per week were superior to one and two days, and two days per week were superior to one for increasing maximal strength (10, 14). One study showed that American football players who trained four or five days per week achieved better results than those who trained either three or six days per week (13).

Frequency for advanced training varies considerably. Advanced weightlifters and bodybuilders use high-frequency training (e.g., 4-6 sessions per week). The frequency for elite weightlifters and bodybuilders may be even greater. Double-split routines (two training sessions per day with emphasis on different muscle groups) are common during training, which may result in 8 to 12 training sessions per week. High frequencies are common in Olympic weightlifters, who have the rationale that frequent short sessions followed by periods of recovery, supplementation, and food intake allow for a better training stimulus. Elite power lifters typically train four to six days per week. It is important to note that not all muscle groups are trained specifically per workout using a high frequency. Rather, each major muscle group may be trained two or three times per week despite the large number of workouts.

> For more practical guidelines on integrating all the program variables throughout the training year, see chapter 12.

SUMMARY POINTS

- Manipulation of the acute resistance training variables is critical to program design. The human body usually adapts to its current workload within one or two weeks. Thus, programs must be continually altered to keep the training stimuli potent and to avoid training plateaus. Any resistance training program can be effective as long as progressive overload, specificity, and variation are incorporated.

- Ways to make workouts more demanding (in accordance with specific goals) include (1) increasing the weights or loads lifted, (2) adding repetitions to the current workload, (3) increasing lifting velocity with sub- to near-maximal loads to enhance the neuromuscular response, (4) lengthening rest intervals to enable greater loading or reducing them to target muscular endurance, (5) increasing training volume within reasonable limits (i.e., 2.5% to 5%), and (6) introducing other advanced training techniques for supramaximal loading (12, 25).

- Without progressive overload (a gradual increase in stress placed on the body), no adaptation will take place. Thus, lifters must strive to progressively train harder over time in order to continue progressing.

- *Specificity* refers to designing programs specifically to targeted goals. Training adaptations are specific to the stimulus. This includes specificity of muscle actions trained, range of motion, energy system utilization, velocity, and neuromuscular recruitment patterns (25). Individualized training programs must target specific components of fitness to maximize performance enhancement.

- Variation, or training periodization (see chapter 11), should be implemented to keep the stimulus novel, thereby forcing the body to adapt. Most often, intensity and volume are periodized. However, all acute program variables can be manipulated to a certain degree. For example, varying exercise selection is an effective way to improve the quality of resistance training workouts. The systematic variation of the training stimulus is mandatory for long-term progression and for reducing the incidence of training plateaus.

5

Power Training

Robert U. Newton, PhD, CSCS*D, FNSCA
Prue Cormie, PhD
William J. Kraemer, PhD, CSCS, FNSCA

This chapter focuses on the most important neuromuscular function in many sport performances, the ability to generate maximal muscular power. *Maximal power* will be defined and its importance to human performance will be discussed. Subsequently, maximal power development and program design will be addressed, including advanced strength and conditioning techniques for developing power output.

Power can be defined as the applied force multiplied by the velocity of movement (65). Since work is the product of the force and the distance moved, and velocity is the distance moved divided by the time taken, power can also be expressed as work done per unit of time (40). Power output for an athlete can range from 50 W, produced during light cycling or jogging, to around 7000 W, produced during the second phase of the pull for the clean in weightlifting (40). The main focus of this chapter is maximal power output, that which can be produced in one or two muscular contractions. This has been termed *maximal instantaneous power* (43); however, for the purposes of this chapter, the term *maximal power* is used.

The ability to explode out of the blocks as the starter's gun fires, jump over a bar 2.45 m high, elude an opponent by rapidly changing direction, snatch 2.5 times your body mass, or drive a golf ball more than 300 m are all exceptional feats of maximal power. Maximal power output is paramount to performance when the aim is to achieve maximal velocity at takeoff, release, or impact (69, 80, 89, 105). This encompasses generic movements, such as sprinting, jumping, changing direction, throwing, kicking, and striking. Therefore, it applies to the majority of sports.

Factors Contributing to Power Output

An athlete's jump when rebounding in basketball shows the importance of maximal power in sport and also allows us to examine the mechanical factors that contribute to power. The height to which an athlete jumps for a rebound is determined purely by the velocity with which he leaves the ground. At the bottom of the movement, the body stops momentarily (figure 5.1). As the athlete extends the trunk, hips, knees, and ankles and leaves the ground, the body is accelerated upward to a maximum takeoff velocity. This velocity is determined by the force that the muscles can generate against the ground multiplied by the time during which the forces are applied, termed *impulse*, minus the impulse due to the body's weight (104).

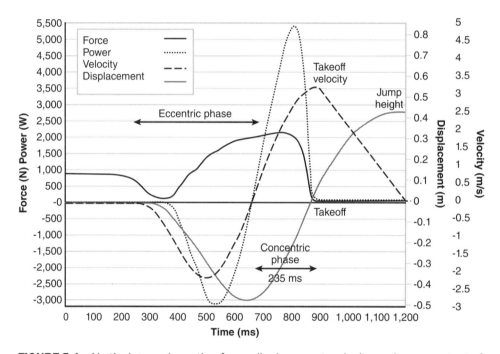

FIGURE 5.1   Vertical ground reaction force, displacement, velocity, and power output of the subject during a countermovement jump. Note that the concentric muscle action is only 235 ms in duration. The resulting takeoff velocity is determined by the sum of the forces that can be produced during this short time period.

Once the athlete has left the ground, he can no longer apply force. The faster the body is accelerated vertically, the shorter the time between the bottom of the movement and takeoff (i.e., 235 ms in figure 5.1). It is here that we can appreciate the importance of maximum muscular power. As an athlete attempts to maximize his power output, the time over which force can be applied to accelerate the body decreases. Therefore, three mechanical properties of the neuromuscular system determine performance:

- The ability to develop a large amount of force in a short period of time, termed the *maximum rate of force development* (mRFD)

- The ability of muscle to produce high force at the end of the eccentric phase and during the early concentric phase

- The ability of muscle to continue producing high force output as its velocity of shortening increases

A number of factors contribute to maximizing these three properties. Discussion of each factor will assist our understanding of the effects of different training strategies and how they may influence training efficiency. Maximal power performance responds to training using a countermovement in which muscles are first stretched and then shortened (stretch-shortening cycle). It responds more fully to specific power training than to heavy resistance training, since power training involves force and velocity, as well as a shorter deceleration phase during which muscle activation decreases. Each component contributing to maximal power production appears to have its own window of adaptation, suggesting that the training program for an athlete should use mixed methods and should target those components with the greatest potential for adaptation—that is, the components in which that athlete is weak.

Stretch-Shortening Cycle

Most powerful activities involve a countermovement during which the muscles involved are first stretched and then shortened to accelerate the body or limb. This action of the muscle is called a *stretch-shortening cycle* (SSC) (66). It involves many complex and interacting neural and mechanical factors, such as activation of the stretch reflex and muscle–tendon interactions. A great deal of research has been directed toward the study of the SSC (10, 11, 37, 42) because it has been observed that performance is greater in SSC movements than when the activity is performed with a purely concentric action (11). For example, differences in jump height of 18% to 20% have been observed between static or squat jumps (SJ) and countermovement jumps (CMJ) (12). An SJ is a purely concentric jump initiated from a crouching position. The CMJ is initiated from a standing position. The athlete performs a quick countermovement, dipping the hips down and then jumping up.

Although several mechanisms have been proposed (10), it would appear that the difference in CMJ and SJ height is due primarily to the fact that the countermovement allows the athlete to attain greater force output at the start of the upward movement. This results in greater forces being exerted against the ground and, subsequently, an increase in impulse ($F \times t$) and acceleration of the whole body upward. The other proposed mechanisms, such as recovery of stored elastic energy, muscle–tendon interactions, and activation of the stretch reflex, appear to play a secondary role in the enhancement of performance by the SSC (10).

Maximal power performance has been shown to respond to training that involves performing SSC movements more rapidly than the athlete is accustomed to with a stretch load of greater magnitude than usual. These activities, termed *plyometrics*, have been found in a number of studies to effectively increase jumping ability and power output (1, 21, 91, 102). Plyometric training results in an increase in the overall neural stimulation of the muscle and, thus, an increase in force output. However, qualitative changes in the muscle activity are also apparent (91). In subjects unaccustomed to intense SSC loads, some studies have shown a reduction in electromyographic (EMG) activity, starting 50 to 100 ms before ground contact and lasting for 100 to 200 ms (91). This is attributed to a protective reflex mechanism by the Golgi tendon organ, which acts during sudden, intense stretch loads that typically reduce the tension in the musculotendinous unit during the force peak of the SSC. After periods of plyometric training, these inhibitory effects (and the observed reduction in the EMG) are reduced (termed *disinhibition*) and SSC performance results are increased (91).

Plyometric training places considerable forces on the musculoskeletal system. Although it has been recommended that athletes have a preliminary strength training base prior to commencing a plyometric training program (e.g., an athlete should be able to squat 1.5 times his or her body weight) (20), low-intensity plyometric drills (e.g., squat jumps, countermovement jumps, lateral jumps, box jumps) can be performed safely without any minimal strength requirement. Keep in mind that plyometrics are often part of the jumping games that children play. The potential for injury is thought to be much higher for depth jumps, which should not be attempted by beginners (89).

Muscular Strength

Strength, the amount of force or torque a muscle can exert at a specified or determined velocity (65), varies for different muscle actions, such as eccentric, concentric, and isometric contractions (68). Often, strength and conditioning professionals and athletes associate the term *strength* with the force that can be exerted during slow-speed, or even isometric, muscle actions. This is often determined using a test of one-repetition maximum (1RM), in which strength is assessed as the maximum weight the athlete can lift once throughout the complete movement. The development and assessment of 1RM strength have received a great deal of research attention, and interested readers may refer to the relevant literature (2, 6, 45). When lifting a maximal weight, the limiting factor is muscle strength at slow contraction velocities. Muscle strength as required in 1RM lifts, however, is needed in a limited number of athletic endeavors (e.g., powerlifting). Most sports require high force output at much faster velocities of movement and the rapid attainment of high force from a relaxed state.

Research findings (22, 46, 101, 102) and anecdotal evidence from strength and conditioning professionals indicate that if an athlete's strength at slow movement velocities increases, then power output and athletic performance also improve. This occurs since maximum strength, even at slow velocities, is a contributing factor in maximal power. In other words, a fundamental relationship exists between strength and power that dictates that an athlete cannot possess a high level of power without first being relatively strong. Research involving heavy strength training programs with untrained to moderately trained subjects has demonstrated that such training results not only in improved maximal strength but also in increased maximal power output (22, 47, 62, 78, 93, 94, 101, 102). Although strength is a basic quality that influences maximal power production, the significance of this influence diminishes somewhat when the athlete maintains a very high level of strength (69). Despite this, the current strength level of athletes will always dictate the upper limit of their potential to generate maximal muscular power because the ability to generate force rapidly is of little benefit if maximal force is low.

When attempting to maximize power output, the concentric phase follows the eccentric phase. As such, it starts from zero velocity. Therefore, the force produced during the latter part of the eccentric phase, the changeover from lengthening to shortening (which includes a phase when the muscle is contracting isometrically), and the subsequent concentric contraction is determined by the maximum strength of the agonist muscles during slow eccentric, isometric, and concentric contractions. If maximal strength is increased, then higher forces can be exerted during this time, resulting in increased impulse, which leads to increased acceleration (22). However, as the muscles begin to achieve high velocities of shortening, strength capacity at slow movement velocity has a reduced impact on the ability of the muscle to produce high force (32, 61, 62). This fact becomes increasingly important as the athlete attempts to train specifically for maximal power development.

Targeting Power Development

Use of slow-velocity, heavy resistance training for the development of maximal power is justified on the basis that power is equal to the product of force and velocity of the muscle action. It has often been reasoned that increasing 1RM strength is sufficient to influence power output. While such reasoning is supported by research involving untrained subjects over short-term training interventions (22), it does not apply to trained athletes who have established a solid foundation of strength (101). If we are to maximize improvements in power performance in such athletes, then we must train both the force and velocity components. Because the movement distance is usually fixed by the athlete's joint ranges of motion, velocity is determined by the time taken to complete the movement. Therefore, if we train using methods that decrease the time over which the movement is produced, we increase the power output. Intimately linked to this concept is the mRFD, or maximal rate of force development.

Resistance Training and Power

In terms of training, several studies have shown improved performance in power activities (e.g., vertical jump) following a strength training program (1, 4, 21, 102). For example, one study demonstrated a 7% improvement in vertical jumps following 24 weeks of intense resistance training (46). Despite these observed improvements, specific power training appears much more effective (47), especially for trained athletes. In one study, subjects performed movements in which they attempted to maximize power output with relatively lighter loads and showed a 21% increase in vertical jumps. These results indicate that specific training adaptations might exist for heavy resistance training versus power-type training. Heavy resistance training using high resistance and slow velocities of concentric muscle action leads primarily to improvements in maximal strength (i.e., the high-force, low-velocity portion of the force–velocity curve; see figure 5.2). These improvements are reduced at the higher velocities. Power training utilizes lighter loads and higher veloci-

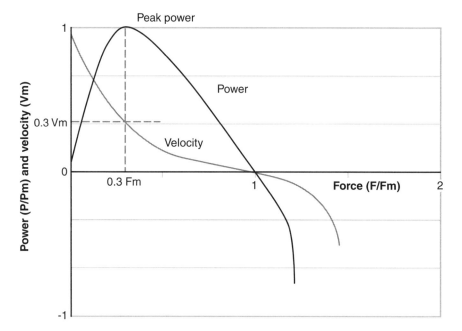

FIGURE 5.2   Relationship among force, velocity, and power for skeletal muscle. *Vm*, *Pm*, and *Fm* are maximum movement velocity, maximal power output, and maximum isometric force output, respectively.

Adapted, by permission, from J.A. Faulkner, D.R. Claflin, and K. K. McCully, 1986, *Power output of fast and slow fibers from human skeletal muscles. In Human muscle power*, edited by N.L. Jones, N. McCartney, and A.J. McComas (Champaign, IL: Human Kinetics), 81-94.

For guidelines on integrating power and resistance training at different stages of the training year, see chapter 12.

ties of muscle action, resulting in increases in force output at the higher velocities. Rate of force development (RFD) is also improved (47).

Although velocity-specific training adaptations are observed, performance changes with training are not always consistent with this principle. The conflict results from the complex nature of powerful muscle actions and the integration of slow and fast force production requirements within the context of a complete movement. Another confounding influence in observing clear, specific training adaptations is the fact that in untrained people, a wide variety of training interventions will produce increases in strength and power. Depending on the training status of the subject, the response may not always follow the velocity-specific training principle (67).

For subjects with low levels of strength, improvements throughout the force–velocity spectrum may be produced regardless of the training load or style used (22, 67). For example, changes in the force–velocity relationship following 10 weeks of training were similar in relatively untrained subjects exposed to either heavy resistance training or ballistic power training (figure 5.3) (22). The changes observed in the heavy strength–trained athletes were driven by improvements in maximal neural activation and muscle thickness. In contrast, the changes observed following ballistic power training were produced by improvements in the rate of rise in muscle activation. Despite the differing nature of adaptations to each training stimuli, both resulted in significant improvements throughout the force–velocity relationship, particularly for maximal power in untrained people (22).

It appears that training adaptations of single factors (i.e., high force, high power) occur only after a base level of strength and power training has been achieved. This notion is supported by the fact that if the athlete already has an adequate level of strength, then the increases in maximal power performance in response to traditional strength training will be poor. More specific training interventions will be required to further improve maximal power output (45). Thus, improvement of maximal power output in trained athletes may require more complex training strategies than previously thought (102).

This contention is supported by research (101) comparing changes in 1RM squat, vertical jump, and flying 20 m sprint velocity during eight weeks of either weight training or plyometric training. Subjects were classified as *weak* or *strong* based on their pretraining 1RM squat. The results demonstrated significant negative relationships between improvements induced by weight training in sprinting, jumping, and pretraining 1RM performance. The authors hypothesized that this was due to the principle of diminishing returns, whereby initial improvements in muscular function are easily attained, but further improvements are progressively harder to

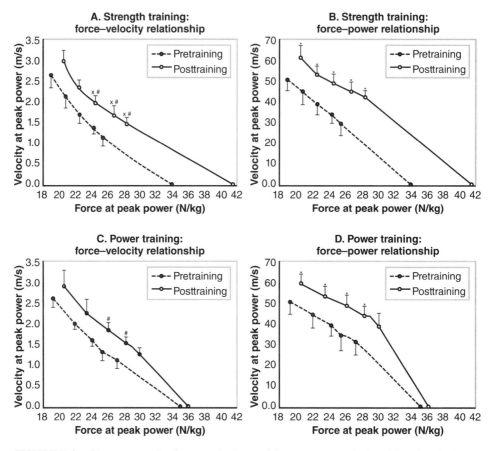

FIGURE 5.3 Changes to the force–velocity and force–power relationships for the jump squat (i.e., a CMJ with a bar held across the shoulders) in response to 10 weeks of heavy resistance training (*a* and *b*) and ballistic power training (*c* and *d*). Significant improvement in force (*x*), velocity (#) or power (*).

Adapted, by permission, from P. Cormie, 2009, *A series of investigations into the effect of strength level on muscular power in athletic movements* (Perth, WA: Edith Cowan University, School of Exercise, Biomedical, and Health Science), 263.

achieve. Unexpectedly, the performance gains from the plyometric training were unrelated to initial strength levels.

Resistance Training and Rate of Force Development

Since time is limited during powerful muscle actions, the muscle must exert as much force as possible in a short period of time. This quality has been termed *maximum rate of force development* (figure 5.4). This may explain to some extent why heavy resistance training is ineffective for increasing power performance in well-trained athletes. Squat training with heavy loads (70% to 120% of 1RM) has been shown to improve maximum isometric strength (i.e., movement velocity equals zero). However, it does not improve the RFD (22, 48) and may even reduce the muscle's ability to develop force rapidly

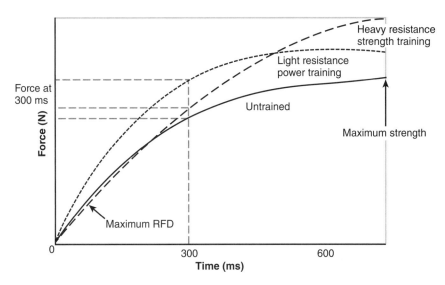

FIGURE 5.4 Isometric force–time curve indicating maximum strength, maximum rate of force development, and force at 200 ms for (1) untrained subjects, (2) heavy-resistance, strength-trained subjects, and (3) light-resistance, power-trained subjects.

Adapted, by permission, from K. Häkkinen, P.V. Komi, and M. Alen, 1985, "Effect of explosive type strength training on isometric force- and relaxation-time, electromyographic and muscle fibre characteristics of leg extensor muscles," *Acta Physiologica Scandinavica* 1985. 125(4): p. 587-600.

(45). On the contrary, an activity during which athletes attempt to develop force rapidly (e.g., maximal jump squat training with light loads) improves their ability to increase force output at a fast rate (22). Specifically, maximal power-type resistance training increases the slope of the early portion of the force–time curve (47), as can be observed in figure 5.4.

Although heavy resistance training in this study increased maximum strength and, thus, the highest point of the force–time curve, it did not improve power performance appreciably, especially in athletes who had already developed a strength training base (i.e., who had accumulated more than six months of training) (45). The reason may be that the movement time during powerful activities is typically less than 300 ms (105). Most of the force increases cannot be realized over such a short period of time. In other words, the athlete does not have the time to utilize the strength gains achieved through heavy resistance training during powerful activities.

Overcoming the Deceleration Phase in Traditional Resistance Training

The results of many studies (7, 102, 106) highlight a further problem with traditional resistance training and power development. It has been observed that when an athlete lifts a maximal weight in a bench press, the bar decelerates for a considerable proportion (24%) of the concentric movement (36), as the weight approaches the end of the range of motion. The deceleration phase increases to 52% when the athlete performs the bench press lift with a lighter resistance (e.g., 81% of 1RM) (36). In an effort to train at a faster velocity that is more specific to sporting activity, athletes may attempt to move the bar rapidly during the lift. However, this also increases the duration of the deceleration phase, since the athlete must still slow the bar to a complete stop at the end of the range.

The problem of the deceleration phase can be overcome if the athlete actually throws or jumps with the weight (82). This type of movement is most accurately termed *ballistic resistance training*. *Ballistic* implies acceleration of high velocity, with actual projection into free space. The common English meaning of the word as defined in the Macquarie Dictionary is "of or pertaining to the motion of projectiles proceeding under no power and acted on only by gravitational force and the resistance of the medium through which they pass" (29). Since projecting the load into free space so that it becomes a projectile is the essential aspect of this type of training that differentiates it from other forms, the term *ballistic resistance training* seems most appropriate.

Previous research has compared the kinematics, kinetics, and neural activation of a traditional bench press movement performed with the intention of maximizing power output and the ballistic bench throw, in which the barbell is projected from the hands (figure 5.5) (82). Significantly better performances were produced during the throwing movement compared with the press for average velocity, peak velocity, average force, average

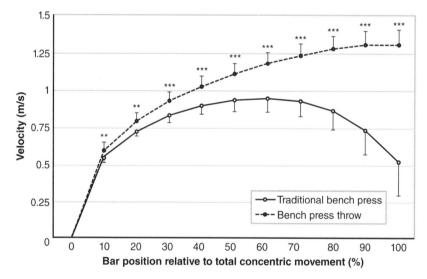

FIGURE 5.5   Mean (±SD) bar velocity in relation to total concentric bar movement for a traditional bench press, performed as rapidly as possible, and a bench throw (**$p < 0.01$; ***$p < 0.001$).

Reprinted, by permission, from R.U. Newton et al., 1996, "Kinematics, kinetics, and muscle activation during explosive upper body movements," *Journal of Applied Biomechanics* 12: 31-43.

power, and peak power. The average muscle activity during the concentric phase for pectoralis major, anterior deltoid, triceps brachii, and biceps brachii was higher (19%, 34%, 44%, and 27%, respectively) for the throw's condition. Further analysis of the velocity and force profiles revealed a deceleration phase during the press, lasting 40% of the concentric movement that was associated with a decrease in muscle activation. It was concluded that performing traditional press movements rapidly with light loads does not create the ideal loading conditions for the neuromuscular system with regard to maximal power production. This was especially evident in the final stages of the movement in which ballistic weight loading conditions—with the resistance accelerated throughout the movement—resulted in greater velocity of movement, force output, and EMG activity.

Plyometric training, weighted jump squats, and weightlifting movements avoid this problem of deceleration by allowing the athlete to accelerate all the way through the movement to the point of projection of the load (i.e., takeoff in jumping, ball release in throwing, impact in striking activities).

Training Methods for Power Development

Methods for developing power in athletes include heavy resistance training (in accordance with the power requirements of the sport), ballistic training (which should constitute a considerable proportion of the training volume), plyometrics, and weightlifting. Resistance training for strength translates to gains in power performance, but probably not immediately. Tapering and recovery are important aspects of a training program that should vary according to the performance demands of the sport.

Heavy Resistance Training

To be powerful, the athlete must also be very strong in the movements requiring high power expression. This relationship becomes more direct as the power requirements of the specific sport gain greater emphasis. As a general rule, the athlete should be able to generate three times the muscle tension required during the actual sporting performance. This corresponds to the observation that the neuromuscular system can generate greatest power output when it is working against a load of approximately 30% of maximal strength.

For example, in a sport for which high vertical jump is crucial (e.g., volleyball or basketball), athletes should be strong enough to squat with a load equivalent to two times their body mass on the barbell. That is, when athletes are jumping with no external load (i.e., body mass only), they are working around a load that is 30% of their maximum strength. In sports like triple jump, long jump, and sprinting, in which the driving action is off a single leg, the leg-extensor strength should be even higher. Keep in mind that a single-leg press or squat of three times body weight is not realistic, since this would be an extraordinary level of strength. However, such a theoretical analysis does indicate the need for very high strength development in athletes who require very high maximal power. For detailed information on assessing and developing strength, the interested reader is referred to texts such as that by Zatsiorsky and Kraemer (107) and to chapter 4 of this text.

Despite the fact that heavy resistance training results in movement velocities lower than those typically encountered in sporting movements (e.g., jumping or throwing) (25, 82), traditional resistance training exercises have been successfully used to improve maximal power output in dynamic, sport-specific movements (1, 7, 22, 71, 93, 94, 101, 102, 106). Although performance of these exercises does require the generation of relatively high power outputs, improvements in maximal power following training have primarily been a result of the physiological adaptations responsible for increasing maximal strength (i.e., increased cross-sectional area and maximal neural drive) (16, 22, 51, 71).

Consequently, in relatively untrained subjects with low to moderate strength levels, maximal power increases significantly following training with traditional resistance exercises but increases more slowly as strength level increases to approach the athletes' genetic potential (45, 50, 80, 101). As a result, increases in maximal power output following heavy resistance training are prominent in the early phases of training or in athletes who demonstrate a relatively low level of strength (i.e., aerobic endurance athletes) (49, 101). Although the use of heavy resistance training is vital in the development of strength and power, further training-induced improvement in maximal power requires the involvement of other, more specific movement patterns.

Ballistic Resistance Training

Ballistic movements (e.g., jump squat, bench throw) eliminate any deceleration phase by requiring athletes to accelerate throughout the entire range of motion to the point of projection (i.e., takeoff or release) (82). Stemming from the continued acceleration throughout the range of motion, concentric velocity, force, power, and muscle activation are higher during a ballistic movement than during a similar traditional exercise for resistance training (25, 82). As a result, many researchers and strength and conditioning professionals recommend including ballistic movements rather than traditional resistance exercises in training programs aimed at enhancing maximal power. These recommendations are based on the fact that ballistic movements are more sport-specific and, therefore, may prompt adaptations that allow for greater transfer to performance.

Supporting such recommendations is research demonstrating significant improvements in maximal power output during sport-specific movements following training with ballistic exercises (3, 22, 23, 70, 73, 76, 81,102,

103). Furthermore, power output is also improved across a variety of loading conditions (i.e., improved power-producing capabilities under both low-load and high-load situations) (23, 76, 81). An eight-week training intervention involving well-trained male volleyball players (squat 1RM / body mass = 1.69) revealed that training with ballistic movements (jump squats) resulted in a significantly greater change in sport-specific vertical-jump performance than training with traditional exercises (squat and leg press) (81). Therefore, training with ballistic movements allows athletes from a variety of backgrounds (i.e., beginner, advanced, or elite) to improve power production in a variety of sport-specific movements.

The precise mechanisms driving adaptation to ballistic power training involving ballistic movements are not clearly defined. It is theorized that these movements elicit adaptations in neural drive, activation patterns, and intermuscular coordination that are specific to movements typically encountered in sports. These adaptations are hypothesized to contribute to observations of enhanced RFD and result in the ability to generate more force in shorter periods of time (22, 23, 47, 70, 76, 81). Hence, the use of ballistic movements in training programs is very effective at enhancing maximal power output in sport-specific movements, as well as power production capabilities, under a variety of conditions (e.g., against a range of loads).

Ballistic movements are typically performed across a variety of loading conditions (i.e., from 0% to 80% 1RM) based on the specific exercise utilized and the requirements of the sport the athlete is involved in. It may be advantageous to perform a heavy set (80% 1RM) immediately before a lighter set (0% 1RM) because of the postactivation potentiation effect. Another method is to perform light and heavy days rather than to mix loads within a session. This scheme is particularly useful for athletes during the competitive season, when lighter days are required following a competition.

Typically, jump squats (i.e., CMJ performed with a bar loaded to a percentage of body weight or 1RM and held across the shoulders) are the primary ballistic resistance training exercises used to improve muscular power in the lower body. For the upper body, bench press throws are particularly effective for boxers or football players who require high force to punch or fend off an opponent. These are performed like a normal bench press, but the bar is thrown and then caught. For the shot put, athletes can use an inclined bench and adjust the angle so that the throw is in the same plane as their put. Pulling movements can also be performed ballistically, with the athlete lying on a bench and pulling the bar rapidly upward. A rubber stopper or foam dampener is required to soften the impact with the bench. Specifically designed equipment is available for ballistic resistance training. Due to considerations of specificity, free-weight bars are being used more frequently with a special power cage that provides bottom stops in case of a missed catch or bungled jump. The equipment may also incorporate braking systems to limit impact forces and instrumentation to record force, power, and velocity of the movements.

Plyometrics

Plyometrics are a training modality involving exercises in which athletes perform rapid SSC movements (99). A great deal of exercises are classified as plyometric, including a range of unilateral and bilateral catch-throw, push-up, bounding, hopping, and jumping variations (99). Typically, plyometric exercises are performed with little to no external resistance (i.e., body mass only or light medicine ball). Overload is applied by increasing the stretch rate (i.e., minimizing the duration of the SSC) or the stretch load (i.e., increasing height of drop during depth jumps) (28). Plyometric exercises can therefore be tailored to train either short (100-250 ms in duration; e.g., ground contact in sprinting, long jump, or high jump) or long SSC movements (duration greater than 250 ms; e.g., CMJ or throw) (89).

As a result of the ability to target both short and long SSCs, as well as the ballistic nature of these movements, plyometric exercises are very specific to a variety of movements typically encountered in sport. Hence, it is not surprising that the use of plyometrics to enhance power production capabilities has been shown to significantly improve maximal power output during sport-specific movements (1, 19, 57, 73, 97, 102). These improvements are, however, typically restricted to low-load, high-velocity SSC movements (97, 102).

The current literature involving the use of plyometric training doesn't provide much insight into the mechanisms driving improvements in maximal power. Similar to ballistic movements, plyometrics are theorized to elicit specific adaptations in neural drive, activation patterns, and intermuscular control that improve RFD capacity (19, 91). Adaptations to the mechanisms driving enhanced performance during SSC movements are also hypothesized to contribute to improved maximal power production following plyometric training (19, 91). Therefore, the high degree of specificity of plyometric training for a range of sporting movements makes training programs that incorporate plyometric exercises very effective at improving maximal power in sport-specific movements.

Weightlifting Movements

Olympic weightlifting movements (i.e., snatch, clean and jerk) and their variations (i.e., power clean, hang clean, power snatch, hang snatch, high pull, hang pull, and push press) are commonly incorporated into power training programs of athletes competitive in all types of sports (34, 35, 92). Similar to ballistic movements, *weightlifting exercises* (see figure 5.6) require athletes to accelerate throughout the entire propulsive phase (i.e., second pull), causing the projection of the barbell and often the body into the air (41, 88). The inherent high-force, high-velocity nature of weightlifting movements creates the potential for these exercises to produce large power outputs across a variety of loading conditions.

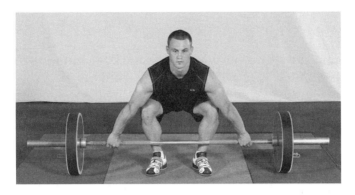

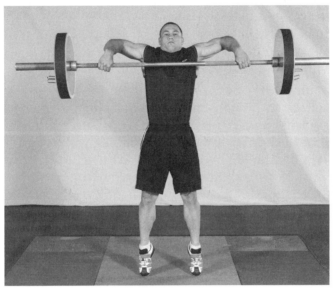

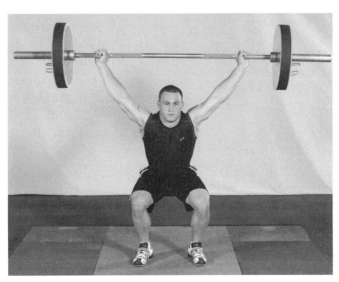

FIGURE 5.6 Olympic weightlifting movements such as the snatch require the athlete to accelerate the barbell throughout the propulsive phase, providing a good stimulus for power development.

For example, power output has commonly been found to be greatest at loads equivalent to 70% to 80% 1RM in weightlifting movements (25, 44, 64). Additionally, the movement patterns required in weightlifting exercises are commonly believed to be very similar to generic athletic movements, such as jumping and sprinting (58). Empirical observations are supported by evidence of similarities in the kinetic features of the propulsive phase in both weightlifting and jumping movements (17, 41). Significant relationships have also been observed between performance in weightlifting movements and power output during jumping ($r = 0.58$-0.93) as well as sprint performance ($r = 0.57$) (18, 59).

Despite the widespread use of Olympic weightlifting exercises and variations to enhance power and the evidence highlighting its specificity to generic athletic movements, little research exists examining the efficacy of power training with these movements. In previously untrained men, Tricoli and colleagues (97) observed significant improvements in static and countermovement jump height, as well as in 10 m sprint performance, following eight weeks of ballistic power training with weightlifting movements. In addition, the improvement in CMJ height was greater than the improvement following eight weeks of plyometric training (97). Power training with weightlifting movements is theorized to significantly improve both maximal power output and, more specifically, power output against heavy loads. Thus, the use of these movements in training is ideal for athletes who are required to generate high velocities against heavy loads (i.e., wrestling, rugby union front row, American football linemen).

The mechanisms responsible for improvements following power training using weightlifting movements have not yet been investigated. The skill complexity involved with such movements, together with the use of heavy loads, are hypothesized to elicit unique neuromuscular adaptations that allow for improved RFD and superior transfer to performance. Therefore, the nature of weightlifting movements, coupled with the specificity of their patterns to numerous athletic movements, creates the potential for Olympic weightlifting movements to be very effective power training exercises.

For practical tips on integrating plyometric and weightlifting exercises into an athletic training plan, see chapter 12.

Translation of Strength Gains to Power Performance

We have already discussed the concept that increasing muscle strength does not necessarily translate immediately to increased power output (with the exception of untrained athletes). Athletes must be given time to practice with the adapted muscle strength (9). This occurs somewhat automatically as part of the periodization of training. Translation can also occur through the performance of complex training. Here, athletes perform heavy resistance training and then, immediately on completing the set, attempt a very sport-specific set of exercises. For example, a set of heavy back squats could be followed by a set of vertical jumps, or a set of heavy split squats could be followed by a 40 m sprint. The most important point to remember is that resistance training may not immediately translate into increased power performance. Therefore, athletes must be given power training exercises that are very close to their sport's movements to assist in this translation.

Tapering and Recovery to Optimize Power Performance

As we have discussed, a wide range of neural and muscular factors must combine optimally to produce maximal power output. Certain training modes affect these components in a negative manner. For example, heavy resistance training alters the architecture of muscle pennation in the opposite direction desired for power production. So, in preparation for power- and speed-oriented events, heavy resistance training must be tapered up to four weeks prior to competition. This is not to say that training is stopped altogether, because this would result in strength decrement and, thus, power loss. The volume of heavy resistance training must be reduced markedly to perhaps one to three sets performed once per week leading up to competition.

This strategy is quite variable depending on the performance demands of the sport. If high strength and power is required, as in American football or rugby, then heavy resistance training must continue right through the preseason and in-season periods. In fact, it is desirable that personal bests in strength be set toward the end of the competitive season in American football, rugby, and other collision-combative sports. This is the phase when the hardest and most important competitions occur.

Selecting Load and Velocity for Power Development

Power output varies dramatically as the load an athlete is required to accelerate during a movement changes (25, 62, 63, 78, 85). For example, peak power output during a jump squat has been shown to range from 6332 ± 1085 W at 0% 1RM to 3986 ± 564 W at 85% 1RM (i.e., a 37% variation) (25). Consequently, the loading parameters used in ballistic power training programs influence the type and magnitude of performance improvements observed as well as the nature of the physiological adaptations underlying the improvements.

Kaneko and colleagues (62) illustrated that different training loads elicited specific adaptations to the force–velocity relationship and, subsequently, power output. Four groups completed 12 weeks of elbow-flexor training (ballistic resistance training) at different loads: 0%, 30%, 60%, and 100%

of maximal isometric force (F_{max}). Although all groups displayed significant improvements in maximal power, the most pronounced alterations in the force–velocity relationship were seen at and around the load utilized during training. For example, the 0% F_{max} group predominately improved power in low-force, high-velocity conditions, while the 100% F_{max} group predominately improved power under high-force, low-velocity conditions (62). Stemming from this seminal research, a range of loading conditions have been endorsed to elicit improvements in maximal power output throughout the literature, including heavy loads, light loads, the optimal load, as well as a combination of loads.

Heavy Loads

Despite the ensuing low movement velocity, training with heavy loads (i.e., ≥ 80% 1RM) has been suggested to improve maximal power output based on two main theories. First, due to the mechanics of muscle action (i.e., force–velocity relationship) and the positive association that exists between strength and power, increases in maximal strength following training with heavy loads results in a concurrent improvement in maximal power production (22, 47, 62, 74, 78, 86, 93, 100, 102). The second theory forming the basis for the prescription of heavy loads is related to the size principle for motor-unit recruitment (51, 87, 90). According to the size principle, high-threshold motor units that innovate Type II muscle fibers are only recruited during exercises that require near-maximal force output (52, 55, 56). Therefore, the Type II muscle fibers, which are considered predominately responsible for powerful athletic performances, are theorized to be more fully recruited (and thus trained) when training involves heavy loads (53, 76, 89, 102). Heavy loads are typically utilized in conjunction with either traditional resistance training exercises or both ballistic and weightlifting movements in an attempt to improve maximal power.

Heavy loads are most commonly prescribed for traditional resistance training exercises with the aim of improving maximal strength. As a result of the subsequent increase in F_{max} following training, the stronger athlete is able to generate greater maximal power output and improved power output throughout the loading spectrum (i.e., based on the inherent force–velocity relationship of muscle) (47, 62, 74, 78, 86, 93, 100, 102). These observations hold true for relatively weak or inexperienced athletes. They are driven by increases in myofibrillar cross-sectional area, especially of Type II muscle fibers, and in maximal neural drive (22, 46, 51, 74, 100).

Changes to maximal power following such training in strong, experienced athletes are much smaller in magnitude (5, 45, 50, 101). Thus, the use of traditional resistance exercise with heavy loads plays an important role in initial improvements in maximal power. However, this role does not typically extend beyond the time in which a reasonable level of strength is reached and maintained (69).

Heavy loads are also commonly used in power training programs incorporating ballistic and weightlifting movements. Although a paucity of research is investigating the adaptations following such training, they are theorized to be different from heavy load training with traditional resistance exercises. Ballistic and weightlifting training with heavy loads would still allow for the recruitment of high-threshold motor units (30, 31). However, improvements in power output are hypothesized to be due to improved RFD capabilities, as well as improved neural-activation patterns and intermuscular coordination (47, 76). These adaptations are theorized to positively influence maximal power output, but they would have their greatest influence at the loads utilized during training (i.e., adaptations specific to load or movement velocity) (62, 76, 78). Thus, heavy-load ballistic and weightlifting training may beneficially influence power output in both novice and experienced athletes.

Unfortunately, little research exists examining the efficacy of ballistic power training with heavy-load ballistic and weightlifting exercises. Tricoli and colleagues (97) reported that weightlifting training using four- to six-repetition maximum loads resulted in significant improvements in maximal jump height and 10 m sprint performance. However, this study involved relatively untrained subjects who also showed a significant improvement in 1RM following the training (97). McBride and colleagues (76) observed improvements in peak power during 55% and 80% 1RM jump squats, but not during a 30% 1RM jump squat following eight weeks of ballistic jump squat training with 80% 1RM. These improvements were associated with improved muscle activity of the vastus lateralis during the 55% and 80% 1RM jump squats, suggesting load- or velocity-specific adaptations (76). Although more research is required to elucidate the effect of heavy-load ballistic and weightlifting training on power production and the mechanisms responsible for performance improvements, such training is theorized to be ideal for athletes required to generate high power outputs against heavy loads (i.e., wrestlers, rugby union front rowers, American football linemen).

Light Loads

The use of light loading conditions (i.e., 0% to 60% 1RM) in conjunction with ballistic and plyometric exercises is commonly recommended and utilized in ballistic power training programs (14, 19, 47, 57, 62, 73, 75, 76, 78, 102, 103). Such training parameters permit athletes to train at velocities similar to those encountered in actual on-field movements. Light loads are recommended, due to the high RFD requirements and the high power outputs associated with such resistances (47, 62, 76).

A great deal of research has demonstrated that training with light loads increases maximal power output during sport-specific movements and improves athletic performance (i.e., various jumping, sprinting, and agility tasks) (14, 19, 23, 47, 57, 62, 70, 73, 75, 76, 78, 83, 102, 103). Furthermore, comparisons between light and heavy loads in equivalent (i.e., same movement pattern) training modalities revealed that maximal power is improved to a greater degree following training with light loads (62, 76). Thus, it is well established that ballistic power training with light loads is very effective at improving maximal power output in sport-specific movements.

Research investigating the mechanisms responsible for these improvements is limited. The high movement velocity, RFD, and power requirements of ballistic power training involving light loads are theorized to elicit adaptations in neural activation patterns and intermuscular coordination that drive improvements (22, 23, 47, 70, 76, 81). Therefore, training with light loads is recommended for athletes who are required to generate high power outputs during fast movements against low external loads (i.e., sprinting, jumping, throwing, and striking) (63). It is important to note, however, that these findings are only relevant when light loads are utilized with ballistic and plyometric exercise. The use of light loads with traditional resistance training or weightlifting movements is not recommended by researchers or commonly used by strength and conditioning professionals because such training would not provide an adequate stimulus for adaptation in either the force or velocity requirements of such exercises. It is not possible to overload the muscle sufficiently using light resistances while stopping the weight at the end of the range of motion (54, 80, 82).

Optimal Load

Throughout the literature, the load that elicits maximal power production in a specific movement is commonly referred to as the *optimal load* (25, 33, 63, 64, 102). Power is maximized at approximately 30% F_{max} in single-muscle fibers and single-joint movements (13, 27, 32, 38, 62, 95, 96, 98). However, the load that maximizes power in multi-joint, sport-specific movements varies depending on the type of movement involved. For example, the optimal load typically ranges from 0% 1RM in the jump squat (24, 25), to 30% to 45% in the bench press throw (85), and up to 70% to 80% 1RM in weightlifting movements (25, 44, 64).

Since improvements in power output are most pronounced at the load used in training (62, 76), training with the optimal load provides an ideal stimulus to elicit an increase in maximal power output for a specific movement. Although the exact mechanisms underlying superior adaptations after training with a specific load remain unidentified, it is theorized that the optimal load provides a unique stimulus due to specific adaptations in neural activation patterns (47, 62, 76). This theory is supported by several investigations demonstrating that training with the optimal load results in superior improvements in maximal power production compared to other loading conditions (62, 76, 78, 102).

While the scientific evidence illustrates that training at the optimal load is very effective for improving maximal power output in a specific movement over short-term interventions (8-12 weeks), this does not necessarily mean that training at the optimal load is the best or only way to increase maximal power over a long-term training program. Furthermore, much of the research in this area has been conducted using homogeneous groups of low to moderately trained subjects, so it is unknown if similar results would be observed when training well-trained or elite athletes. Even so, ballistic power–training programs in which movements are performed at the optimal load are excellent for improving maximal power output in a specific movement.

Combining Loads

Ballistic power training using light loads improves the high-velocity region of the force–velocity relationship (i.e., power at high velocities against low loads). The use of heavy loads enhances the high-force portion of the curve (i.e., power at low velocities against heavy loads) (32, 46, 47, 60, 62, 76, 78). The theory behind the use of a combination of loads in a ballistic power–training program is to target all regions of the force–velocity relationship in an attempt to augment adaptations in power output throughout the entire curve. Thus, it is argued that training with a combination of loads may allow for all-round improvements in the force–velocity relationship, which result in superior increases in maximal power output and greater transfer to performance than either light- or heavy-load training (95, 96).

Research has established that significant improvements in maximal power output and various athletic performance parameters occur following training with a combination of loads (1, 23, 53, 70, 73, 81, 84, 95, 96). What's more, results from some of these investigations suggest that improvements in maximal power and athletic performance are more pronounced in combined light- and heavy-load training programs compared to programs involving training at a single load or other load combinations (1, 23, 53, 95, 96). However, most of these studies did not control for the total work completed by various groups (1, 53, 95, 96). Thus, it is difficult to delineate whether the loading parameters or the differences in total work performed contributed to their observations.

When the total work done during training was equivalent, Cormie and colleagues (23) reported no differences in the improvement of maximal power output or maximal jump height between a light-load-only program and a combined light- and heavy-load program. However, the combined training group also displayed improvements in power and jump height throughout a range of loaded jump squats and improved both F_{max} and dynamic 1RM. No such improvements were observed in the light-load-only group (23). These results suggest that the combination of light and heavy loads elicits greater all-round improvements in the strength/power profile than training with a light load only.

However, each of the research investigations relevant to this topic were conducted on relatively inexperienced, weak subjects. Typically, they involved a combination of ballistic power and strength exercises (i.e., jumping and heavy squatting), rather than a combination of ballistic power exercises with light and heavy loads (i.e., 0% and 80% 1RM jump squats). As a consequence, it is unknown if these findings apply to well-trained athletes who already maintain a high level of strength. Additionally, it is not clear if a combination of loads surrounding the optimal load (i.e., 0% to 60% 1RM) may be more beneficial at enhancing maximal power in subjects who are well trained. Further research is also required to determine if adaptations are influenced by whether the combination of loads are used within a single set (i.e., complex training), a single session, or in separate training sessions.

Velocity Specificity

The theory of velocity specificity in resistance training suggests that adaptations following training are maximized at or near the velocity of movement used during training (15, 26, 61, 62, 72, 77, 79). However, a conflicting school of thought exists in which training adaptations are theorized to be influenced to a greater degree by the intention to move explosively regardless of the actual movement velocity (5). These conflicting theories have led to confusion surrounding the appropriate selection of loads and exercises to utilize during ballistic power training. Therefore, the development of an effective power training program must include consideration of the actual and intended velocity of movement involved with training exercises.

The controversy surrounding the critical training stimulus for velocity specific adaptations—actual versus intended movement velocity—has received much attention from researchers and strength and conditioning professionals (5, 39). Research evidence indicates that the intention to move explosively influences adaptations to training. It is vitally important during ballistic power training, irrespective of the contraction type, load, or movement velocity of the exercises used (5, 39). However, the bulk of the literature indicates that velocity-specific improvements in maximal power are more likely elicited by the actual movement velocity utilized during training (8, 15, 26, 46, 47, 61, 62, 72, 76-79). Therefore, the intention to move explosively and the actual movement velocity are both vital stimuli required to elicit neuromuscular adaptations driving performance improvements following training. In order to maximize the transfer of training to performance, it is imperative that athletes train with loads that allow for similar movement velocities to those typically encountered in their sport. Additionally, athletes should attempt to perform these exercises with the goal of generating maximal force as rapidly as possible.

SUMMARY POINTS

- The exquisite movements that make sport so exciting, such as the slam dunk or the blistering burst of speed in football, require very high power outputs and the optimization of a wide range of neural, muscular, mechanical, and skill components.

- The mechanisms that contribute to maximal power production are many and relatively complex. They include the rate of force development and action of the stretch-shortening cycle, as well as baseline muscular strength.

- The use of a variety of training methods (high load, slow velocity with low load, high velocity) is best, in which the various factors contributing to the target performance are determined and assessed, and then specific training phases are implemented, with frequent follow-up testing.

- Although maximal strength is very important, development of this component alone will decline in efficiency as the training age of the athlete increases. More sophisticated training methods incorporate heavy- and light-load ballistic training, plyometrics, and weightlifting. Even unloaded or overspeed techniques are of benefit.

- The two key concepts of this chapter are specificity (in terms of matching the target activity in velocity, range, and type of movement) and variation of loading (in terms of resistance, volume, and intensity) to continue to elicit gains in power performance.

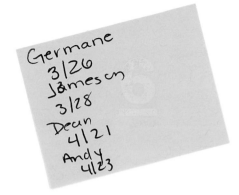

Anaerobic Conditioning

Jay R. Hoffman, PhD, CSCS*D, FNSCA

Physiological adaptations resulting from exercise are specific to the type of training program employed. Thus, it becomes imperative that athletes and strength and conditioning professionals adhere to the basic principle of training specificity. For athletes to achieve the desired physiological adaptations, they need to train the energy system that is predominantly recruited for their sport. Exercise programs for anaerobic athletes must focus on developing the anaerobic energy system. These adaptations are necessary for athletes to maximize their ability to perform high-intensity activity with rapid recovery between each exercise bout (e.g., repeated sprint ability).

In designing an effective training program, the strength and conditioning professional must understand the physiological demands that the athlete experiences during competition. Examples of sports that rely primarily on the anaerobic energy system include the team sports of American football, basketball, and ice hockey, and individual sporting events such as track and field, swimming, and cycling (specifically, the sprinting events). Other sports, such as soccer, field hockey, lacrosse, and team handball, rely on both the aerobic and anaerobic energy systems. However, the substitution patterns in those sports necessitate a greater reliance on the aerobic energy system to maintain prolonged activity. This chapter reviews the physiological adaptations from anaerobic conditioning, discusses program development, and provides specific examples of anaerobic conditioning programs.

Physiological Adaptations From Anaerobic Conditioning Programs

Physiological adaptations are specific to the type of training program employed. The adaptations commonly generated from anaerobic programs are as follows:

- Increase in the transformation of Type II fibers to a more glycolytic subtype
- Significant elevations in glycolytic enzymes (phosphofructokinase, phosphorylase, lactate dehydrogenase)
- Increase in maximum blood-lactate concentrations
- Reduced blood-lactate concentrations during submaximal exercise
- Improved buffering capacity

These adaptations, which are the basis for preparing athletes for competition, focus primarily on transformation of muscle-fiber subtype and metabolic alterations, including enzymatic changes and an enhanced buffering capacity (5). It is important to differentiate training programs that enhance anaerobic power development from conditioning programs that enhance anaerobic conditioning. Generally, the latter enhances anaerobic capacity, which is athletes' ability to maintain high-intensity exercise for a prolonged period of time (e.g., a competitive game). Other chapters in this book detail methods to enhance anaerobic power.

Transformation of Muscle-Fiber Subtype

Muscle fibers are generally classified as being fast-twitch (Type II) or slow-twitch (Type I). The difference between the two classifications relates to force characteristics, contraction speed, and fatigue rate. Fast-twitch fibers have high force capacity and a high speed of contraction, but fatigue quickly. In contrast, slow-twitch fibers have a slower contraction rate and a lower force capability, but are fatigue resistant. Thus, athletes who wish to excel in high-power sports, such as basketball, American football, or speed skating, would benefit from a higher percentage of fast-twitch fibers.

The proportion of Type I (slow-twitch) to Type II muscle fibers appears to be genetically determined. Their expression appears to be set early in life. Although a few studies have suggested that conditioning programs can alter the proportion of Type I to Type II muscle fibers (7, 9, 10, 18), the overwhelming majority of investigations have been unable to see any alterations in fiber-type composition as a result of conditioning programs. It is generally believed that training can only accomplish transformations within a fiber type. That is, within each fiber type (slow-twitch or fast-twitch), several different subtypes exist that respond to the exercise stress. These subtypes form a continuum that represents greater or lesser characteristics of that particular fiber type. Fiber subtypes become more glycolytic (anaerobic) or oxidative (aerobic), depending on the training stimulus that occurs. Interestingly, the growth in understanding of fiber subtypes in the past few years has resulted in the realization by sport scientists that the subtype IIx is more representative of a "couch potato." This fiber subtype can be transformed quite rapidly into a more active subtype of the Type II fiber subtype through an exercise program (5, 12).

High-intensity exercise appears to be a potent stimulus for transforming the fiber subtype Type IIx to Type IIa (12, 19-21). Most of the population of Type IIx fibers has been reported to have converted to Type IIa fibers following 20 weeks of training (21). Fiber subtype transformations from IIx to IIa are also seen in athletes performing a combined high-intensity resistance training and endurance training program (12). Interestingly, subjects who were only performing endurance exercises also tended to increase the proportion of Type IIa fibers, but they significantly elevated their Type IIc fibers (the most oxidative of the Type II subtypes, and most conducive for enhancing prolonged exercise).

Fiber subtype transformations appear to occur quite rapidly (within two weeks) during participation in physical conditioning programs. However, these adaptations may be transient. During periods of inactivity or detraining, fast-twitch fiber subtypes will transform from Type IIa back to Type IIx (21), but resumption of the training program will transform the fiber subtypes back to their trained state in a relatively shorter period of time. These studies highlight the dynamic nature of skeletal-fiber transformations.

Metabolic Adaptations

Three energy systems provide fuel for exercise. The phosphagen energy system is primarily used to fuel high-intensity exercise (maximal effort) for very short durations (<30 s), the glycolytic energy system fuels sustained high-intensity (an intensity at which the demand for oxygen is greater than the ability to supply it) exercise for to 2 to 3 minutes, while the oxidative energy system fuels prolonged activity of low intensity (when the demand for oxygen is met with an ability to supply it). All three energy systems are always activated, but the mode of exercise determines which of these energy systems is dominant. The first two energy systems do not require oxygen; hence, they are termed the *anaerobic energy system*. The latter energy system does require oxygen and is termed the *aerobic energy system*.

Athletes training in anaerobic sports, such as hockey, basketball or American football, must use drills or exercises at the intensity of movement that stresses the appropriate energy system. To stress the anaerobic system, high-intensity activity should be focused on the specific energy system used during competition. For example, the sport of American football consists of repeated high-intensity activity that averages 5 seconds per play, with approximately 25 to 30 seconds of rest between each play (5). The anaerobic conditioning program should consist of drills and recovery periods that are similar in duration to the activities that occur during the game. In addition, strength and conditioning professionals will likely extend the duration of the sprints or drills during specific times in the training year to elicit further physiological adaptations (e.g., enhanced buffering capacity), which are discussed later in this chapter and in chapter 12. Conditioning programs that focus on specific energy systems cause adaptations that result in a more efficient utilization of energy from that particular system. Often times, this is scientifically evaluated by examining enzymatic changes within the muscle.

Phosphagen Energy System

To improve the functioning of the phosphagen energy system, adaptations would have to increase phosphagen concentrations within the muscle by increasing concentrations of either adenosine triphosphate (ATP) or creatine phosphate (CP). Another way would be to enhance the recovery of this energy system between bouts of exercise. However, research findings are not consistent regarding athletes' ability to cause physiological adaptations to this particular energy system to make it more efficient during competition or training. This is probably the primary reason why sport supplementation (specifically creatine supplements) has been so effective in the past 15 to 20 years—these supplements can affect the phosphagen system even though it is difficult to manipulate it with training.

Research has shown that short-duration (~5-6 s), high-intensity exercise causes little to no change in resting phosphagen (ATP or CP) concentrations, or in enzymes of the phosphagen energy system (i.e., creatine kinase) (1, 15, 23). Even during high-intensity exercise of longer duration (>10 s), the enzymatic changes in the phosphagen energy system are not consistent. During 30 seconds of continuous knee extensions, significant elevations in both creatine kinase and myokinase (enzymes of the phosphagen energy system) were seen following seven weeks of training (1), while others were unable to find any significant change in the concentration of these enzymes following six weeks of training (15 and 30 s maximal sprints on a cycle ergometer) (8). However, another study (16) showed that two weeks of sprinting (15 s maximal-effort cycling sprints) performed every day resulted in a significant increase (44%) in creatine kinase, clearly demonstrating a rather rapid adaptation to high-intensity training. It does appear that training adaptations to the phosphagen energy system can occur, and that these changes may occur within two weeks of training. Differences among studies are likely related to training status, experience, duration of sprint, and length of training program.

Glycolytic System

As duration of high-intensity exercise increases, the energy required to fuel this exercise is derived primarily from the glycolytic energy system. Training studies using bouts of exercise between 15 and 30 seconds or longer have shown significant elevations in the glycolytic enzymes, such as phosphofructokinase, phosphorylase, and lactate dehydrogenase (6, 8, 14, 16). Elevations in these enzymes may enhance the efficiency of the glycolytic energy system. Parra and colleagues (16) have shown that these changes can occur within two weeks of training in previously untrained athletes. Interestingly, evidence suggests that the intermittent nature of high-intensity activity with sufficient recovery provides a greater stimulus to glycolytic enzyme adaptations than continuous exercise does (4). In addition, intermittent exercise, such as high-intensity interval training (10 sets of 10 s sprints with a 1:4 work-to-rest ratio for 15 weeks in competitive athletes) not only enhance anaerobic power to a greater extent than continuous exercise does, but may also enhance $\dot{V}O_2$max to the same magnitude that 20 to 25 minutes of continuous exercise does (22).

Oxidative Enzymes

The exercise stimulus causing an elevation in concentrations of glycolytic enzyme concentrations also appears to significantly increase mitochondrial enzyme activity (oxidative enzymes) (2, 23). These changes enhance the efficiency of the mitochondria that may be responsible for slowing the use of muscle glycogen and reducing lactate production at a given intensity of exercise. This may have important implications for the anaerobic athlete by helping preserve muscle glycogen and potentially limiting fatigue. An increase in the concentration of these enzymes is more prevalent when the duration of high-intensity exercise exceeds 3 minutes (3). In addition, the magnitude of the increase in these enzymes does not reach the concentrations typically seen following prolonged aerobic endurance training. However, the implications of an increase in oxidative enzymes from anaerobic training programs suggest that anaerobic athletes may be able to generate some improvements in their aerobic capacity (13, 22, 24). This may have some important implications for enhancing exercise recovery.

Buffering Capacity

High-intensity exercise results in a lowering of muscle pH, contributing to the onset of muscle fatigue. The burning sensation that is often felt by athletes who are performing prolonged sprints is a reflection of acid buildup within the muscle fibers and blood that forces them to slow down or stop the exercise. Training programs that stress the anaerobic energy system change the ability of the muscle to tolerate high concentrations of metabolic acidosis. One of the basic adaptations to anaerobic conditioning is an improved buffering capacity that allows the muscle to withstand high concentrations of acid buildup. Buffers that are produced within the muscle, such as bicarbonate and muscle phosphates, help maintain the acid–base balance within the exercising muscle. During training (8 weeks), the buffering capacity within the muscle may increase 12% to 50% (17). This depends on the conditioning level of the athlete and the design of the training program. Regardless, this adaptation has an important role in delaying fatigue during high-intensity exercise and in increasing the tolerance of trained athletes to accumulate large concentrations of acid, due to an improved buffering capacity within the skeletal muscle.

Developing Anaerobic Conditioning Programs

An appropriate conditioning program should be based on a needs analysis of the athletes and their specific sport demands (see chapter 1). The primary movement patterns, duration of these movements, the number of movements, and the work-to-rest ratio are all critical variables that must be identified to prescribe appropriate exercises. Each sport may be quite different. Even within a sport, variability of movements may exist among different positions. Differences in the requirements for each position (e.g., goalie versus forward in ice hockey, lineman versus wide receiver in American football) result in varying physiological demands that require different training programs. With a thorough understanding of the activity demands of the sport, a greater specificity in the types of exercises and in the work-to-rest ratio can be employed to maximize the effectiveness of the training program.

Timing and Duration of the Program

The most frequently asked question concerning anaerobic conditioning programs is when to begin. This question is not simple to answer, primarily due to the fact that there is no uniquely correct answer. Much of this question is related to the concepts of periodization and program implementation, which are discussed in great detail in chapters 11 and 12, respectively. However, nothing in the exercise prescription should ever be based on happenstance. Implementation of the anaerobic conditioning program should be based on scientific evidence and best practices. When considering the time course of physiological adaptations that occur through training, strength and conditioning professionals can calculate the approximate time needed to begin preparing their athletes to reach peak anaerobic conditioning. It is also imperative for strength and conditioning professionals to understand what their players have been doing in the off-season. They must take this information into consideration when determining the onset of training, proper intensity and volume of training, and manipulation of work-to-rest ratios.

For more on integrating anaerobic conditioning into an athlete's annual training plan, see chapter 12.

Team Sports

Matching the work and rest intervals of the sport is an important consideration in maximizing the effectiveness of an anaerobic conditioning program. For example, American football can be separated into a series of plays. These are numbers of series and plays observed in a season of NCAA Division III football (5):

Total number of plays observed: 1,193

Total number of series observed: 259

Average number of series per game: 14.4

Average number of plays per series: 4.6

Percentage of series of 6 plays or greater: 31.2%

Percentage of series of 10 plays or greater: 8.1%

During each game, each team had an average of 14.4 offensive series and 4.6 plays per series. Each play has been reported to last for an average of 5.49 seconds (ranging from 1.87 to 12.88 s) in college football (11). Between plays, each team has a maximum of 25 seconds to begin the next play. However, this play clock does not begin until the referee has set the ball. Thus, the rest interval between plays generally exceeds 25 seconds. In limited reports, the average time between plays in a college football game is 32.7 seconds (11). The average time per play and rest time between plays allows for a more precise development of the work-to-rest ratio needed for anaerobic exercise prescription. According to the preceding data regarding time for each play and the rest interval between plays, it appears that a work-to-rest ratio of 1:5 could be used in off-season conditioning programs for football. Players could perform short-duration sprints that simulate the movement patterns of an actual football game.

This conditioning program for football will begin between 6 and 10 weeks prior to training camp. The football program is longer than the one for basketball, since basketball players often have pick-up (summer league) games. In contrast, football is not a sport that can be played in the off-season. The type of drills and progression of volume and intensity are similar to those displayed in table 12.13 (p. 280). However, specific adaptations can be made for American football players. For example, it appears that college football players get between four and five plays per series and that plays last approximately 5 seconds. Considering that there are about three or four series per quarter, a conditioning program can be developed that simulates a football game, with realistic work-to-rest ratios. In addition, a range of sprinting distances can be incorporated that simulate the varied runs frequently seen in a game.

For more on anaerobic conditioning for team sports and a sample anaerobic training program for basketball, see chapter 12.

Individual Sports

The development of a conditioning program for team sports, such as basketball, American football, or hockey, is quite different than the exercise prescription for athletes participating in an individual event, such as sprinting. Unlike team-sport athletes, who perform various types of movements at variable intensities, sprinters are often required to run a single sprint at maximum ability during a competition. Although they may compete in several different races, the requirements will be similar for each one. The training program for sprinters is primarily focused on developing power, improving running technique and speed, and increasing speed endurance. This latter goal is the focus in their anaerobic conditioning program.

The importance of this is seen in the splits for a 100 m sprinter. The goal of the sprinter is to reach peak running velocity as quickly as possible and to maintain running velocity throughout the length of the sprint. This is known as *speed-endurance*. Table 6.1 shows the splits for Usain Bolt, the Olympic record holder in the 100 m sprint. These results clearly show his ability to maintain his velocity until the final 10 m of the race. However, those who recall that great sprint will remember that he appeared to let up toward the end since he was so far ahead in the field. These splits clearly demonstrate his peak conditioning level in preparation for these games.

The training program for the sprinter is different from that of the basketball or American football player. The anaerobic conditioning program for team-sport athletes is primarily concerned with preparing them for repeated bouts of high-intensity activity with limited rest

 For a sample anaerobic conditioning program for a sprinter, see chapter 12.

TABLE 6.1   Splits for 100-Meter Sprint for Usain Bolt at the 2008 Olympic Games in Beijing

Distance (m)	Time (s)	Time for interval (s)	Speed (km/h)
10	1.85	1.85	19.4
20	2.87	1.02	35.3
30	3.78	0.91	39.6
40	4.65	0.87	41.4
50	5.50	0.85	42.4
60	6.32	0.82	43.9
70	7.14	0.82	43.9
80	7.96	0.82	43.9
90	8.79	0.83	43.4
100	9.69	0.90	40.0

intervals. In contrast, the sprinter's training program is more concerned with the quality of each sprint than with improved fatigue rate.

Anaerobic Conditioning Exercises

A number of exercises can be used as part of a conditioning program that prepares anaerobic athletes for competition. Often, these types of drills are described as enhancing speed-endurance. They were traditionally used to enhance or maintain speed during long-duration sprinting events. These drills have also been described as *metabolic conditioning*, which is a broader term for anaerobic conditioning or anaerobic endurance. In addition, these drills are appropriate for athletes participating in a variety of sports with significant anaerobic components, such as American football, basketball, soccer, lacrosse, and hockey. Although ice hockey players and speed skaters would benefit from performing such drills on the ice, the physiological adaptation that occurs from dry-land training for these athletes would carry over to their sport. Swimmers who compete in sprinting events should focus on anaerobic conditioning in the water.

Interval Sprints

This is an excellent category of conditioning for developing anaerobic capacity. This drill can be performed on a 400 m track or on any measured course. Typically, the athlete sprints the straight part of the track and jogs or walks the turns (see figure 6.1). This results in a 100 m sprint, followed by a 100 m jog. This combination is continued for the length of the workout. The length of the workout and the rest period (jog or walk) depends on both the conditioning and performance level of the athlete. At the beginning of the training program, the number of intervals may be one or two laps and will progressively increase as the conditioning level of the athlete improves. (Chapter 12 discusses program integration in more detail.) The distance for the intervals can also be varied. For instance, shorter intervals (e.g., 40 m) or longer intervals (e.g., 200 m) can be used as well.

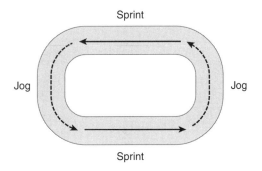

FIGURE 6.1 Running pattern for interval sprints.

Fartlek Training

This type of conditioning can be performed on either a track or a cross-country course. The athlete alternates short bursts of sprinting with jogging.

The length of the sprint can be alternated between short and long distances, with appropriate adjustments made to the rest interval between each sprint. Generally, the same relative work-to-rest ratio can be maintained for both long and short sprints. A major difference between Fartlek runs and intervals is that in the Fartlek runs, the sprints are of varying lengths. During interval training, the length of the sprint is consistent for the workout.

Repetition Sprints

For this drill, the athlete performs maximum sprints for a given distance. The distance can be either short (20-40 m sprints) or long (100-400 m sprints). Following a passive rest, the athlete repeats the sprint. The number of repetitions and the work-to-rest ratio depend on the athlete's conditioning level.

Repetition Sprints From Flying Starts

This drill is similar to the previous one, except that the athlete begins each sprint from a running start, accelerates over 20 m, and then sprints the required distance. Again, the number of repetitions and the work-to-rest ratio depend on the athlete's conditioning level.

Repetitive Relays

This drill uses a group of athletes who form a relay team (see figure 6.2). Athlete A sprints to and tags athlete B, who accelerates to athlete C. Athlete C sprints to athlete D. This process continues for the length of the track. Athletes will remain in the position of the person that they replaced. It is possible to make this drill quite competitive by having relay teams compete against other groups of athletes. The number of repetitions depends on the conditioning level of the athletes. The work-to-rest ratio is controlled by the number of members of the relay team. For instance, assuming that each member of the relay team is similar in speed, then a group of five relay members would result in a 1:4 work-to-rest ratio.

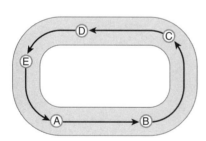

FIGURE 6.2 Setup and running pattern for repetitive relays.

Rolling Sprints

This drill is performed with at least four athletes who are jogging or running slowly in a line around the track (see figure 6.3). On the strength and conditioning professional's signal, the last athlete sprints to the front of the line. As that athlete reaches the front of the line, the strength and conditioning professional signals again. Now, the athlete in the last position sprints to the front. This continues for the duration of the run. To increase the intensity of the run, the strength and conditioning professional can reduce the time between signals or add more runners to the group.

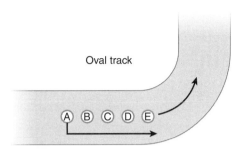

FIGURE 6.3 Setup for rolling sprints.

SUMMARY POINTS

- Adaptations to anaerobic training programs include transformations of muscle-fiber subtype, metabolic adaptations to enzymes, and buffering capacity.

- Although the number of Type I and Type II muscle fibers does not change through training, fibers within each category can change to a different subtype that is more aerobic or anaerobic, depending on the training stimulus.

- Most metabolic adaptations to training affect the glycolytic energy system, which provides energy for intense activity lasting less than 3 minutes.

- In team sports, such as American football, basketball, ice hockey, or soccer, athletes perform repeated bouts of high-intensity activity with limited rest periods between each bout. Thus, conditioning should be focused on preparing the athletes for these sport-specific demands.

- In contrast, sprinters focus more on speed-endurance in order to experience minimal fatigue toward the latter stages of the sprint.

- One of the primary differences between the training programs of these athletes is that sprinters are interested in the quality of each individual sprint, while basketball and football players are primarily focused on the ability to maintain the quantity of high-intensity activity common to their sport.

- Anaerobic conditioning exercises utilize varying intervals of intense effort and rest. The intervals should be determined by the conditioning level of the athlete and by the work-to-rest ratios observed in the sport.

7

Endurance Training

Joel T. Cramer, PhD, CSCS*D, NSCA-CPT*D, FNSCA, FISSN, FACSM

Abbie E. Smith, PhD, CSCS*D, CISSN

Aerobic endurance exercises and competitions are popular and are available to almost everyone. The popular belief is that those who train long and hard perform well. However, this is not always the case. Although training is obviously important, performance is not solely dictated by training volume and intensity. Reaching performance goals in aerobic endurance sports requires an understanding of multiple factors, including the basic physiology behind endurance performance, exercise economy, principles of aerobic endurance training, performance psychology, and overall lifestyle. While this chapter focuses on designing aerobic endurance training programs, it will also address and discuss these peripheral factors as they pertain to the basic variables of program design.

Understanding the basic physiology of aerobic endurance exercise and the expected training adaptations can shed light on the importance of program design. These are some of the physiological processes and markers that respond to aerobic endurance training:

- *Aerobic metabolism* refers to the production of energy from the breakdown of carbohydrates and fats in the presence of oxygen. Aerobic metabolism can produce an abundant amount of energy, but it does so at a much slower rate than anaerobic metabolism (14).

- *Anaerobic metabolism* refers to the production of energy from the breakdown of carbohydrates in the absence of oxygen. Although anaerobic metabolism produces energy at a faster rate than aerobic metabolism, it is less efficient, producing less energy relative to the amount of carbohydrate used and resulting in an accumulation of hydrogen ions and lactate (14).

- *Cardiovascular endurance* refers to the response of the heart and vasculature to aerobic endurance training. As fitness improves, cardiac output increases to an increase in stroke volume (25). Furthermore, during exercise, vasodilation occurs in the active muscles (25). These two factors result in an increased blood flow to the working muscles. An increase in capillary density in response to aerobic endurance training leads to additional blood flow and delivery of oxygen to the muscles.

- *Maximal oxygen consumption ($\dot{V}O_2$max)* is related to cardiorespiratory fitness. It refers to the greatest amount of oxygen that can be used at the cellular level of working muscles (1). The capacity for oxygen consumption relies primarily on the ability of the heart and circulatory system to deliver oxygen and the ability of the working muscles to use the oxygen. Therefore, an improvement in cardiovascular endurance should lead to improved cardiorespiratory fitness and $\dot{V}O_2$max.

- *Lactate threshold* is a fatigue threshold representing an abrupt increase in lactate above baseline concentration. The lactate threshold is often used as a marker of the anaerobic threshold because it represents an increasing reliance on anaerobic mechanisms (1).

The primary energy system that contributes to the transfer of energy during aerobic endurance exercise is the aerobic energy system. However, training at an intensity greater than the lactate threshold and relying mostly on anaerobic metabolism can increase the threshold (16). This allows for an increased capacity for aerobic metabolism. In other words, athletes can perform at a higher intensity and still rely mostly on the aerobic energy system.

Factors in Aerobic Endurance Performance

A number of factors contribute to aerobic endurance performance, including exercise economy, exercise prescription derived from scientifically based training principles, psychological preparation that motivates the athlete, and a lifestyle that leads to training success and adequate recovery. These factors all interact to develop the endurance component of training. The next sections focus in more detail on these aerobic endurance training factors.

Exercise Economy

Exercise economy refers to the metabolic demand of submaximal exercise (26). As athletes become more economical during tasks like running, cycling, or swimming, endurance performance also improves. There are many ways to improve exercise economy, but specificity of the exercise modality should be the main focus. For example, if the goal is to improve running times, then training for that event should consist mostly (if not completely) of running. The goal is to become as efficient at running (i.e., to burn the least amount of calories as possible over a given distance) as physiologically possible. This will allow more calories (energy) to be available during the race, delaying the fatigue process.

In addition to training the body to perform as efficiently as possible at a specific event, other factors can affect running economy, such as stride length (6), body weight (8), and air resistance (23). A comfortable, natural stride length seems to be the most efficient for most runners. However, if overstriding is an issue, runners may want to work on adjusting their stride to become more economical. Body weight should be kept at low but healthy levels based on athletes' body type and body composition. For example, excessive muscle mass may not allow for the optimal efficiency in aerobic exercise. Finally, although air resistance is a little more difficult to control, athletes can improve their economy by wearing tight-fitting clothing that does not catch the wind and by drafting behind other competitors, particularly during a race or time trial.

Training Principles for Aerobic Endurance Training

Optimal performance in aerobic endurance events is based on being able to perform at the highest intensity for a given distance. Therefore, one might expect that the best training consists of exercising at a high intensity for as long as possible. However, well-designed aerobic endurance training is more complex. A variety of training techniques, when combined to form a structured training plan, can lead to optimal performance. An aerobic endurance training plan should include workouts of varying intensities and durations, each having specific benefits to overall endurance performance. As mentioned previously, specificity of modality is very important. For example, if the athletic goal is a running competition, then the athlete should perform mostly running workouts. If a biking competition is the goal, then biking should be the main form of exercise. In addition, supplemental activities, such as resistance training (28) and nutrient timing (20), can be important in reaching performance goals.

Performance Psychology

Psychology plays a large role in aerobic endurance performance. Athletes can be in top physiological shape, but if they are not prepared mentally, their performance will most likely be hindered. Anxiety is commonly experienced before a competition. Although some may think that anxiety is detrimental, it may actually benefit performance (32). Practicing techniques to reduce anxiety before a competition may actually be more harmful than helpful to performance. However, substantial anxiety can have a negative effect on performance. Therefore, athletes should mentally prepare for the anxiety that will most likely accompany that competition so that their emotional state won't negatively influence their performance.

Mental state is also a factor during competition. Two strategies utilized during an endurance competition are *association* and *dissociation* (27). Association consists of being very aware of the physiological sensations of exertion, such as muscular pain, muscular fatigue, hydration, body temperature, and respiration. This technique seems to optimize efficiency and pace. Dissociation is the opposite, consisting of the use of techniques to distract the athlete from the physical pain of the competition (27). Dissociation is linked to an increase in the risk of injury and an increased likeliness of *hitting the wall*, or performing below expectations (36). Therefore, it seems to be more beneficial to be aware of the physiological sensations of an endurance competition, no matter how unpleasant they may be.

Lifestyle

Optimal performance in aerobic endurance competition requires dedication in training and overall lifestyle to bring about optimal recovery from training. Recovery is a very important part of aerobic endurance training. In fact, research shows that athletes with higher aerobic fitness levels can recover faster than people with lower aerobic capacities (17). These results suggest that building base levels of aerobic fitness is essential, not only for performance, but also for recovery. Adequate sleep and sufficient intake of high-quality nutrients are key components to recovery. Since the goal is to get as much benefit from each workout as possible, athletes must optimally recover each day to be ready for the next workout.

Aerobic Endurance Training Variables

Specificity of training has become a refined tool among all sporting events. The dynamics of an aerobic endurance training prescription should incorporate specific details regarding the intensity, duration, volume, and mode of training for the athlete. Additionally, combining these elements over a chronic training period has resulted in physiological adaptations associated with aerobic endurance training (30).

Intensity (Load)

Training intensity can be both a qualitative and quantitative measure of how much effort is utilized during a training session. Intensity measurement varies according to sport and mode of training. For instance, a runner may define intensity by a speed (i.e., miles per hour), while a cyclist may classify intensity with a load (i.e., watts). Despite varying classifications, the same principles can be used to prescribe intensities for all athletes. The minimal training-intensity threshold to improve fitness is also the same for all activities, approximately 40% to 50% of $\dot{V}O_2$max or 55% to 65% of maximum heart rate (HRmax) (30). Additionally, physiological adaptations are specific to the intensity of training. High-intensity training is specifically implemented to improve cardiorespiratory fitness and oxygen utilization (31).

Generally speaking, a quantitative measure of intensity can be obtained using heart rate values and pace training. Using heart rate as a method to measure exercise intensity is one of the most common training strategies for aerobic prescription. Physiologically, heart rate is directly related to cardiorespiratory fitness (4). Therefore, it can be used to recommend intensity levels as a percent of an athlete's maximal fitness level. The most accurate way of assessing cardiorespiratory fitness is in a laboratory setting. However, predicting an athlete's HRmax with age-prediction formulas such as the one provided here can be useful in an athletic setting.

$$\text{Predicted HRmax} = 220 - \text{age}$$

Exercise pace can also be used to measure exercise intensity. This technique uses the results of past competitions (e.g., average minute/mile pace) to establish training intensities. For example, when training at distances longer than competition lengths (e.g., long, slow distance, or LSD), the intensity should be less than the goal pace for competition. Similarly, when performing shorter tempo activities, the pace should be faster than competition pace. This holds true for all aerobic endurance activities, such as cycling, running, and swimming.

For example, if a runner's goal is to run a 5K (3.1 miles) race in 22 minutes, then he must run at a pace of 7.1 minutes per mile (4.4 min/km). If the goal is to run the race in 20 minutes, then he must run at a pace of 6.5 minutes per mile pace (4.0 min/km). To set appropriate goals, a stopwatch (and heart rate monitor if possible) should be used while training to evaluate the athlete's performances. If the athlete is consistently able to run at a pace of 7.1 minutes per mile during training, then a 22-minute race time for 5 km should be easily attainable. Similarly, if heart rate is between 55% and 65% (or even as much as 75%) of age-predicted HRmax while training at that pace, the athlete should be capable of a 22-minute race time for the 5K.

Ratings of perceived exertion (RPE) are an additional valid tool for monitoring exercise intensity. The 15-point Borg scale has been shown to be correlated with blood lactate, heart rate, and $\dot{V}O_2$max responses to exercise (3, 30). RPE has been identified as a correlate of heart rate; however, once that relationship has been identified for an athlete, RPE may be used in place of heart rate, creating another nonlaboratory method for tracking intensity.

Duration and Volume

Exercise *duration* and *volume* are often inaccurately used interchangeably. Although the two terms are related, exercise *duration* refers to the length of time of a training session. It is influenced by intensity. In contrast, training *volume* incorporates both intensity and duration of a training session. For example, volume is often calculated in resistance training as the number of sets performed multiplied by the number of repetitions performed multiplied by the weight lifted (1). The same method is often applied to aerobic endurance training volume by multiplying the duration of exercise by (1) the distance traveled and (2) the exercise intensity (either the average pace or heart rate during a training session).

Regardless of the number used to represent aerobic endurance training volume, tracking volume can be an important variable to monitor. The general perception with aerobic endurance athletes is that physiological adaptations and improvements in performance rely on a greater intensity and duration of training. However, recent research suggests that when exercise is performed above a minimum intensity threshold, the total volume becomes the quintessential component in developing fitness (30). Essentially, when researchers have compared long-duration, low-intensity training programs with short-duration, high-intensity training among competitive aerobic endurance athletes, improvements in fitness are comparable. As with any training goal, the intensity and increase in volume should be based on the individual athlete and the specific sport. Aerobic endurance athletes are at the highest risk for staleness, overreaching, and overtraining. Manipulating and fluctuating training volume may help to avoid overuse injuries and overtraining.

Aerobic Endurance Training Strategies

The structure of any training program is instrumental for athletic success, injury prevention, and individual confidence. As with any sport, a variety of training methods can be implemented to promote the greatest physiological adaptations. However, it is essential that training programs be designed to be specific to the sport, season of competition, and the individual needs of the athlete. Aerobic endurance training programs in particular require thought and creativity, due to the broad range of activities that fall under the umbrella of aerobic endurance. Creative use of the principles of aerobic endurance training program design should focus on reducing the risk of overtraining and enhancing endurance performance.

New research in the lab and on the field has utilized a complex strategy of strength, speed, and stamina to demonstrate the importance of training multiple physiological components, debunking the idea that long, slow distance is the only way to train. This evidence suggests that combining traditional long-duration training with moderate-intensity training and short-duration, high-intensity training may yield the same (if not better) results in performance adaptations. Although these three primary training strategies are all important to a balanced training program, specificity and variety are key to an enjoyable experience and a successful outcome.

Long-Duration, Moderate-Intensity Training

The most common type of training identified with aerobic endurance sports, often referred to as *long, slow distance (LSD)* training, is characterized by moderate intensities (i.e., 60% to 70% of $\dot{V}O_2$max or HRmax) maintained for long periods of time. Typically, the training distance is greater than the race distance by at least 30 minutes (9). Moderate-intensity training (i.e., LSD training) generally constitutes a major portion of an aerobic endurance athlete's training volume. This is sometimes referred to as *base training*. It allows athletes to participate in a relatively large training volume without imposing a high level of stress on the musculoskeletal system. In addition, base training helps enhance the basic cardiorespiratory and cardiovascular adaptations that are expected to occur with aerobic endurance exercise (7, 18). Such adaptations are necessary to allow for progressions in intensity, duration, and volume during training as the competition phase approaches. Building a base level of aerobic capacity also improves the ability to recover between training sessions (17). Prolonged activities have been reported to induce muscle glycogen depletion and to acutely increase the rate of fat metabolism, while chronically leading to an increase in stroke volume, mitochondrial density, and a more efficient oxidative capacity (7, 18). Furthermore, some aerobic endurance athletes have suggested that continuous long-duration activities equal to or greater than competition lengths may have psychological benefits.

Moderate-Duration, High-Intensity Training

This type of training is usually completed at intensities higher than race pace, which may correspond to an intensity at or slightly above the lactate threshold. An athlete's lactate threshold (LT) is associated with an exercise intensity at which lactate begins to accumulate and available aerobic energy sources can no longer keep up with the high rate of energy demand. This ultimately leads to fatigue (29). Training at this intensity can be completed at a constant, steady pace that is often called *pace/tempo training*. Pace/tempo training is done at intensities near the LT. It lasts about 20 to 30 minutes, inducing both aerobic and anaerobic physiological adaptations (9).

At this same intensity, an interval training approach may be utilized that consists of a series of short working episodes separated by brief recovery bouts. Aerobic/anaerobic interval training, which is commonly called *Fartlek training* (1), is primarily used to establish a sense of the race pace, increase the LT, and augment the body's ability to maintain higher intensities for longer periods of time. Specifically, Fartlek training involves periods of moderate training (~70% $\dot{V}O_2$max) combined with short, fast bouts (or hill running) at higher intensities (~85% to 90% $\dot{V}O_2$max or HRmax). Fartlek training can be applied to all sports by combining LSD training and moderate-duration, pace/tempo training. For example, a cyclist may choose to sprint a distance the length of one city block and coast the next block, continuing in a cyclical fashion.

Short-Duration, High-Intensity Training

Interval training has become very popular as a time-efficient training strategy for aerobic endurance athletes. Interval training involves intensities at or above $\dot{V}O_2max$, typically lasting between 30 seconds and 5 minutes (10). For an aerobic endurance athlete, the rest times between intervals are typically equal to or less than the work time itself, which keeps the work-to-rest ratio at 1:1 or 2:1. A variety of work–rest combinations can be used throughout different points of an athlete's season. The primary benefit of interval training comes from the increased volume of training at intensities that otherwise could not be sustained for prolonged periods of time.

Much research has been devoted to the short-term and chronic benefits of interval training (15, 37). Similar to traditional aerobic endurance training, interval training can result in improvements in cardiorespiratory and cardiovascular fitness, blood volume, LT, and muscle-buffering capacity (16). These factors are necessary for improving performance and are similar to those adaptations seen with LSD training. Therefore, if similar adaptations in aerobic endurance performance can be achieved using interval training for 20 minutes versus LSD training for 45 to 60 minutes, then interval training is clearly more efficient. It also results in less stress on the body (34).

Resistance Training

Research supporting the implementation of resistance training in an aerobic endurance training program has expanded as an efficacious strategy for preventing injury and increasing strength, power (i.e., kick at the end of a race), and stamina (28). As with any program, a resistance training program should be designed to enhance the sport-specific goals of the athlete. Athletes and strength and conditioning professionals typically implement strength training as a method to alter body composition, rehabilitate injuries, and improve muscle balance, speed, and local muscular endurance (22). Traditional resistance programs for aerobic endurance athletes have been designed using low-intensity exercises (<67% 1RM), high repetitions (>12), short rest times (30-60 s) for two or three sets. These can be performed one or more days per week, depending on the training season (1). Although this type of workout improves muscular endurance, more recent evidence suggests explosive-strength training is a more effective method for improving running economy and performance (i.e., 5K/10K) (28).

Various aspects of resistance training, such as specific exercises chosen, workout structure, resistance used, volume (repetitions and sets), rest intervals between sets, and training frequency, can be manipulated to mold the strength training program to best meet the athlete's goals. For example, incorporating the squat exercise into an aerobic endurance athlete's training program may reduce the risk for lower body injury, which is common to endurance athletes. It may also increase the athlete's strength and power ability for the sprint during the last stage of a race.

Periodization for Aerobic Endurance Training

Training programs should be designed to maximize performance and minimize fatigue and overtraining during high-volume training periods leading up to competition. Dividing training into phases by systematically altering volume and intensity and providing for adequate regeneration and peak performance around the most important competitions is a common strategy referred to as *periodization* (2). Periodization will be covered in detail in chapter 11, but generally, the training season is divided into a monocyclic design, including a preparatory time (preseason), competitive segment (in-season), transition (postseason, or active rest), and an off-season (35).

Training Phases

Traditionally, training sessions are organized as a set of various cycles (i.e., micro, meso, and macro). A *microcyle* refers to one training session or a group of training sessions. *Mesocycles* are groups of several microcycles centered around the competition phase. *Macrocycles* are a series of mesocycles planned in an annual or semiannual progression (24, 35).

The preparatory, or preseason, mesocycle centers on increasing training intensity and sustaining a moderate to high training volume. Competitive, or in-season, training incorporates competition and important race days, developing a training plan that leaves the athlete rested at peak times. The postseason transition phase allows for active recovery by decreasing the intensity and volume to eradicate any staleness or injury. Although an off-season is not as common among today's aerobic endurance athletes as it used to be (because most athletes compete year-round), it remains an important aspect of any training program. An off-season phase is implemented to establish a cardiorespiratory base, slowly increasing training intensity and duration as the athlete becomes fitter. Notably, a gradual increase in training duration (5% to 10% weekly) should be followed to prevent injury and overtraining (38).

For additional practical considerations in creating an annual training plan for aerobic endurance athletes, see chapter 12.

Tapering Strategies

The concept of tapering has evolved with new strategies for aerobic endurance athletes to reduce volume but achieve peak performance at a time that is most crucial. Tapering involves the alteration of training frequency, duration, and intensity, and the length of time within the reduced phase. More recently, exercise intensity has become the key component in an effective taper. Athletes who maintain activities of moderate intensities ($\leq 70\%$ $\dot{V}O_2$max) demonstrated a decrease in performance following a taper phase. Alternatively, reducing training duration but maintaining a high intensity ($\geq 90\%$ $\dot{V}O_2$max) has proven to be effective in stimulating gains in performance (33). The taper phase should typically last between 7 and 16 days for an aerobic endurance athlete to achieve peak performance (35).

Recovery

Possibly the most overlooked aspect of aerobic endurance training is recovery. Due to the high-volume and sometimes high-intensity aspects of aerobic endurance training, overtraining is a significant risk to aerobic endurance athletes. Overtraining is the result of too much stress, both physiological and psychological, and not enough rest (13). *Overtraining* has been defined as prolonged fatigue and underperformance that follows a heavy period of training or competition. It lasts at least two weeks and is determined by decreases in performance (5). Along with performance decrements, symptoms of overtraining include increased susceptibility to infections (5), weight loss, changes in sleep patterns, drowsiness, irritability, loss of appetite, loss of motivation, depression, anxiety, poor concentration, and high resting, recovery, and morning heart rates (11).

Overreaching is a form of short-term overtraining. Symptoms of overtraining can be reversed with planned rest periods (12). Overreaching can occur when an athlete increases intensity or volume of training to optimize training adaptations and performance. This is usually followed by a period of relative rest or tapering to allow for supercompensation (5). Those practicing an overreaching phase are at a risk for overtraining. Therefore, they must carefully monitor any of the possible symptoms. Recovery from overtraining may take up to five weeks of rest, during which detraining, or a decrease in fitness, will occur. Due to this detraining effect, it may take up to three months to return to full training following a rest period (21). As a result, it is clear that recovery must be carefully planned into a training program, especially during an overreaching phase, to avoid prolonged periods of decreased training.

A simple way to help avoid overreaching and overtraining for novice athletes is to slowly build base levels of fitness (i.e., increase aerobic capacity). LSD training is helpful while staying within the confines of 55% to 65% of HRmax while training. During this time, physiological adaptations, like weight loss, increases in leg and hip strength, and improvements in economy will all help to improve performance and decrease the risk for overtraining. Athletes with higher fitness levels recover faster than those with lower fitness levels (17). Thus, establishing a high base level of fitness is critical for long-term performance and recovery.

In addition, for both novice and experienced athletes, a sound dietary strategy is also critical for glycogen repletion and muscle recovery (19). A recent study showed that consumption of both protein and carbohydrate is important for the replenishment of lost glycogen from the muscle, as well as for muscle repair and rebuilding (19). The timing of these nutrients is also important. They should be consumed as soon as possible after a workout (19), and if possible, during the workout (20) to maintain intensity.

> For sample aerobic endurance training programs for the marathon, triathlon, and 5K races, as well as for swimming and rowing, see chapter 12.

SUMMARY POINTS

- The primary mode of training for aerobic endurance athletes should be the mode in which they compete (e.g. running, cycling, swimming). Specificity of training is important to improve exercise economy and overall performance.

- Calculations of training volume for aerobic endurance athletes should take intensity, duration, and distance into account. Intensity can be monitored by using heart rate or by comparing exercise pace to past competition results.

- New research has established that combining traditional, long-duration training with moderate-duration and intense, short-duration methods, such as pace/tempo training, Fartlek training, and interval training, yields the same or better results for performance. Resistance training may also be a valuable addition for aerobic endurance athletes.

- Tapering is the reduction of training volume prior to competition in order to improve performance. The tapering phase typically lasts 7 to 16 days.

- Due to the volume and intensity of many aerobic endurance training plans, overtraining is a significant risk to endurance athletes.

8

Agility Training

Lee E. Brown, EdD, CSCS*D, FACSM, FNSCA
Andy V. Khamoui, MS, CSCS

Agility can be defined as quick, full-body changes in direction and speed or simply the ability to change direction (2). Any casual observer of sport can describe the importance of such a skill to athletic performance. Most, if not all, field or court sports require agility for competition. For example, the extensive lateral movements in tennis required to sustain a rally and the frequent cutting motions in soccer, American football, and basketball clearly depict the prevalence of agility in sport.

On the playing field, an athlete typically performs rapid changes of direction in response to a stimulus. For instance, an American football player notices an oncoming opponent and, to avoid being tackled, reacts by cutting one way and running in the other direction. Long rallies between tennis players occur because they have the ability to adjust and change direction to cover the court as needed. This suggests a two-part model of agility: a visual and decision-making component in addition to a physical component (2, 20). This chapter focuses primarily on the physical components of agility. As a result, it examines training as it relates to developing the physical properties of improving change-of-direction ability, rather than highlighting visual decision-making processes (e.g., reaction time).

Factors in Agility Performance

Designing an agility training program requires an understanding of how the body functions or acts while performing changes in direction. The act of changing direction can be described generally as a stop-and-go event that requires the athlete to stop the body (braking force) and restart movement (propulsive force) with minimal time between the two phases. As a result, training should target this quick stop-and-go ability.

Further, since agility requires athletes to propel their own bodies on the field or court, body mass influences change-of-direction ability. Newton's first law states that an object at rest or in motion maintains its current state unless acted on by some external force that causes it to move or stop. Newton's first law has also been called the *law of inertia* because inertia refers to an object's resistance to change (i.e., being moved or stopped). This directly relates to an object's mass, since an object with greater mass also has greater inertia. We all know this intuitively based on our experiences in everyday life. For instance, trying to pick up a box full of textbooks poses a greater challenge than grabbing a box of tissues because the textbooks have greater mass and, correspondingly, greater resistance to being moved (i.e., inertia).

This is relevant to the ability to change direction because athletes with greater body mass also have greater inertia. Therefore, stopping while in motion will be more difficult for them. To successfully perform stop-and-go events, these athletes need the physical tools to overcome the inertial resistance inherent with large body mass. Note that athletes with larger body mass typically also have greater muscle mass. This additional contractile tissue may assist them in overcoming inertial resistance.

In addition to the movement concepts just described, a basic understanding of the internal biochemical processes that provide fuel for activity is essential. These internal processes include the phosphagen, anaerobic, and aerobic energy systems. Their contributions to providing fuel are based on the intensity and duration of an activity. A maximal-effort event of short duration, such as a 100 m sprint, primarily utilizes the phosphagen system. At the other end of the spectrum, aerobic processes provide fuel for longer duration events of lower intensity, such as a distance run. The contribution of the anaerobic system increases in activities 2 to 3 minutes in duration at intensities below maximal, such as a 400 m sprint. In short, the contribution of each energy system depends on the nature of the activity. Changes of direction in sport and during test assessments can last less than 5 seconds, more than 10 seconds, and everywhere in between. This implicates a primary role of the phosphagen and anaerobic systems in providing fuel for change-of-direction activities. The section on specificity further discusses the role of energy systems in training considerations.

The remainder of the chapter is devoted to addressing methods of assessment as well as training considerations, including specificity, transfer of training, agility drills, and program design.

Assessing Agility

Before implementing an agility training program, baseline measures of change-of-direction ability should be assessed so that progress may be tracked over time. Numerous agility tests exist, but each differs in terms of the length of time needed to complete the test, the number of directional changes, and the primary direction of force application (e.g., lateral, front to back) (2). Ideally, the test should be representative of what might occur during a typical competition in terms of movement patterns. The following tests have been used to assess change-of-direction ability:

- *T test.* This assessment requires the athlete to move in a T-shaped pattern (see page 43). It requires lateral and front-to-back movements, and is often used as a drill and assessment for athletes in basketball and American football. For various norms, see table 8.1.

- *5-10-5 shuttle.* The 5-10-5 shuttle consists of rapid directional changes in a linear plane (see page 4). It is commonly used as an assessment in American football, basketball, soccer, and most other field and court sports. This test has also been referred to as the *pro-agility test.* It is used as part of player assessment in the NFL combine. The setup for this test is very simple since it only requires three cones that are placed 5 yards (5 m) apart in a straight line. For various norms, see table 8.1.

- *Illinois test.* The Illinois test (see page 45) lasts considerably longer than the T test and 5-10-5 shuttle, covers more space, consists of a greater number of changes in direction, and requires the athlete to turn in different directions and run at different angles (19). In essence, this test consists of straight sprinting and weaving around obstacles. For various norms, see table 8.2.

Training for Agility

Following the initial assessment of agility, the athlete can undertake a training program to develop change-of-direction ability. The subsequent sections address important aspects of agility training, including specificity, examples of drills, and the manipulation of program-design variables to produce optimal outcomes. The section on transfer of training also provides a rationale for exercise selection. The following section covers the concept of specificity as it relates to agility training.

Specificity

Specificity refers to training with the purpose of attaining a particular outcome. Athletes therefore utilize training programs that allow for the greatest transfer to their sports. Specificity of training can be applied in terms of energy systems, muscle groups, and movement patterns. For example, a lineman in American football might incorporate resistance exercises that target upper and lower body strength and power in addition to short-sprinting ability because those characteristics are needed for the position.

Specific training related to agility development should consider spatial aspects of the sport. In other words, the amount of space that an athlete covers within a given sport should be identified and applied in a training program. A basketball player will only be able to move within the confines of the court. Likewise, a soccer player can only roam within the space limitations

TABLE 8.1 Norms for T test and 5-10-5 Shuttle by Sport, Population, and Gender

Sport	Population	Gender	T tests	5-10-5 shuttles
Recreational	University	M	10.49 ± 0.89	–
		F	12.52 ± 0.90	–
Baseball	National Association of Intercollegiate Athletics (NAIA)	M	10.11 ± 0.64	–
Basketball	NCAA Division I	M	8.95 ± 0.53	–
	Guard		8.74 ± 0.41	–
	Forward		8.94 ± 0.38	–
	Center		9.28 ± 0.81	–
American football	High school (age 14-18)	M	–	5.02 ± 0.24
	NCAA Division I		–	4.53 ± 0.22
	Offensive and defensive linemen		–	4.35 ± 0.11
	Wide receivers, defensive backs		–	4.35 ± 0.12
	Running backs, tight ends, linebackers		–	4.6 ± 0.2
	NCAA Division III		–	4.6 ± 0.2
	Offensive linemen		–	4.8 ± 0.2
	Defensive linemen		–	4.8 ± 0.2
	Offensive skill positions		–	4.5 ± 0.2
	Defensive backs		–	4.6 ± 0.2
	NFL-drafted rookies		–	–
	Rounds 1 and 2		–	4.38 ± 0.29
	Rounds 6 and 7		–	4.45 ± 0.29
Soccer	Elite youth	M	–	–
	Under 14		11.6 ± 0.1	–
	Under 15		11.0 ± 0.2	–
	Under 16		11.7 ± 0.1	–
	NCAA Division III	M	–	4.43 ± 0.17
		F	–	4.88 ± 0.18
Volleyball	NCAA Division I	F	11.16 ± 0.38	–
	NCAA Division III		–	4.75 ± 0.19

Data from Hoffman 2006.

TABLE 8.2 Illinois Test Norms in Seconds for Males and Females

Category	Males	Females
Excellent	<15.2	<17.0
Good	15.2-16.1	17.0-17.9
Average	16.2-18.1	18.0-21.7
Fair	18.2-18.3	21.8-23.0
Poor	>18.3	>23.0

Reprinted from Roozen 2004.

of the field. Therefore, agility drills that exceed the dimensions of the court or field or surpass the typical space covered by the athlete lack specificity. The importance of sport specificity cannot be overstated. An attacking soccer (football) player may be required to perform frequent changes of direction while maintaining control of the ball; therefore, specificity of training advocates soccer drills that integrate dribbling and ball control. Similarly, a basketball player needs to be agile while dribbling in order to advance the ball downcourt and, at the same time, avoid the opposing team. To train for agility within the context of basketball, athletes must integrate dribbling in conjunction with change-of-direction drills.

Consideration of the energy requirements of a given sport when training for agility is also important, since changes of direction are performed intermittently during an ongoing event. Specifically, agility movements are typically performed in a suboptimal state, because other components of the sport require energy expenditure (e.g., jumping, tackling, straight sprinting). Therefore, it may be useful to conduct change-of-direction training within a similar sport-specific environment by integrating agility drills throughout a practice session.

The surfaces where the athlete will train should be taken into consideration. A few studies have documented different physiological responses of athletes while testing or competing on different surface types (5, 17) that indicate the terrestrial environmental influences on performance. For example, one study measured blood-lactate levels, heart rate, and running speed in soccer players during an identical running test on three different surfaces: a treadmill, natural grass, and synthetic turf (5). Levels of lactate, which forms as a result of vigorous muscular work and produces a burning sensation in muscle, were greater during the test on synthetic turf than on the other surfaces. In addition, testing on the synthetic turf produced greater heart rates and lower running speeds, indicating a higher degree of exercise intensity (difficulty). A comparable study using tennis players found greater lactate levels and heart rates when athletes played on a clay court than on a hard court (17).

Collectively, these results highlight the influence of surface types on the body during physical activity. Surface types during training should be similar to those athletes will encounter during competition. Field-sport athletes should perform agility drills on a field of natural grass or a field turf, depending on the playing surface they encounter during competition. Similarly, court-sport athletes should perform agility training on the surfaces they use in competition, such as a hardwood floor for basketball or the various surface types for a tennis player.

Transfer of Training

The coach or athlete interested in developing agility ultimately wants to know what types of exercises to use. Several training studies have been conducted in an effort to identify the best approach for enhancing agility performance. These studies have typically examined the effect on agility performance of training programs that consist of traditional lower-body resistance exercises (e.g., Olympic lifts, back squats, deadlifts, lunges, or jump training), straight sprinting, or specific change-of-direction drills.

Few studies have demonstrated improvements in agility performance following a traditional lower-body resistance-training program that consists of Olympic lifts, squats, deadlifts, and lunges (6, 11-13, 21). In fact, the majority did not observe significant improvements in agility when athletes performed lower-body resistance exercises exclusively. However, studies evaluating the value of strength training in conjunction with extensive agility training have produced favorable results (3). In one study (15), subjects performed jump-squat training (i.e., squatting down and jumping up with a bar on the upper back) with a load of either 30% or 80% of the athletes' back squat 1RM (weight lifted in a single, maximum effort). Performance in the T test improved in both training groups, with greater improvements occurring in the group with 80% 1RM than in the one with 30%.

This sort of training may be beneficial because of the movements that occur during changes in direction. As the introduction describes, agility can be characterized as stop-and-go events that consist of braking (stop) and propulsive (go) forces. Performing the jump squat with additional load targets these actions at greater intensities than athletes are normally accustomed to, which leads to favorable adaptations when they perform rapid changes in direction.

The other jumping study that improved agility performance required subjects to perform several variations of jumps, including horizontally (jumping forward), laterally (side to side) on one leg, and laterally on both legs (16). Time to complete both the T test and Illinois agility test decreased following the jump-training period. These types of jumps may improve change-of-direction ability because similar movement patterns and physical characteristics are used in both the jumps and the agility tests. The physical requirements for performing lateral and horizontal movements in the T test and Illinois agility test are the same physical components recruited during lateral and horizontal jumping. Therefore, it seems logical that the benefits provided by these types of jumps could improve agility performance when incorporated into a training program.

A small number of studies have also looked at the effect of straight-sprint training on agility performance (14, 22). One investigation observed improvements in agility (14), while the other did not find improvement in change-of-direction performance (22). Based on these results, the effectiveness of training that strictly uses straight sprints for agility has not been fully established. On the other hand, training studies consisting of agility drills have consistently improved change-of-direction performance (3, 4, 7, 8, 18). Specifically, these studies integrated general agility training (sprinting with change of direction) or agility drills with actual training sessions for rugby, volleyball, and soccer athletes. Therefore, it appears that the concept of specificity holds true, since the greatest, most consistent gains in agility performance have been documented after change-of-direction training. In other words, to develop agility, athletes need to train with agility drills.

In summary, traditional lower-body resistance exercise alone may not be an optimal means of developing agility. Further, the effectiveness of straight-sprint training on agility performance has not been well established. In contrast, jump training, including loaded jump squats and horizontal and lateral jumps, holds promise. The strength and conditioning professional may integrate jumping exercises into an athlete's resistance training program to improve agility performance if desired. The benefit of agility-specific drills on change-of-direction ability seems to have strong support. As a result, agility training can be recommended as an appropriate training mode for improving change-of-direction speed.

Agility Drills

The various agility drills presented in this section utilize premarked distances (lines), cones or domes, and specialized equipment, such as ladders. They also differ in distance covered, duration, number of directional changes, and movement patterns. These characteristics, which alter the complexity of each drill, should be considered when selecting drills for a given population.

Just as in any other form of exercise, proper technique should be practiced at all times. Throughout the entire drill, the athlete's head should stay in a neutral position, with the eyes looking straight ahead. Athletes often hyperextend the neck or tuck the chin down due to fatigue or habit. This should be corrected in order to maximize technique, reduce risk of injury, and allow the athlete to pick up on task-relevant cues presented during practice and competition. Any changes in direction should be initiated from the top down. This means that the head turns in the intended direction first, followed by the rest of the body. Another way to think about this is for the athlete to lead with the eyes to the intended target or direction, and then let the body follow. During the actual change of direction (braking phase), lowering the center of mass will allow the athlete to stop and go much more quickly.

Finally, effective use of the arms greatly benefits the ability to perform change-of-direction tasks, since the arms provide balance and help rotate the body, allowing directional changes to occur (1). For example, suppose an athlete performs a single change of direction during a 5-yard (5 m) shuttle. After he initiates the foot plant (braking phase), the outside arm (same side as planting foot) will come across the trunk, enabling the athlete to rotate the body and move in a new direction. During this process, the athlete should keep the arms near the body to minimize the resistance to rotation (rotational inertia), which occurs by swinging the arms away from the body (1). In other words, a greater concentration of mass closer to the point of rotation (torso) allows rotation to occur with greater ease. This is accomplished by keeping the arms close to the body. These cues should enable the athlete to perform agility movements much more effectively.

CARIOCA

PURPOSE

Develop balance, flexibility in the hips, footwork, and lateral speed

PROCEDURE

The athlete should do the following:

- Start in a two-point stance
- Step with right foot over the left leg (*a*)
- Move the left foot to the left (*b*) behind the right leg
- Step with the right foot behind the left leg (*c*)

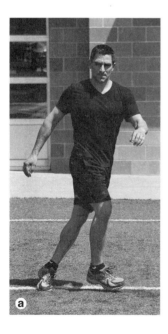
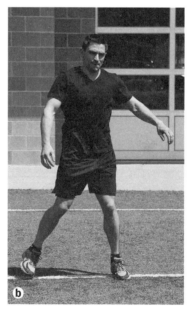
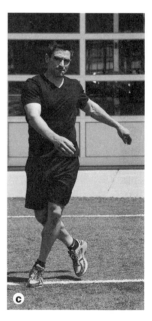

DOUBLE-LEG LATERAL HOPPING

PURPOSE
Develop explosiveness and change-of-direction ability in the lateral direction

PROCEDURE
In a marked-off area 1 yard (1 m) wide, the athlete should do the following:

- Start on the left side of the marked-off area
- Push off to the side with both legs, making sure to clear the marked-off area
- After landing, quickly explode back across the area to the starting position
- Perform 5 to 10 consecutive repetitions in a rapid fashion (across and back counts as one repetition)

COMPLEX VARIATIONS
In a marked-off area 10 yards (10 m) long and 1 yard (1 m) wide, the athlete should do the following:

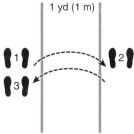

- Start at one end and hop the length of the area in a zigzag pattern (diagonally) to the other end
- Perform hops with single leg only

HEXAGON

PURPOSE
Improve agility

PROCEDURE
Mark off a hexagon with sides about 2 feet (61 cm) long, although this can vary. The athlete should do the following:

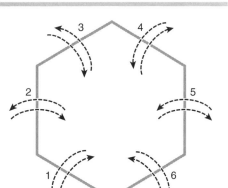

- Begin in the middle of the hexagon facing a determined direction
- While facing that direction, jump with both feet outside each side of the hexagon
- Perform this pattern both clockwise and counterclockwise while being timed

COMPLEX VARIATIONS
- Use single-leg hops
- Vary the size of the hexagon

20-YARD SHUTTLE

PURPOSE

Improve ability to change direction, footwork, and reaction time

PROCEDURE

The athlete should do the following:

- Start in a two-point stance straddling the starting line
- Turn to the right, sprint, and touch a line 5 yards (4.6 m) away with the right hand
- Turn back to the left, sprint 10 yards (9 m), and touch the far line with the left hand
- Turn back to the right and sprint 5 yards through the starting line to finish

COMPLEX VARIATION

20-yard combination agility drill. The athlete performs different skills on each leg of the line drill (e.g., skipping, carioca, bounding, etc.).

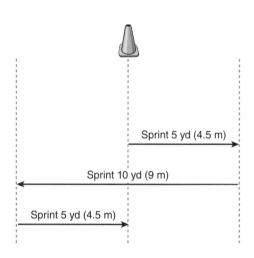

60-YARD SHUTTLE SPRINT

PURPOSE

Improve agility and conditioning

PROCEDURE

The athlete should do the following:

- Start in a two-point stance
- Sprint forward 5 yards (4.6 m) to the first line and touch it with either hand, then turn and return to the starting line
- Sprint forward 10 yards (9 m) to the second line and touch it with either hand, then turn and return to the starting line

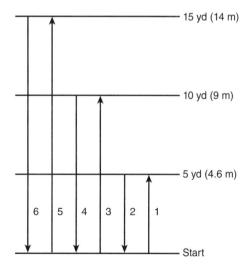

- Sprint forward 15 yards (14 m) to the third line and touch it with either hand, then turn and return through the starting line

100-YARD SHUTTLE SPRINT

PURPOSE

Improve ability to change direction, footwork, and reaction time

PROCEDURE

The athlete should do the following:

- Start in a two-point stance on the starting line
- Sprint 5 yards (4.6 m) to the first line, touch it with the right hand, return to the starting line, and touch it with the left hand
- Sprint 10 yards (9 m) to the second line, touch it with the right hand, return to the starting line, and touch it with the left hand
- Sprint 15 yards (14 m) to the first line, touch it with the right hand, return to the starting line, and touch it with the left hand
- Sprint 20 yards (18 m) to the second line, touch it with the right hand, return to the starting line, and touch it with the left hand

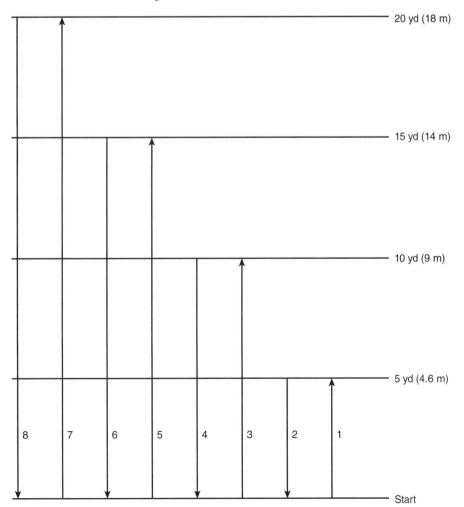

40-YARD LATERAL SHUFFLE

PURPOSE

Improve agility, conditioning, and flexibility in abductors and adductors, develop strength

PROCEDURE

The athlete should do the following:

- Start in a two-point stance, straddling the starting line
- Shuffle 5 yards (4.6 m) to the first line, touch it with the right foot, shuffle back to the starting line, and touch it with the left foot
- Shuffle 10 yards (9 m) to the second line, touch it with the right foot, shuffle back to the starting line, and touch it with the left foot
- Shuffle 5 yards to the first line, touch it with the right foot, and shuffle back to the starting line

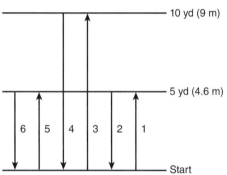

15-YARD TURNING DRILL

PURPOSE

Improve ability to change direction, flexibility in hips, and footwork

PROCEDURE

The athlete should do the following:

- Start in a two-point stance
- Sprint forward 5 yards (4.6 m) to cone 1 and make a sharp right turn around it
- Sprint to cone 2, located 5 yards to the right of the start and on the diagonal from cone 1, and make a left turn around it
- Sprint 5 yards through the finish

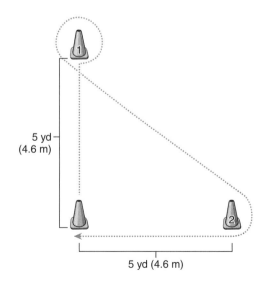

COMPLEX VARIATIONS

The athlete should do the following:

- Put the inside hand on the ground when making turns
- Change the distance between the cones
- Make turns on command, not at the cones

20-YARD SQUARE

PURPOSE

Improve ability to change direction, body position, transitions between skills, and cutting

PROCEDURE

The athlete should do the following:

- Start in a two-point stance
- Sprint 5 yards (4.6 m) to cone 2 and make sharp right cut
- Shuffle right 5 yards and make a sharp cut back at cone 3
- Backpedal 5 yards to cone 4 and make a sharp left cut
- Shuffle to the left to cone 1

COMPLEX VARIATIONS

The athlete should do the following:

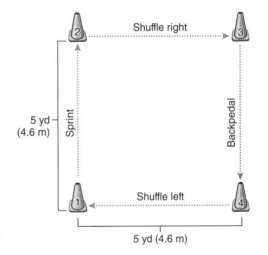

- Start from different positions (for example, lying down, from a four-point stance, and so on)
- Change the distance of the cones to match the demands of his sport
- Change the skills employed during each leg to meet specific needs
- Cut with the inside or outside leg
- Cut on the outside of the cone or circle around the cones
- Put the inside hand on the ground during turns

FIGURE EIGHTS

PURPOSE
Improve ability to change direction and reaction time

PROCEDURE
The athlete should do the following:

- Position two flat cones 5 to 10 yards (4.6-9 m) apart
- Start in a two-point stance
- Run a figure eight between the cones, placing the inside hand on each cone while making the turn

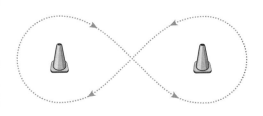

COMPLEX VARIATIONS
The athlete should do the following:

- Change the distance between the cones
- Change the radius of the turns
- Start the drill from various positions (for example, lying down, sitting, a four-point stance, and so on)

Z-PATTERN RUN

PURPOSE
Improve transitional movement and turning ability

PROCEDURE
The athlete should do the following:

- Position three cones on two lines 5 yards (4.6 m) apart such that the cones on line 1 are at 0, 10, and 20 yards (0, 9, and 18 m), and the cones on line 2 are at 5, 15, and 25 yards (4.6, 14, and 23 m)
- Start in a two-point stance
- Sprint diagonally 5 yards to the closest cone, plant the outside foot, and run around the cone
- Continue to sprint diagonally to each cone and run around it

COMPLEX VARIATIONS
The athlete should do the following:

- Start from different positions (for example, lying down, a four-point stance, and so on)

- Change the distance of the cones to match the demands of the sport
- Change the skills employed during each leg to meet specific needs
- Cut with the inside or outside leg
- Put the inside hand on the ground during turns

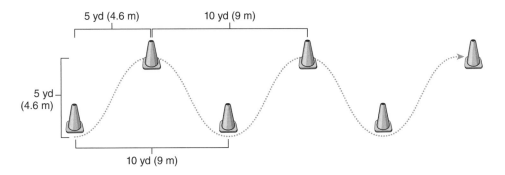

ICKEY SHUFFLE

PURPOSE

Enhance coordination and improve lower body quickness

PROCEDURE

The athlete should do the following:

- Start on the left side of the ladder
- Step laterally with the right foot and place it inside the first square of the ladder, then place the left foot inside the same square
- Step laterally with the right foot to the right side of the ladder, then place the left foot in the second square
- Bring the right foot into the square with the left foot
- Step laterally to the left side of the ladder and place the right foot into the third square
- Repeat this pattern

To add complexity to ladder drills, athletes should look up during the drill and avoid looking at their feet. All drills should be performed both forward and backward.

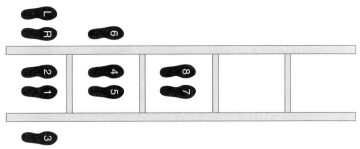

IN-OUT SHUFFLE

PURPOSE

Improve agility, balance, coordination, and quickness

PROCEDURE

The athlete should do the following:

- Start in a two-point stance
- Begin standing sideways to the ladder, with the ladder in front
- Step straight ahead into the first square with the left foot
- Follow by putting the right foot into this same square
- Step back and diagonally with the left foot until it is in front of the second square to the left
- Follow with the right foot until it is in front of the same square
- Repeat this sequence throughout the ladder
- Ensure that each foot hits every box

COMPLEX VARIATIONS

The athlete should do the following:

- Perform the same pattern with each foot in a separate box
- Use every other box and increase the length of the lateral step
- Perform the drill backward (that is, start with the ladder behind)

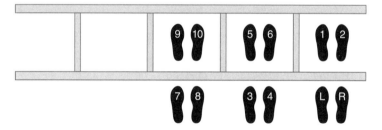

SIDE RIGHT-IN

PURPOSE

Improve agility, balance, coordination, and quickness

PROCEDURE

The athlete should do the following:

- Start in a two-point stance
- Begin standing sideways to the ladder
- Step with the right foot into the first square

- Step forward with the left foot over the first square to the other side of the ladder
- Step laterally with the right foot into the second square
- Step backward with the left foot, landing in front of the second square
- Step laterally with the right foot into the third square
- Repeat this sequence down the ladder

COMPLEX VARIATION

- *Side left-in.* The athlete should perform the drill, starting with the left foot and using the opposite foot (as compared to the preceding instructions).

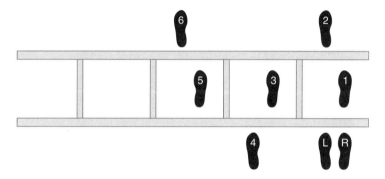

SNAKE JUMP

PURPOSE

Improve agility, balance, coordination, hip flexibility, and quickness

PROCEDURE

The athlete should do the following:

- Start in a two-point stance, straddling one side of the ladder
- Keeping both feet together, perform a series of quarter-turn jumps
- The direction the feet should point for each jump is as follows: straight ahead, right, straight ahead, left, straight ahead, and so on
- Rotate the hips with each jump

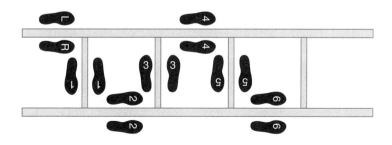

CROSSOVER SHUFFLE

PURPOSE

Increase flexibility and power in the hips, improve ability to change direction

PROCEDURE

The athlete should do the following:

- Stand to the left of the ladder
- Cross the left foot over the right to step into the first square of the ladder
- Laterally step with the right foot to the right side of the ladder
- Immediately cross the right foot over into the second square
- Laterally step with the left foot to the left side of the ladder
- Repeat the process down the ladder
- Remember: Only one foot is in the ladder at any one time.

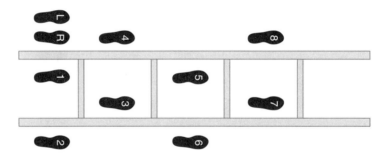

The above drills and diagrams, with the exception of double-leg lateral hopping are reprinted, by permission, from Brown LE, Ferrigno, VA. *Training for Speed, Agility, and Quickness*. 2nd ed. Champaign, IL: Human Kinetics; 2005. For many more drills and additional information on agility training, readers are encouraged to consult this text and its accompanying DVD.

Agility Program Design

After an initial assessment of change-of-direction ability, the athlete can begin a training program to develop agility. Any training program, whether it is intended to develop strength, speed, or aerobic endurance, requires short- and long-term planning to maximize gains while minimizing fatigue and plateaus. This planning and development requires the manipulation of what sport scientists and practitioners call *program variables*. These consist of selection, order, frequency, intensity, volume, and rest periods for exercises performed during a given training session (table 8.3). Whenever possible, recommendations are provided for the prescription

For practical tips on integrating agility training and other forms of training in the context of an athlete's annual plan, see chapter 12.

TABLE 8.3 Summary of Acute Program Variables for Agility Training

Program variable	Guidelines
Exercise selection	Consider: • Movement patterns • Distances encountered in competition

Exercise order	*Novice*
	    Least to most complex
	Advanced
	    • Least to most complex or
	    • Most complex with decreased intensity to start

Frequency	• 2-3 times per week • Can increase or decrease based on training status of athlete
Intensity	Maximum or near maximum

Volume	~5 drills (adjust accordingly based on individual readiness)
	Novice
	    ~5-10 repetitions per drill
	Advanced
	    5-25 repetitions per drill

Rest	• Work-to-rest ratio of 1:4 to 1:20 • Adjust accordingly based on athlete training status and complexity of drill

of program variables based on training studies that successfully improved change-of-direction ability. It will be assumed that the positive results from these studies occur from effective planning and implementation of program variables.

Exercise and Drill Selection

The selection of individual drills should be based on what an athlete might encounter in a game situation. For instance, soccer players cover vast amounts of ground during the course of a game. Movement patterns performed by a typical field player include long sprints integrated with changes of direction when timing a run into open space so that teammates have an outlet to play the ball into. Therefore, the 40-, 60-, and 100-yard shuttle sprints, as well as the 40-yard lateral shuffle and the 55-yard sprint backpedal, would be appropriate training drills. The player performing a long shuffle drill (e.g., 40-yard lateral shuffle) would not run 40 yards straight, but might make eight change-of-direction runs of 5 yards each. These drills provide change-of-direction tasks in conjunction with comparable distances a soccer (football) player might cover. A similar approach could be taken for a wide receiver or a running back in

American football. Thus, the selection of agility drills should be made after identifying both the characteristics of the sport and differences among positions within the sport.

It should be noted that an athlete's initial training level will factor into the selection of exercises. A novice or deconditioned athlete will likely require an initial series of basic drills to get accustomed to the demands of training before progressing to more complex routines.

Exercise Order

The order of agility drills within a training session largely depends on the training status of the athlete or population being trained. In general, a novice will perform less complex exercises (those of shorter duration and with fewer directional changes) prior to doing more complex ones (those longer in duration and with more directional changes). This allows the beginner to become familiar with the movement patterns and physical characteristics needed to perform change-of-direction tasks. Advanced athletes could use this same exercise order, with the less complex drills serving as a warm-up to get them ready for more advanced exercises. The advanced athlete may also go directly into complex drills at the start of the session, but perform initial repetitions at a lower intensity before going into maximal-effort repetitions.

Frequency

Frequency refers to the number of training sessions performed during a given unit of time. Improvements in change-of-direction ability have been demonstrated in as little as twice per week for 4 weeks (2). The most common training frequency administered in successful training studies is two or three times per week (2). The duration of these training programs ranged from 6 to 14 weeks in length, with the most common period being 8 to 10 weeks (2). In any case, a consistent agility training program at a frequency of two or three times per week over the course of several weeks appears to be necessary for improvements in change-of-direction ability. Chapter 12 discusses the integration of agility training into the yearly training program.

Intensity

A practical definition of *intensity* is the effort of a given exercise. Other modes of training usually prescribe intensity as a percentage of some maximum value obtained during an assessment of the training parameter. For example, resistance-exercise intensity is usually quantified as a percentage of one-repetition maximum (1RM). In aerobic exercise, it's quantified as a percentage of maximum heart rate (HRmax) or oxygen uptake ($\dot{V}O_2$max). Agility training, on the other hand, does not utilize manipulations in intensity the way a resistance or aerobic exercise program might. Athletes perform agility drills at maximum or near-maximum effort and speed to develop change-of-direction ability because by definition, this stop-and-go event must occur very quickly, with minimal downtime between the two phases.

Volume

Because intensity in agility exercises does not vary, volume is the program variable that must be manipulated to adjust the difficulty of the program. Volume represents the total quantity of exercises performed in a training session. It can be calculated by adding the number of repetitions performed per drill. A single repetition constitutes completion of a drill one time through (i.e., a complete sequence). If an athlete performs 5 repetitions of ladder drills and 5 of cone drills, the total volume performed is 10 repetitions or sequences. To increase volume, an athlete can perform more repetitions per drill or increase the number of drills performed during a training session.

Unfortunately, the optimal volume to bring about the best gains has not been identified in the scientific literature. There has also not been much research on the topic. Completing approximately 5 to 25 repetitions of five drills has been accepted as adequate training, with adjustments made for initial levels of fitness and the nature of the drills (i.e., complexity, difficulty) being performed (9). For example, the 100-yard shuttle sprint might be performed a total of 3 to 5 times because of the longer distance covered, while the 20-yard shuttle could be performed for 20 times total (two sets of 10 repetitions). A beginner may perform only 5 to 10 repetitions of a drill when first starting a new agility program, depending on the difficulty of the drill. In addition, the number of drills performed can also be adjusted based on individual readiness. The same number of repetitions does not need to be performed for each drill, and priority should be given to weak areas.

Rest

Recovery periods should be provided between repetitions and drills so that technique can be maintained. A work-to-rest ratio between 1:4 and 1:6 should provide adequate recovery (9). For example, a drill lasting 15 seconds would use recovery intervals of 1 to 2 minutes. Adjustments can also be made to enable adequate recovery, based on an athlete's current fitness level and on the complexity of the agility tasks being performed. Athletes who are less fit may require longer recovery periods during a training session. Likewise, those using more difficult or challenging drills may require longer rest times. In fact, work-to-rest ratios as large as 1:20 are not uncommon, since the athlete should be ready and able to give a maximal effort on each repetition.

Structure of Training Programs

A common agility-training session consists of components similar to other training modes, such as a general warm-up, specific warm-up, main session, and cool-down. The general warm-up consists of low-intensity exercises that use large muscle groups (jogging) to raise core body temperature and prepare the athlete for training. The specific warm-up also serves as preparation, but it is more specific to the objectives of the training session. This can be accomplished by performing a few agility drills at a lower intensity (walk through) to get the body primed for the change-of-direction tasks constituting the bulk of the training session. The cool-down, which consists of low-impact activity, can be thought of as a reverse warm-up that gradually brings the body back to preactivity levels.

For sample agility-training programs that target fast footwork in close quarters, changes of direction over varying distances, and the agility requirements of basketball players, see chapter 12.

SUMMARY POINTS

- The frequent changes of direction performed in most field- and court-based sports highlight the importance of agility. Agility involves quick changes of direction and speed. Therefore, it relies on the capacity to very quickly stop the body (braking force) and restart movement (propulsive force).

- Like most other performance parameters, agility can be improved through a well-planned training program that utilizes acute program variables and the concept of specificity.

- The development of skilled change-of-direction ability requires agility-specific interventions. Therefore, athletes should train with agility drills.

- Agility drills should be selected to match the distance athletes will cover in a game situation and the types of changes in speed and direction they are required to make.

- To improve change-of-direction ability, agility drills need to be performed two or three times a week over the course of at least several weeks.

- Agility drills must always be performed at high intensity to be effective. The difficulty of agility training sessions can be manipulated through the number of drills performed and the length of rest intervals.

Speed Training

Jay R. Hoffman, PhD, CSCS*D, FNSCA
John F. Graham, MS, CSCS*D, FNSCA

Speed can be defined as the ability to run a specific distance in a particular time. Speed is known as an important contributor to success in sport performance. A number of studies show that speed is often the deciding factor between starters and nonstarters in team sports (4, 5, 15). The most important factor influencing speed for athletes is genetic makeup. Athletes with long limbs and a high percentage of fast-twitch muscle fibers have both a physiological and a biomechanical advantage for being faster than athletes with shorter limbs and a lower percentage of fast-twitch fibers. However, running speed also depends on skill and technique that, when flawed, can be improved. As such, if athletes can improve their running technique and increase their strength and power, it is possible that they can also improve their speed. Many experts in the strength and conditioning profession have provided support for this concept (3, 7, 10, 18, 21, 22, 24, 29).

Speed training is an integral part of the preparation of athletes participating in sports where speed is a significant factor in performance outcomes (e.g., American football, baseball, basketball, lacrosse, and soccer) (2, 10, 14, 21, 22, 26, 27). Speed training enables athletes to use maximal force during sport-specific speed movements and patterns (22, 25, 28). It influences and benefits the muscles and muscle groups that link eccentric muscle actions with concentric muscle actions, or the *stretch-shortening cycle* (SSC) (6, 19). A SSC occurs when a muscle or muscle group is stretched and then immediately shortened (much like a rubber band).

Stretch-shortening actions make use of two events: tension and length–impulse response to the motor neural system, and inherent muscle–tendon activity (6, 19). Short-term SSC actions tend to enhance muscle performance, speed, acceleration, and power through elastic energy, whereas long-term adaptations reduce muscle stiffness and increase neuromuscular activation (6, 19, 26). The SSC is often recognized as a link between power and speed that enables athletes to increase both performance variables (17, 19, 24). See chapter 5 for more detail on the functions of the SSC.

Factors in Speed Performance

The ability to accelerate from the start may vary considerably among athletes. Some Olympic-caliber sprinters can continue to accelerate through the 70 m mark in a 100 m sprint. Although the ability to accelerate is important, the rate at which this acceleration occurs may have even greater importance. The goal for all athletes is to reach peak velocity (which involves maximizing acceleration) as quickly as possible. Running velocity is influenced by strength and power, which is why athletes who have set goals to become faster should be committed to both a resistance training program (see chapter 4) and targeted speed training.

As long as athletes can still accelerate, they will gain speed. Only if they begin to decelerate will they slow down. To maintain sprinting speed, athletes need to focus on improving their speed-endurance. Speed-endurance is not a factor for short-distance sprints, such as the 40 m sprint, in which athletes should accelerate throughout the racing distance. However, this becomes very relevant for sprint distances of 100 m or greater. Here, speed-endurance becomes a factor for determining sprinting success.

Stride Rate and Stride Length

Speed is the interaction of stride rate and stride length. The stride contains two steps, or *foot strikes*, which can be defined as the points of contact between the foot and the ground (see figure 9.1). *Stride rate* is the number of steps that are taken with each leg during the distance of a run. If a sprinter in a 100 m run takes 25 foot strikes with his or her right leg and 24 foot strikes with his or her left leg, it equates to 49 strides. If the sprinter runs the 100 m in 11.0 seconds, he or she would have a stride frequency of 4.45 strides per second. Elite sprinters have a stride rate of about 5 strides per second (23).

As the stride rate increases, the amount of time spent on the ground (called the *support phase*) is decreased, while the time spent in the flight phase is increased. If the stride rate of an athlete increases, but his or her stride length remains constant, his or her running speed will increase. Similarly, if the athlete's stride rate remains constant but his stride length is increased, his or her running speed will also increase.

During a sprint, both stride rate and stride length increase, causing running velocity to increase as well. As an athlete comes off the blocks in a race or out of stance in a drill, the initial change in speed is the result of

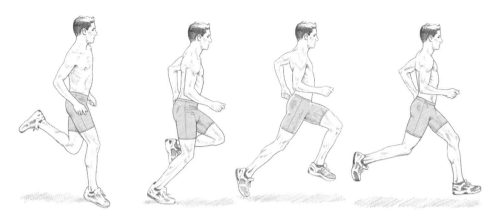

FIGURE 9.1 A stride in running includes two foot strikes, as shown here.

Adapted, by permission, from J. Puleo and P. Milroy, 2010, *Running anatomy* (Champaign, IL: Human Kinetics), 20.

an increase in running stride. The sprinter is using short, choppy strides to overcome the inertia of not moving. The stride length begins to increase as the sprinter accelerates. As running velocity increases further, increases in both stride length and stride rate contribute to the higher running veloci- ties. However, stride length increases up to running velocities of about 8 m/s (11). As speed is increased even further, a slight decrease in stride length is seen, with a sustained increase in stride rate. The contribution of both stride rate and stride length to sprinting speed will change at different running velocities. Stride rate appears to be more important in determining the runner's maximum velocity than stride length is (23).

Both stride rate and stride length appear to be quite variable among ath- letes. Stride length depends on an athlete's height and leg length (23, 24). Tall athletes with greater leg lengths generally have longer strides. Stride rate is also quite variable, with large differences seen between trained and untrained runners (23, 24). Trained sprinters can achieve a greater stride rate than untrained runners can. They reach their maximum velocity much earlier than untrained runners do. Improvements in power performance appear to increase the acceleration ability of athletes by decreasing the ground contact time of each stride and increasing the impulse production during each takeoff (9, 23, 24).

Muscle Fiber-Type Composition

As discussed earlier in this chapter, muscle fiber-type composition has a critical role in determining running speed. Muscles are comprised of two types of fibers. Type I fibers, also referred to as *slow-twitch, oxidative fibers,* provide low force output and slow conduction speed, but are fatigue resis- tant. They are beneficial to athletes who participate in aerobic endurance events. Type II fibers, also referred to as *fast-twitch, glycolytic fibers,* have a high force output and fast contraction speed, but are easily fatigued. These fibers are beneficial for athletes who participate in explosive sports that require speed and power performance.

Each of these fibers has subtypes. Fiber subtypes have the basic characteristics of the fiber type (slow-twitch or fast-twitch), but can be altered based on the training stimulus or lack of stimulus. That is, fibers may become more oxidative or glycolytic depending on the type of training program. However, athletes cannot change the fiber-type composition, so although Type I fibers may become more anaerobic or glycolytic through sprint or interval training, they will never acquire many of the characteristics generally associated with Type II fibers. Most people are born with an equal number of Type I and Type II fibers. Although training can help athletes reach their maximum potential, their fiber-type distribution will affect the events they can excel in. This is why it is not easy to develop elite athletes. They are generally born, not made!

Muscle architecture also appears to have an important role in speed ability. The combination of muscle thickness, fascicle length, and the resulting pennation angle has been suggested to influence speed performance (1, 20). Muscle fibers that have a greater pennation angle generate more force, and muscle fibers with a smaller pennation angle have demonstrated a characteristic to shorten faster, thus helping athletes increase speed (1, 20).

Sprinting Mechanics and Technique

Technique training for sprinting can be divided into five areas: starting, acceleration, drive phase, recovery phase, and deceleration.

Starting

Athletes start from a variety of positions, including stationary or moving. Athletes in sports such as baseball and softball generally initiate all speed movements in a two-point stance from a stationary position, while those in other sports (e.g., field hockey, soccer, basketball, and lacrosse) may also initiate movement in a two-point stance but from an active movement (jog, shuffle, or backward run). American football offers a variety of starting positions, including a stationary three- or four-point stance for linemen and fullbacks, a two-point stationary stance for quarterbacks, receivers, and running backs, a stationary or moving two-point stance for linebackers and defensive backs, and a moving or stationary two-point stance for players on special teams.

When beginning a speed movement from a two-point stance, the athlete should be in a comfortable position, with feet shoulder-width apart or slightly narrower, body weight equally distributed on both feet, and the arms bent at 90° angles, with the hand on the lead-leg side next to the buttock and the other hand at the side of the face. The athlete's center of gravity should be above the front foot, with the front leg bent at nearly 90°. Before initiating movement, approximately two-thirds to three-fourths of the body weight should be shifted to the lead leg. The start should occur with both feet applying force to the ground and an explosive movement forward. The rear foot should leave the ground first with a fast forward swing and the rear arm should propel forward (10, 16, 29).

The start from a three- or four-point stationary stance should occur with the athlete in a comfortable position. The body weight should be evenly distributed between hands, feet, and knees, the arms should be in a straight alignment shoulder-width apart, and the head and back should be aligned. Prior to initiating the start, the athlete should align the center of gravity above the lead leg, bend the front leg to nearly a 90° angle and the rear leg at nearly 125°, move the hips shoulder-width apart or slightly wider, and straighten both arms and place them slightly in front of the hands. The start occurs with an explosive driving force from both feet, with the rear leg moving first with a forward swing. At the same time, the alternate arm should move actively (10, 16, 29).

The moving start transpires with the athlete moving at a easy walk or jog, with only a slight forward lean. During the start, the athlete should apply force to the ground with both feet and explode forward, with the rear foot leaving the ground first with a fast forward swing and the arm propelling forward (10, 16, 29).

Acceleration

During the acceleration phase, the body gradually straightens and the strides lengthen. As the ball of the foot makes contact with the athletic surface, the foot should be in a dorsiflexed position. The athlete should look down and limit torso flexion at the waist. Acceleration differs from maximal velocity (drive and recovery phase) in the following ways: Stride length is increased over the acceleration period and front-side mechanics are stressed (e.g., leg action that occurs in front of the body) (6, 10, 23, 29).

Drive and Recovery Phases

The drive phase of each stride begins when the ball of the lead foot creates forceful contact with the surface and ends when the foot leaves the surface. The athlete's center of gravity should be slightly behind the lead leg at the initial point of contact. The forceful contact of the ball of the dorsiflexed lead foot is extenuated by extension of the hip, knee, and ankle. The short period of surface contact should continue until the athlete's center of gravity passes over and in front of the lead foot. When the ball of the lead foot leaves the ground, the drive phase is completed (6, 10, 23).

The recovery phase of each stride begins as the ball of the lead foot separates from the ground and continues until the foot returns back to the ground. Keeping the foot dorsiflexed, the athlete should flex the knee and pull the heel toward the hip rapidly. This allows for a faster swing of the recovery leg due to a mechanical advantage, since the leg is closer to the hip's axis of rotation. Once the heel reaches its maximum height, the athlete should drive it forward, with the intent of passing the dorsiflexed foot above the opposite knee. As he or she begins to straighten the leg in preparation for ground contact, the athlete should focus keeping the foot in a dorsiflexed position and driving to the surface with powerful hip and knee extension (6, 10, 23, 27).

While moving through the drive and recovery phases, athletes should consider the following factors. The head should be kept in its normal alignment with the trunk and the torso and shoulders should be kept steady to avoid rotation. The body angle should remain between 80° and 85°, and the muscles of the head, neck, shoulders, and upper extremities should remain relaxed. The arm swing should start with the lead arm bent to 70° (opposite the trail leg), with the hand beside the cheek on that side, and end with the rear arm bent to 130° (opposite the lead leg) and positioned slightly past the hip on that side (6, 23). With appropriate positioning, the sprinter will display an upright trunk, level head, and maximal hip height during a maximal-effort run.

Deceleration

Successful deceleration and stopping in sports allows athletes to transition between acceleration or maximal velocity to change direction, based on what the action dictates. The key to deceleration and changing direction without coming to a complete stop is to flex the ankles, hips, and knees as each foot contacts the ground. This extends the time that force may be absorbed and distributed throughout the body, allowing athletes to reduce speed and make a change in direction or come to a stop (10).

Speed Program Design

For more on implementing speed programs and integrating speed training with other forms of exercise in the context of an athlete's annual plan, see chapter 12.

This section describes how to design a sprint training program, which should always be incorporated into an athlete's yearly conditioning program. This section focuses on specific program design and provides examples of exercises.

Surfaces and Footwear

Before beginning the training program, it is important to decide the facility to be used (i.e., indoor court, grass field, or track) and the type of shoes to be worn. Athletes should perform their speed training workouts on a surface similar to the one they compete on. For instance, basketball players should perform their sprint training on a basketball court and ice hockey players should perform their sprint training in an ice rink. Athletes should also select footwear intended for speed training and competition. For those playing in an outdoor venue, natural grass remains the preferred surface. However, new grasslike synthetic fields, with similar shock-absorbing qualities, provide an equivalent running surface. Footwear like screw-in and molded cleats are designed for use on grass and grasslike synthetic fields. Surfaces should be flat and level with no obstacles (sports equipment, immovable natural objects, or groundskeeping equipment). Regardless of the surface and footwear worn, athletes must ensure their footwear is comfortable, well-fitted to their feet, and tied snug to avoid unnecessary movement of the foot that may cause injury.

Speed Training Exercises

Fundamental speed drills assist the progression of proper form and technique in speed training, with benefits that lead to improved acceleration, maximal velocity, and speed-endurance development. Fundamental speed drills provide a forum for speed techniques to be broken down into smaller segments and perfected at reduced speeds so that they may be transferred to maximal acceleration, velocity, and speed-endurance training. Prior to implementing the speed drills into the training program, strength and conditioning professionals should know the purpose of each drill and should be able to demonstrate the drill with proper form and technique. In addition, they should monitor athletes for proper form and technique during drill performance. Ideally, the drills should be performed when athletes are fully recovered and not fatigued from other types of training or sport practice. Table 9.1 shows an example sprint training workout using some of the drills described in the following sections.

TABLE 9.1   Sample Sprint Training Workout

Drill	Reps	Distance or time
Arm swing drill	2-4	10 s
Form starts (push-up starts)	2	11 steps for distance
	2	5 yd (4.5 m) in 3 steps
	2	10 yd (9 m) in 5 steps
	2	15 yd (14 m) in 7 steps
Downhill overspeed running	4-6	30 yd (27 m)
Uphill runs	4-6	20-30 yd (18-27 m)

HEEL-UPS

PURPOSE
Enhancement of foot speed

MOVEMENT
A 20-yard (18 m) course is marked out. The athlete should run the length of the course on the ball of the foot, pulling the heel of the lower leg up to touch the buttocks with each step. After a short recovery (30-45 s), the athlete repeats the exercises, moving back to the original starting position. The athlete should do the following:

- As the leg bends, bring the knee up and forward
- Keep the head in its normal alignment with the trunk
- Keep the torso and shoulders steady and avoid rotation
- Maintain a body angle between 80° and 85°
- Relax the muscles of the head, neck, shoulders, and upper extremities
- Begin arm swing with the lead arm bent to 70° and the hand beside the cheek on that side (opposite the trail leg)
- End the arm swing with the rear arm bent to 130° and the hand slightly past the hip on that side (opposite the lead leg)

ARM ACTION (SEATED)

PURPOSE
Proper arm movement

MOVEMENT
The athlete should do the following:

- Assume a long seated position with the knees locked
- Begin with one arm bent in front of the face and the other arm back (*a*)
- Swing the arms from the shoulder
- Hammer the arm down and back, just barely scraping the knuckles on the ground (*b*)
- Keep a hand in front of the face at all times
- Perform a hammering action down and back with the other hand

The drill is correct if the butt bounces off the ground. This results from the momentum of the arm movement.

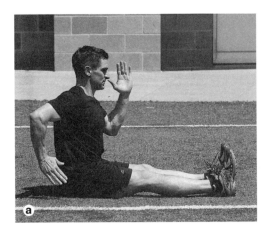
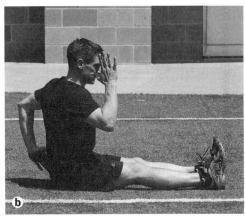

ARM ACTION (STANDING EXCHANGE)

PURPOSE
Proper arm movement

MOVEMENT
The athlete should do the following:

- Begin with one arm flexed in front of the body with the thumb up
- Hold the other arm behind the body with the elbow flexed and the thumb up
- Exchange the position of the arms in a karate chopping action
- Emphasize driving the arm down and back in a hammering action
- Pause to accentuate the exchange

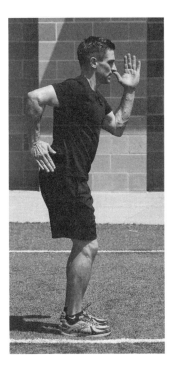

LEAN AND FALL RUN

PURPOSE

First-step quickness and running position

MOVEMENT

The athlete should do the following:

- Stand tall with the feet hip-width apart (not wider)
- Balance body weight over the middle of the feet
- Lean forward from the waist (*a*)
- Keep the upper body quiet
- Fall forward from the center
- Naturally let the foot take a step and come down under the hip (*b*)
- Keep the first step short
- Continue a running movement for about 10 to 20 yards (9-18 m) (*c*)
- While moving into the sprint, push back against the ground to make each step progressively longer

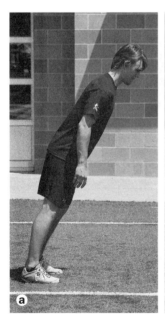
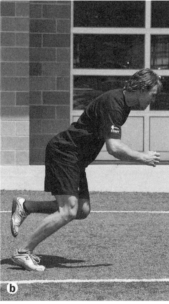
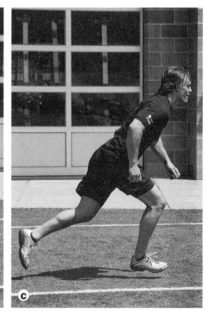

DROP AND GO

PURPOSE

First-step quickness and position

MOVEMENT

A partner is needed for this drill. The sprinter should do the following:

- Execute a lean and fall and allow the partner to catch (*a*)
- Hold that position for a one count, then let the partner step aside and release
- Accelerate out of the forward lean (*b*)
- Maintain posture and alignment
- Be quick with the arms to put force into the ground

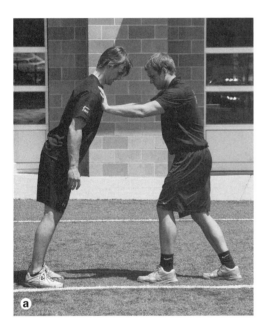
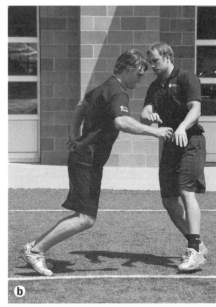

JUMP AND GO

PURPOSE

First-step quickness and position

MOVEMENT

The athlete should do the following:

- Begin with feet shoulder-width apart
- Draw back the arms, then drive them upward and forward
- Jump off with both feet
- Land on a single foot
- Drive off that leg and sprint

BOUND INTO RUN

PURPOSE

First-step quickness and position

MOVEMENT

The athlete should do the following:

- Use a two-foot jump for takeoff (*a*)
- Drive one leg forward and push the ground away as the lead leg comes into contact with the ground (*b*)
- On landing, drive upward and forward with the opposite arm and leg (*c*)
- Swing the trail leg through and reach for the ground
- Execute four bounds into a sprint

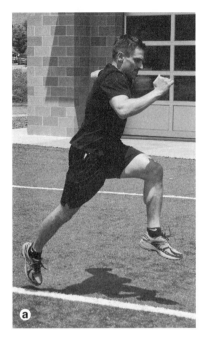 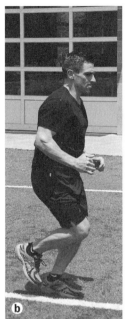 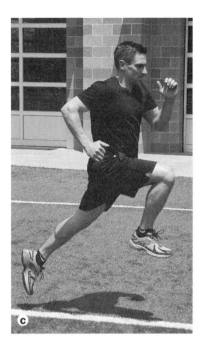

SCRAMBLE OUT

PURPOSE

First-step quickness and position

MOVEMENT

The athlete should do the following:

- Lie facedown with the hands at the sides in a push-up position (*a*)
- Scramble out, emphasizing triple extension of the ankle, knee, and hip (*b*)
- Maintain a powerful arm drive

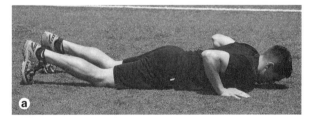

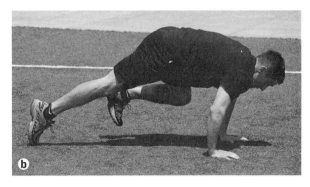

TWO JUMPS AND GO

PURPOSE

First-step quickness and position

MOVEMENT

The athlete should do the following:

- Begin with feet shoulder-width apart
- Drop into a quick countermovement by flexing the ankles, knees, and hips
- Draw the arms back at the beginning of the jump, and then drive them upward and forward
- Jump off with both feet using this technique and land on both feet
- Jump off again with both feet but land on one leg
- Drive off that leg and sprint for the remainder of the distance

PUSH-UP STARTS

PURPOSE
First-step quickness and position

MOVEMENT
The athlete should do the following:

- Assume a push-up position (*a*)
- On the command, move into a sprinting position with a four-point stance (*b*)
- Start to sprint

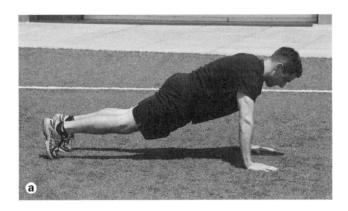

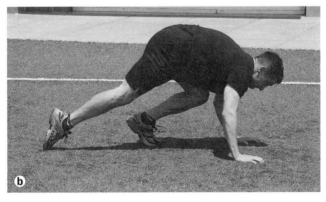

Resisted Speed Training

Resisted speed training involves the athlete pulling a fellow athlete or implement that provides resistance. Resisted speed drills force athletes to recruit an increased number of muscle fibers, resulting in an augmented neural activation (8, 21). This elevated response helps athletes increase speed when the resistance is removed through increased stride length and power output. Resistances used should not decrease the athletes' standard speed by more than 10%. Greater resistance may actually damage running technique, negating any potential benefit from resisted running.

Recommendations for Resisted Running Drills

- Recommended distance: 10-40 yd (9-36 m)
- Sets and repetitions: 3-4 sets of 4-8 reps
- Recovery: 90-120 s

LIGHT SLED PULLS

PURPOSE

Increase speed strength, power, and stride length

MOVEMENT

The athlete should do the following:

- Attach a lightweight sled with an adjustable harness or waist strap
- Utilize proper speed form and technique (as outlined in the speed technique section of this chapter)
- Sprint for 10 to 40 yards (9-36 m) (*a*)

When athletes perform this drill, a strength and conditioning professional should observe their form, technique, and speed in covering the yardage. If the strength and conditioning professional notices that the athlete's form or technique is faulty or that the time to complete the distance is longer than their standard time by more than 10%, the resistance may be too heavy and should be reduced.

A tire, bag, or a partner (*b*) holding a cord can also be effective as a resistance device. Recently, some nonmotorized treadmills have been marketed that provide controlled resistance. Resistance must be at a level that allows athletes to maintain proper running form.

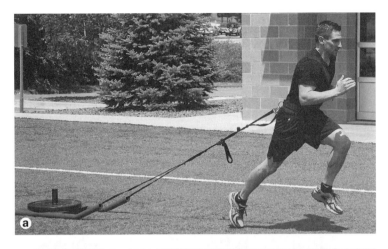

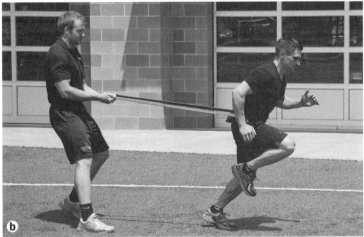

HILL RUNNING

PURPOSE

Provide an effective overload to improve explosive power and running speed

MOVEMENT

The athlete sprints up a slight hill for a set distance, not to exceed 100 yards (91 m). The athlete should do the following:

- Emphasize good running form with maximum knee drive and elbow pump
- Begin at a short distance and increase distance over time
- Choose a hill with a slope between 6° and 10° (Anything greater than this causes a reduction in stride length and compromises training results.)
- Perform each sprint at 100% effort

Assisted Speed Training

Assisted speed training uses an implement (sport cord) or contrast to help athletes run faster than they normally would. By training with assisted speed, athletes can increase stride frequency and length more than is generally possible (8, 21). The objective behind this form of training is for athletes to run faster than they would under routine circumstances by using an artificial mechanism to increase both stride rate and length. When incorporating assisted running into a speed training program, attention should be taken to ensure that athletes do not exceed 110% of their maximum running speed. If not, stride length may be overextended, resulting in deceleration and a decrease in stride frequency (12, 13).

THREE-PERSON TUBING ACCELERATION DRILL

PURPOSE

To enhance stride frequency and length and quick leg recovery in first couple of steps for the one athlete being towed and to enhance starting power and stride length for the two athletes being resisted

MOVEMENT

The strength and conditioning professional should do the following:

- Group three athletes of identical or nearly equal speed together. (The closer the athletes are to each other in speed, the more effective the drill will be.)
- Attach the three athletes together with three adjustable waist belts and two 8-foot (2.4 m) elastic resistance cords.
- Position the two athletes being resisted 4 yards (3.6 m) in front of and 4 yards to the right and left of the athlete being towed, forming a *V* shape.
- When the three athletes are lined up to begin the drill, connect each of the athletes being resisted to the athlete being towed with a sport cord.
- To ensure that the athletes line up in the same position each time, place dome cones in a *V* shape at both ends of the field. (The front cones at each end should be separated by 25 yards, or 23 m.)
- When arranging the cones, make certain that the cones at each end are directly in line with each other to ensure that the athletes run in a straight line.
- Before beginning the drill, ensure that all three athletes are in a good running position and are ready to begin.
- To begin the drill, give two consecutive commands by voice or whistle.
- On the first command, have the two athletes who are towing (resisted) begin running at full speed toward the cones 25 yards in front of them

in a straight line. (For maximum benefit to all three athletes, these two athletes must remain the set distance apart and must run in a straight line. Because the athlete being towed remains still for a moment, these athletes are pulling against resistance at the beginning of their sprint.)

- On the second command (immediately following the first), have the athlete being towed (assisted) begin running at full speed to the cone directly downfield. (Since this athlete begins the sprint with a pull from the other athletes, he will experience an overspeed effect.)

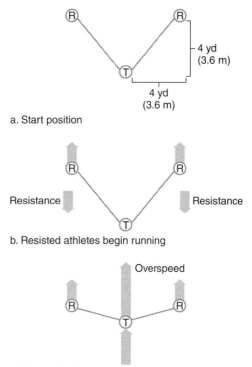

a. Start position

b. Resisted athletes begin running

c. Towed athlete begins running and experiences an overspeed effect

The athletes should do the following:

- Aim to pass the two athletes who are towing (role of assisted athlete)
- Keep the sport cords tight and parallel to the ground throughout the drill
- Decelerate once they have reached the front cones at the other end of the drill (The two athletes towing will sprint 25 yards and the athlete being towed will sprint 30 yards.)
- Perform the drill from each of the three positions 2 to 4 times (6 to 12 total repetitions)

DOWNHILL RUNNING

PURPOSE

Enhance acceleration through the use of overspeed training

MOVEMENT

The athlete sprints down a slope similar to that used for uphill running (6° to 10°).

CONE JUMPS AND SPRINT

PURPOSE

Increase explosive power and acceleration

MOVEMENT

Athletes should do the following:

- Stand facing a series of six consecutive cones that are 6, 12, or 18 inches high (15, 30, or 26 cm) and are placed 3 to 6 feet (1-2 m) apart
- On a verbal or whistled command, begin jumping forward over the cones (More advanced athletes may jump forward over two cones and backward over one until all six cones have been jumped.)
- After jumping over the sixth cone, sprint 15 to 20 yards (14-18 m) forward to a cone directly in front
- Loop the cone or touch it with the hand
- Sprint back to the sixth cone

The strength and conditioning professional may do the following:

- Increase the intensity of the drill by increasing the height of some or all six cones, increasing the distance between cones, or increasing the distance of the sprints
- Increase volume by adding a second repetition of the drill
- Use bags or other elevated implement (However, the implement should be soft and able to give when stepped on to avoid unnecessary injuries.)

SUMMARY POINTS

- Speed is a critical component in training programs for sport performance.
- Speed training should focus on running technique, acceleration to maximal velocity, and speed-endurance.
- Special consideration should be given to the utilization of proper form and technique.
- Athletes should not progress to more advanced drills until they have mastered fundamental speed drills.

10

Balance and Stability Training

Nejc Sarabon, PhD

From the perspectives of achieving superior, sport-specific technique and diminishing the possibility of injury development, prevention-training modalities should be used. In this context, sensorimotor training (also called *proprioceptive training*, *functional joint-stability training*, and *balance training*) can be a useful tool. Its positive effects improve joint stability during functional movements, static and dynamic balance, and movement awareness, or kinesthesia. Injury prevention can help athletes perform a sufficient quantity of training to maintain adequate sport preparedness. On the other hand, improved kinesthesia is important for developing self-awareness, improving precision, and achieving more efficient movement at lower energy cost.

Sensorimotor training as we know it today was first introduced for the rehabilitation of diseases and injuries to the locomotor and central nervous systems. From the beginning, its goals have been directed toward restoring neuromuscular function, reestablishing functional joint stability, and improving balance, based on automatic (reflex) corrective responses.

In addition to the closely controlled reflex by the central nervous system and volitional motor control, other factors affect joint stability and balance. Important factors include the anatomical shape of joints that impose restraints on movements, the nature of the applied load, and passive soft tissue structures, such as ligaments and the joint capsule. These should be considered in rehabilitation when injury of joints and their surrounding soft tissue structures are involved. All these factors define joint stiffness and stability in a specific situation according to the movement environment. All measures should be taken to increase joint stability in cases where the risk of injury is highest, especially in sports.

Balance and joint-stability training have been proven to have positive effects on sensorimotor function in rehabilitation and sports (6). Their positive effects should be used to reestablish motor-system function after injury or to improve sport technique by decreasing susceptibility to injury. Strength and conditioning professionals and therapists are responsible for the application of training. Nevertheless, creativity is welcomed in exercises that enable interesting and effective training, even if athletes are unfamiliar with them or the exercises present a new training modality.

Program Planning and Periodization

When planning training for balance or functional joint stabilization, specific directives should be provided based on the athlete's goals. Examples include prevention of injury, development of athletic ability, and rehabilitation. When choosing a training protocol for sports, the exposure of different body parts and their susceptibility to injury should be considered. See chapter 1 for more about considering injury risk during needs assessments.

Training for balance and functional joint stabilization is usually an integral part of demanding protocols for sport training or rehabilitation. However, their ability to increase jumping power, strength, or strength-endurance is limited (5). Most of the available research on the use of balance and stability training for strength and muscle activation has examined untrained subjects. In these studies, no advantage is seen during short (three- to six-week) training programs (1, 3, 7). When training competitive athletes, traditional resistance training or plyometric training modalities should be of primary consideration for developing strength and power. In competitive sports, the role of balance and joint-stability training for preventing injury, especially later in the season, may be more relevant. In the latter part of the season, stress accumulates and athletes' exposure to injury increases. These training modalities can also be used during the first part of the season, since they have a positive effect on injury prevention during all training periods.

Literature inspecting balance training and functional joint-stabilization training focuses on their acute and chronic effects on the sensorimotor system. Adaptations to training for balance and functional joint stabilization initially occur quickly. Similar to other training modes, the rate of improvement is reduced as training progresses. As such, it can be suggested that balance training and functional joint-stabilization training should be used throughout the season to achieve and maintain a higher level of neuromuscular function. The following recommendations help athletes achieve sufficient adaptations of the neuromuscular system:

- Balance training programs should be at least four weeks in length. Athletes should continue training throughout the competitive season to maintain improvements.

- To preserve the acquired level of the neuromuscular function, at least three workouts should be used per week. These require additional training units to enable improvements.

- At least one set of each exercise should be used, since this causes acute adaptations. Although it is recommended that athletes perform more than just one set, the upper limit is not reported in literature.

- At least four repetitions are needed to achieve positive long-term adaptations.

- One repetition should last at least 20 seconds.

Although these basic guidelines for achieving distinguishable adaptations can be extracted from research articles, their application into practice remains insufficient. This is because the quantity of their usage is determined by fatigue, level of physical preparedness, complexity or intensity of the exercises, previous experience, and (in rehabilitation) state of injury. Responsibility lies with the athlete, the strength and conditioning professional, and the therapist to determine the appropriate training volume that both assures positive adaptations and minimizes overstress and possible negative effects, especially in rehabilitation.

Safe Progression for Balance Exercises

The major concern with balance and joint-stabilization exercises is to avoid potentially dangerous movements that depend on the preparedness of the athlete or patient and on the state of the healing tissue. Slow progression should be followed toward extreme ranges of motion or movements where joint stability is compromised or susceptibility to injury is increased. For the majority of joints, extreme ranges of motion are usually susceptible to injury, since both muscle force and neuromuscular control are diminished. For example, combined abduction and outer shoulder rotation or increased ankle inversion are positions in which the shoulder and ankle joints are relatively unstable and are susceptible to injury. These ranges of motion should be avoided in early stages of rehabilitation. Another example is patellofemoral pain syndrome, where movements in 30° to 60° range of knee flexion should be avoided to avoid overstressing the articulation surface of the patella. Here, compressive force is at its highest, which stresses the patellar cartilage. Perturbing forces in extreme positions should be introduced gradually. Athletes who are healthy but untrained should follow the same principle, slowly moving to more vulnerable and unstable ranges of movement.

The speed of movement should be increased slowly to enable good control over joint stability. Higher velocities of movement in early stages, when the subject is still unaccustomed to the movement pattern, can cause diminished control of movement. For example, performing torso stabilization while sitting in an almost static, erect position on an exercise ball can be dangerous if the additional movements presented by the strength and conditioning professional are too fast. This results in ineffective reflexive stabilization of abdominal muscles and possibly unsafe amplitudes of movement.

In programs for sport-injury prevention, rate of movement should slowly progress toward the speeds used in the sport, enabling joint stabilization during fast, sport-specific actions. For example, stabilization exercises of the shoulder joint for throwing athletes should progressively move toward more explosive movements, enabling adaptation of the neuromuscular system to appropriately stabilize the joint during pitching, throwing the ball in cocked position, and ending a throw. In addition to a progressive increase in the speed of movement, athletes should work on eccentric and explosive strength, preparing the soft tissue of the joint and the musculoligamentous area to cope with increased stress.

Bigger forces can be introduced with training, but not until the subject has mastered balance or functional-joint-stabilization tasks. Acquiring an appropriate movement strategy is more efficient if the load applied is not too high. This holds especially true in case of rehabilitation programs.

For uninjured athletes, training for balance and functional joint stabilization should always be challenging. Active involvement of both the athletes and their neuromuscular systems enables conditioning. If an exercise does not demand corrective movements, training will be ineffective, since the neuromuscular system is not required to react and adapt to perturbation or reestablish joint stability and body equilibrium.

Progression from less to more demanding tasks is suggested. For example, a progression from monoaxial to multiaxial balance board is recommended. Athletes should also progress from a bigger to a smaller support surface and incorporate longer work intervals, additional tasks, and a higher frequency of oscillation into their routines. When athletes master a movement, the strength and conditioning professional should upgrade it or introduce a new, unfamiliar movement. Since adaptations of the neuromuscular system are induced by increasing the demand of conducting a task, this rule should be followed.

Stability Training for Joint Systems

By following the directions presented here when planning training for balance and functional joint stabilization, appropriate exercises and training quantity can be chosen. Since different joint systems are usually stressed in training, some specifics should be considered. The following sections describe these in more detail.

Torso and Core

The human torso consists of the spine, pelvis, hips, abdomen, and the rib cage. It is one of the most important systems, enabling human motion in daily and sport activities. As such, it is a base for upper and lower limb movement and enables transfer of energy and force from the legs to the arms. For example, in its final stage, the javelin throw demands a synchronized movement of the legs and torso to transfer additional power from the lower body to the shoulder girdle, arms, and, finally, to the javelin. On the other hand, a strong and stable torso enables humans to perform elevation of heavy loads and rotational movements, preventing possibly harmful movement and stress to the spinal column. It is the center of the functional kinetic chain, enabling movement of the body and different body parts. The muscles surrounding the abdominal cavity produce a corset that stabilizes the upper body, particularly the spine.

In popular literature, torso stability has also been called *core stability*, stressing its central role in human movement. Torso stability exercises should be used in rehabilitation. Stabilization of the spinal column involves the abdominal muscles, especially the transversus abdominis, part of the internal oblique, the diaphragm, and the pelvic floor muscles. Their contraction results in an increase in intra-abdominal pressure, supporting the rib cage and pelvis. This results in decreased compressive and torsion stress, especially on the lumbar spinal column.

Studies of patients (including athletes) show that coordinating the muscles that stabilize the spinal column may be effective for treating lower back injuries (2). The combination of strength and balance training attempts to reestablish appropriate torso strength and stability. The primary issues associated with activation patterns of multiple trunk muscles among people suffering from back injury are as follows:

- Decreased sense of position and repositioning of the torso
- Delayed stabilizing muscle response
- Diminished or even missing preactivation of torso muscles in rapid distal movements, causing lower back pain
- Impaired recruitment of the torso musculature during fast and explosive movements
- Increased body sway

Training Guidelines

When considering functional joint stabilization and balance training of the torso, athletes should apply limb movements that demand reflexive stabilization of the trunk muscles. These movements may be either anticipated or spontaneous. When applying anticipated perturbations, reflexive preparatory responses are trained. This is especially important in everyday activities and in sport-specific movement techniques. On the other hand, unexpected perturbations demand reflexive, nonpreparatory trunk stabilization, which aids in the prevention of injury during unexpected impact from external forces.

Perturbations can be applied through two main systems. One system involves standing on an unstable platform, enabling the transfer of movements to the pelvis and trunk and demanding compensatory activity in order to effectively counterbalance the body. This lower limb approach can be achieved by extending the legs or kneeling. On the other hand, perturbations can be transmitted to the torso through stiff upper limbs. The arms should be almost totally extended to avoid active amortization of perturbing movements in the elbows.

These two approaches can be merged together in the next stages of training development, causing unpredicted movements to be derived from the lower and upper limbs. The choice of hand or leg strategy should be used according to the athlete's needs. Athletes who move against gravity must have an exceptionally stable torso during movement. As with other sports, perturbation movements can be transmitted through the upper limbs, stressing torso stability. This is required in sports such as tennis, rugby, and wrestling. Both principles should be used in a stability program.

The main rationale in exercises where perturbing movements are applied through extended hands or legs is that forces will be compensated for by pelvic and spinal motion. An increase in the frequency and amplitude of the applied movements depends on the athlete's preparedness. If the disturbance exceeds the athlete's abilities, other body parts will compensate, relieving the musculature of the trunk and spine and consequently defeating the purpose of the training.

As mentioned previously, translatory movements are those that demand an active hip strategy involving torso stabilization and movement. To achieve translatory movements, balance boards and exercise balls can be used. Since the hip musculature is of great importance and can be influenced by deconditioning or injury, additional stress can be placed on it by varying the stance width and symmetry of foot placement. A narrower foot placement slightly increases gluteal activity. To achieve an even greater activation of the unilateral hip musculature, asymmetrical foot placement should be used on a balance board, extensively stressing gluteal muscles of the leg closest to the axis. Maximal gluteal activity can be achieved by using a single-leg stance. This might be of importance for runners suffering from iliotibial band syndrome, patellar tendon pain, or a catching sensation on the lateral side of the hips, where the underlying biomechanical problem can be caused by inappropriate coordination of the hip musculature.

When working with injured athletes, strength training should slowly be integrated as the torso stabilization program progresses. Pushing movements can slowly be introduced, demanding stability and strength at the same time. Sport-specific movements should be used to achieve the highest positive transfer of torso stability. Some studies suggest that torso stability is increased in the activities the athletes are trained in. For example, high-level golf players have specifically improved torso stability during the golf swing.

Exercises

In all trunk stability exercises, special attention must be paid to the activation of the torso musculature. This increases upper body stability and muscle responsiveness. Fundamentally, three basic concepts of trunk stability exercises can be used: (1) from the legs toward the torso, (2) from the hands towards the torso, and (3) a combination of these two approaches.

LEGS-TO-TORSO APPRROACH: KNEELING ON AN EXERCISE BALL

The athlete should maintain a straight back, push the hips forward, and direct the gaze forward. For a variation, the arms may be placed akimbo (hands on hips with elbows bowed outward) or in abduction, depending on the athlete's ability to maintain balance. The same principles can be followed using other balance boards and standing with straight knees.

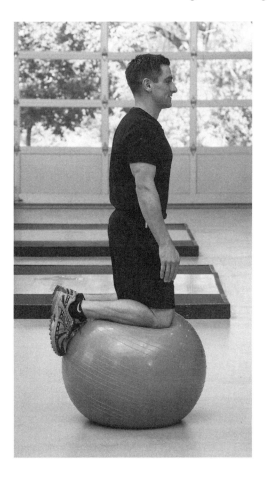

HANDS-TO-TORSO APPROACH:
PUSHING SIDEWAYS WITH AN EXERCISE BALL

The athlete should stand with legs positioned pelvis-width apart and with flexed knees to sustain a stable position, and then rotate the torso to push the ball against a wall (*a*). After the ball contacts the wall, the athlete should hold the elbows still, transferring the energy to the torso. The athlete should try to continue with the intended movement isometrically (*b*).

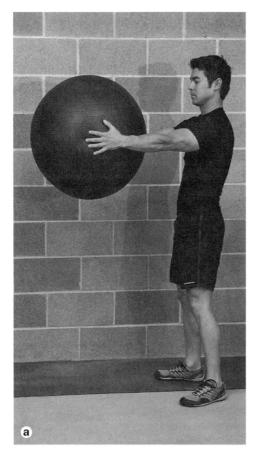
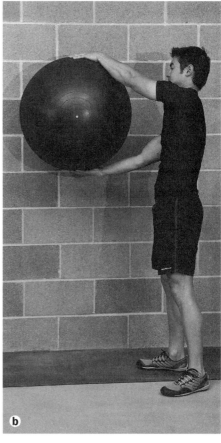

COMBINED APPROACH

The athlete assumes a two-leg stance on a balance board, extending the knees and holding weights in extended hands. The legs and hands should be straight, transferring disturbances to the torso.

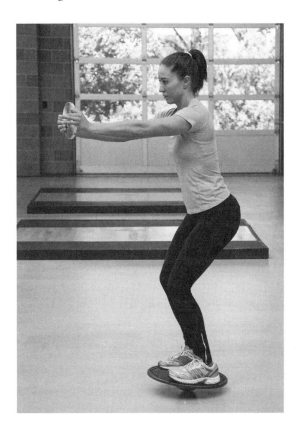

Knee

The knee is a relatively simple hinge joint. A major portion of its movements occur as rotations around the mediolateral axis, resulting in flexion and extension. During these motions, some anterior or posterior translation accompanies the axial rotation. If anteroposterior translation exceeds the functional limits (such as when landing from a jump), the movement stresses the passive stabilizers of the joint. In some cases, this results in laxity or even partial or full ligament rupture. This is especially important during rehabilitation of injured ligaments, since these translational forces can damage recovering ligaments, especially the cruciate ligaments, if reconstructed. As such, during rehabilitation, closed kinetic chain exercises are a safer choice since they cause less strain on ligamentous structures. If open kinetic chain exercises are used, caution should be exercised to avoid excessive anterior or posterior translation of the tibial plateau. During closed kinetic chain exercises, force is directed at a more perpendicular angle in relationship to the articular surface of the tibia. In contrast, in open kinetic chain exercises, force is usually directed parallel to the articulating surfaces, causing additional stress in the anteroposterior direction.

Nevertheless, both open and closed chain exercises should be used for the functional joint stabilization of the knee in both injured and uninjured athletes, since movements of the lower limbs are performed in both open and closed chain conditions. An example is during the support and swing phases of the running cycle.

Functional stabilization programs of the knee joint should start with simple exercises that cause only stabilizing responses to flexor and extensor movements. Anteroposterior translational forces should be used slowly in minor amplitude to stress the knee joint as much as possible. They should not stress major body reactions and balancing strategies. During these exercises, excessive valgus movements should be avoided. When these movements are mastered, rotational movements can be used. During these movements, all possible knee joint movements take place. This progression is especially useful in rehabilitation settings when neuromuscular function is compromised. When training athletes, the same principle can be used, especially if an additional load is applied.

Training Guidelines

To enable progressive emphasis on joint stability, several interventions can be used. Transitioning from a two-leg to a single-leg stance is used to stress an individual knee joint. Athletes and strength and conditioning professionals should remember that some movement strategies should be trained according to specific sport demands. Sometimes exposing athletes to intense exercises in a two-leg stance is functionally more appropriate than exposing them to exercises with a single-leg stance. For example, in skiing, functional joint stabilization and continuous balancing are primarily established with a two-leg stance. Additional load is applied to imitate radial forces during turns. Asymmetrical squats may be useful to mimic the asymmetric leg position during turns. During a basketball game, single-leg landing maneuvers often result in knee injury, demonstrating the need for single-leg exercises for knee joint stabilization.

Exercises can be made progressively more challenging, both in terms of strengthening and balancing, to enable superior stabilization of the knee joint. This has the effect of functionally improving movements at higher movement velocities or at higher perturbing forces, such as what occurs during a smaller curve radius during skiing or during a direct hit from an opponent in American football.

Various balance boards and foam pads can be used. From the perspective of biomechanics, foam is an unnatural surface, since the velocity of displacement decreases with amplitude. In contrast, the velocity increases during displacements on balance boards. Functionally, balance boards may be more appropriate for use in sports, while foam is more suited for the early rehabilitation period.

For functional joint stabilization of the knee and for general balance training, a variety of balance boards can be used. To assure progression, boards that enable movements only in the mediolateral axis, such as T-boards, should be used. The height of the board has an important effect, since as it increases, the translatory movement increases as well. Since translatory movements demand large-scale body reactions, the specific effect on knee joint stabilization is questionable. Balance discs can be used early in rehabilitation as well. The intensity of the exercise can be increased by using discs with smaller diameters. Smaller support surfaces increase destabilizing movements. If only one board is available, a softer surface can influence the mechanical characteristics of balance boards, enabling progression.

The adaptation from exercise to improved performance is most effective if the movement is similar to those used in sport. From this perspective, exercises should mimic the movements seen in the sport. When training the legs and knees, different stances can be used to simulate the positions used during competition.

Exercises

Three rudimentary groups of stability exercises exist for developing general stability of the lower extremities, with the main stress placed on the knee: (1) closed kinetic chain exercises with fixed foot placement, (2) dynamic transition from the unsupported phase to closed chain stabilization using steps and jumps, and (3) combination of rhythmic stabilization in open kinetic chain exercises.

BALANCING ON A T-BOARD

The hip musculature can be additionally stressed by asymmetric foot placement. Position can be varied between the frontal plane (*a*) and the sagittal plane (*b*). A diagonal stance (*c*) increases body sway by upgrading exercise intensity in the sagittal plane.

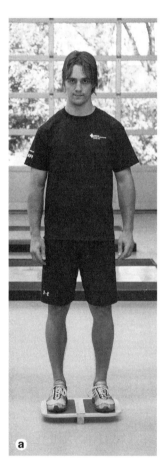
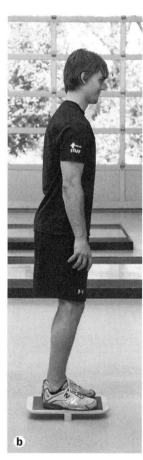
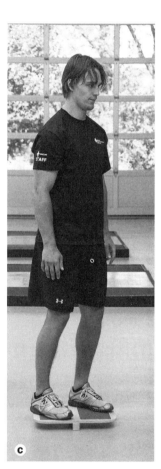

SINGLE-LEG STANCE ON A BALANCE BOARD

The geometry of the balance board can be varied to stress different axes and directions of movement. Basically all standing exercises can be performed on different balance boards, depending on the goals set before exercising.

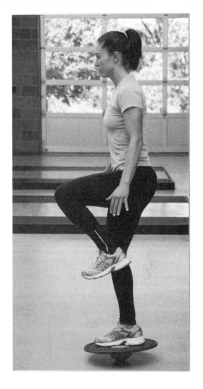

SQUATTING ON A BOSU BALL

This exercise combines the demands of strength and high balance. The depth of the squat can be varied. Other strength and coordination exercises (ball handling, ball passing, and so on) can be applied in a similar way.

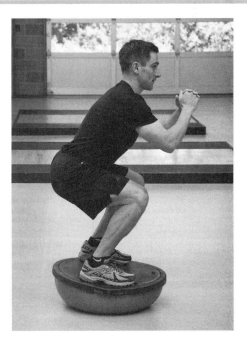

BALANCE PAD LUNGE

This exercise can be performed with or without additional loads. The athlete should keep the back straight and should look forward throughout the drill (*a*). When stepping on the balance pad, the athlete should maintain this position to reestablish balance, and then slowly return to the starting position. The lunge (*b*) should be performed in every direction.

During jumping exercises, balance pads or balance boards can be used for landing. The latter is especially useful for two-leg landings. Rotation during the flight phase can be added to increase the intensity during one- or two-leg jumps. When landing, the athlete should try to establish a stable stance, which is an important part of jumping exercises. Jumps are the final stage of training for functional joint stabilization and balance, and must be considered as such, especially in rehabilitation settings.

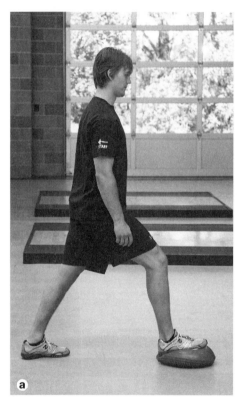

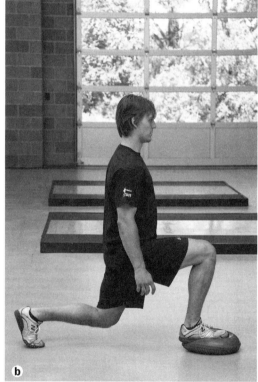

SINGLE-LEG LANDING ON A BALANCE PAD
AFTER A FORWARD JUMP

The athlete starts by facing the balance pad (*a*), then jumps forward, landing on one leg on the pad (*b*). Athletes can jump in different directions to stress specific directions of joint or body movement. Backward and diagonal jumps can be used in the same manner. Different levels of body rotations in the flight phase are also a good way to increase intensity under sport-specific conditions.

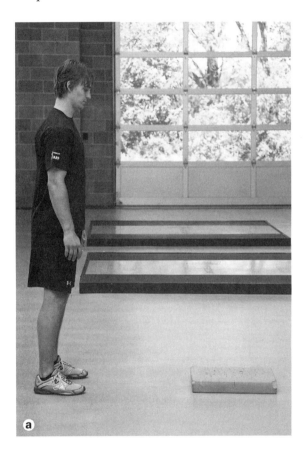
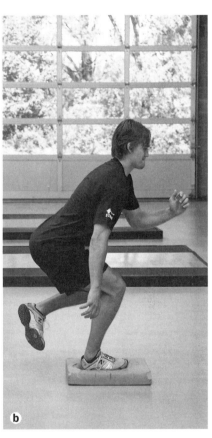

WALK OR RUN OVER A POLYGON OF BALANCE PADS

The speed of movement can be slowly increased, stressing stability during foot placement in the short support phase of running.

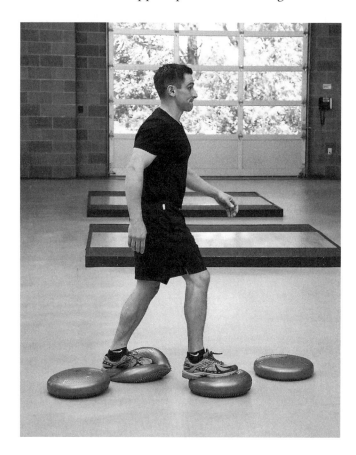

RHYTHMIC STABILIZATION

Rhythmic stabilization may be applied through the hands (*a*), a rope (*b*), or elastics during the back swing of the step while walking or running. The same principle of applying disturbances can be used in different leg positions during the swing phase. Additionally, athletes should gradually progress to dynamic leg movement by using slow movements and imitating the swing phase of the walking or running stride.

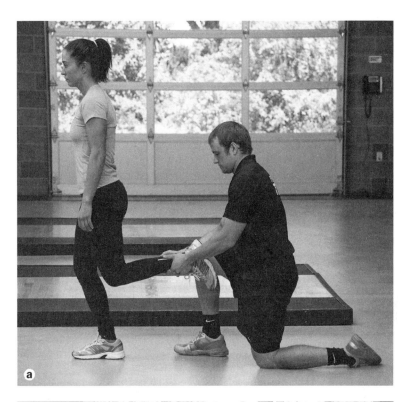

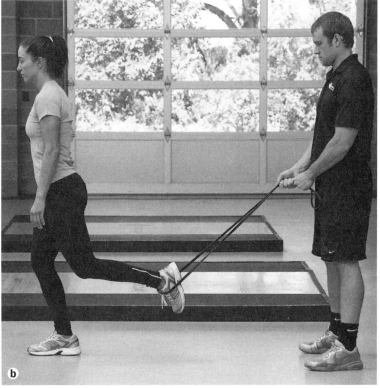

Ankle and Foot

The human foot and ankle are a complex interplay of bones that are connected into a multijoint system, working together as one functional unit. The foot and ankle are the first to come into contact with the ground during upright locomotion. They are stressed by the weight of virtually the whole body, plus the inertial forces that result from landing. Appropriate functioning of the foot and ankle enables absorption of these high-impact forces during ground contact and decreases loading on other ligament structures and joints of the body. The rotational axes of the ankle and foot enable different movements, consequently adapting the foot to the shape of the ground. Different joint systems have specific axes of rotation that are important in functional-joint-stabilization training. Since specific injuries relate to the tissues or muscles responsible for movement around and along a specific axis, balance exercises are usually limited to monoaxial boards. The basic movements of the ankle joint are plantar flexion (figure 10.1a), dorsal flexion (figure 10.1b), inversion (figure 10.1c), and eversion (figure 10.1d).

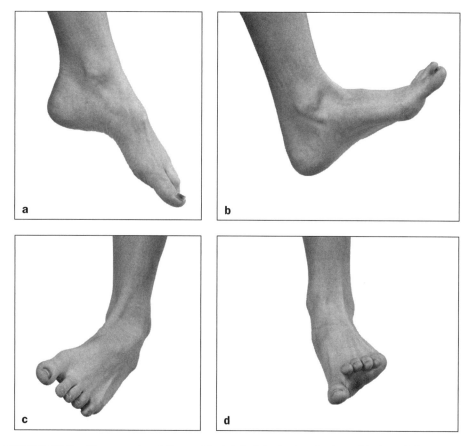

FIGURE 10.1   Movements of the ankle joint: (a) plantar flexion, (b) dorsal flexion, (c) inversion, and (d) eversion.

If the foot and ankle joints are functioning appropriately, the foot shape shows specific plantar arches. The three different arches are the medial longitudinal arch, the lateral longitudinal arch, and the transverse front-foot arch. They are supported by specific bone and joint structures, the muscular system, and the connective tissue. They can be influenced by training, fatigue, injury, or disease. Their role is to act as shock absorbers during ground contact, especially in the initial support phase in running, as well as in cutting maneuvers in sports like tennis, basketball, or others that stress the foot and ankle joints in inversion and internal rotation.

The ankle is injured more in sports than any other joint (4, 8). The most common ankle injury is a lateral ankle sprain, sometimes resulting in chronic ankle instability. For this reason, preventive means specifically for functional joint stabilization have been implemented in sports. Some attention has been given to factors that contribute to ankle instability as a way to help avoid injury. Some argue that extremes of ankle stiffness and flexibility can influence susceptibility to injury, especially if the ligament apparatus is stretched and its stiffness decreases. On the other hand, evertor and invertor muscle strength has been shown to influence ankle joint stability, with eccentric invertor strength being the most important factor to address.

Training Guidelines

Monoaxial balance boards are usually used to stress specific movements, especially inversion and eversion. The amplitude of the movement should not exceed the limits defined by pain or flexibility. The range of motion can be slowly increased, but only after pain, swelling, and motor control have been normalized (during rehabilitation from injury). Progression to multiaxial balance boards is recommended to slowly stress the complex movement of the ankle joint.

When starting with functional joint-stabilization training, low balance boards should be used, decreasing translational movements and stressing compensatory movements of the foot and ankle. Gradually, balance boards of greater height can be used. However, strength and conditioning professionals should keep in mind that higher boards demand elevated strength of the musculature stabilizing the foot and ankle joint. The majority of exercises should be performed in a closed kinetic chain, especially when training for locomotion, since joint stiffness is increased.

During rehabilitation, balance mats can be used. Because of their mechanical properties, movements should be relatively constant, since the velocity of displacement does not increase with increased amplitude. This makes balance mats a safer choice in rehabilitation protocols. To enable progression, foam of different consistency can be used. Softer mats are more demanding.

Exercises for functional stability of the ankle joint are usually performed barefoot to enable movement in all joints of the foot and ankle. To elevate the intensity, progression to agility or footwork exercises is recommended. Functional movements from sports, like side stepping and cutting maneuvers, can slowly be added under controlled conditions. As the velocity of the movement increases, so does the stress on the foot and ankle joint. Before using agility exercises, athletes should jump on an uneven surface to enable the motor system to adjust to plyometric work. Special attention should be given to stressing evertors and invertors during exercises for functional joint stabilization. Exercises that require eversion or inversion on soft hemispheres are useful.

Additional loads can be used when athletes master specific exercises. Joints should be slowly introduced to environments where stability must be maintained under greater forces. Exercises can be directed toward sport-specific movements, imitating special movement strategies such as side-stepping maneuvers, landing on uneven surfaces, and so on.

Exercises

These figures show two basic stability exercises for the ankle joint. These may be modified or progressed as described in the preceding section.

SINGLE-LEG STANCE ON A BALANCE PAD

Note that difficulty can be increased by changing the hardness of the balance pads.

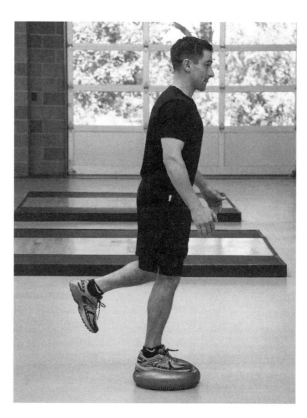

SINGLE-LEG STANCE ON A RUBBER HEMISPHERE

During balancing, eversion and inversion can be used to stress the invertor and evertor muscles of the ankle.

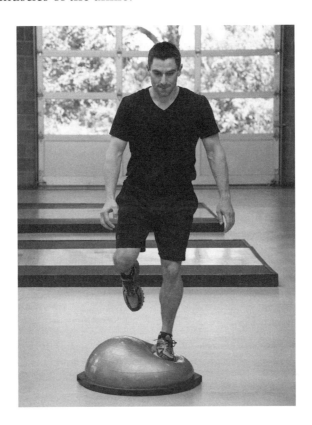

Shoulder

The shoulder girdle is a complex multijoint system. Basic joint mechanics enable a high level of mobility, which challenges joint stability. The most proximal joint in the system is the scapulothoracic joint, forming the base for other hand movements. The scapula lies on the thorax, enabling gliding movements in mediolateral and inferosuperior directions and in a combination of the two as rotational movements. Additionally, the scapula can rotate around its longitudinal axis. Muscles enabling its movements consist of elevators (upper fibers of the trapezius, the levator scapulae, and the rhomboids), retractors (medial fibers of the trapezius and the rhomboids), depressors (the latissimus dorsi and the lower fibers of the trapezius), and protractors (the serratus anterior and the pectoralis minor and major).

The glenohumeral joint is a ball-and-socket joint, which allows movement in all directions. The humeral head, which is shaped like one-third of a sphere, lies in the glenoid fossa, which enables the rotational behavior.

However, since the glenoid fossa is relatively shallow, it is prone to instability. The muscles controlling its movement are the abductors (the deltoid and the supraspinatus), the external rotators (the infraspinatus and the teres minor), the internal rotators (the subscapularis, the teres major, and the pectoralis major), and the adductors (the subscapularis, the pectoralis minor and major, the latissimus dorsi, and the teres minor and major). Three important muscles (the infraspinatus, the supraspinatus, and the teres minor) insert at the superior part of the humeral head at the greater tuberosity, usually called the *rotator cuff*. This insertion of muscles can impinge on superior structures like the acromion, the coracoacromial ligament, or the coracoid, especially in overhead activities.

The basic concern during injury rehabilitation and injury prevention for the shoulder joint should be the normalization of the scapular movement, which is also called *scapulohumeral rhythm* when combined with glenohumeral movements. If scapular movements are not optimal, excessive movements in the glenohumeral joint occur, since compensation potentially leads to impingement or other types of injury.

Neuromuscular control mechanisms of glenohumeral stability affect the quality and effectiveness of functional joint stabilization. As described previously, scapulothoracic and glenohumeral muscle stabilizers have to work in coherence. The previous section describes the force interactions of the following muscles: (1) the subscapularis versus the teres minor and infraspinatus, (2) the deltoid versus the lower rotator cuff, (3) the rotator cuff tendons as dynamic capsular stabilizers, (4) and the trapezius and serratus anterior in full glenohumeral abduction.

Training Guidelines

Exercises for shoulder joint stabilization can be performed in either an open or closed kinetic chain. Usually both are needed, but the specifics of the sport should be kept in mind. The following guidelines will help athletes, sport and conditioning professionals, and therapists structure and implement a program for functional joint stabilization.

Early in the rehabilitation process, exercises should be performed in the mid-range of shoulder movement, slowly continuing toward the ends of the range of motion of problematic or unstable joints. The same principle should be followed to influence and improve feeling in a certain position. Mid-range muscle receptors are of primary importance. To achieve good scapulothoracic stabilization, exercises facilitating synergistic parascapular contractions should be used, such as punches, push-ups, and press-ups against higher resistance.

As previously mentioned, the shoulder joint is a complex structure. Its soundness is enabled by different subcomponents of the stability apparatus. These components can be mobilized by different perturbation types (direction of the perturbing force, amount of applied force, and repeatability). These disturbances should be close to those encountered in the athlete's sport. For example, throwing athletes can use oscillatory disturbances in the late cocking phase to stimulate the change from the eccentric to the concentric part of the throw, additionally stressing active stabilizers.

In impingement syndromes, exercises should be performed with minimal adduction of the humerus. If possible, active adduction should be performed. This can be achieved by holding a towel between the upper arm and the torso. In compromised shoulder stability, exercises in the scapular plane should be used, since active stabilizers are most effective in ensuring joint stiffness. In rhythmic stabilization exercises, it is very important to additionally stress the preparatory and reactive muscle activity in order to improve functional joint stabilization.

Slow progression in plyometric exercises is valuable, since they can help the neuromuscular system better cope with stress during throwing or hitting. As such, they train eccentric muscle activity, enabling better eccentric control. They also increase sense of joint position in the late cocking phase, which is usually performed in the extremes of lateral rotation, and increase muscle stiffness, enabling better use of elastic energy and counteraction to extensive perturbations. During latter stages of rehabilitation and in injury prevention programs, exercises should mimic sport-specific movements, including their position (overhead extreme lateral rotation, elevated stress in contact position in spiking or hitting a ball with a racquet) and function. Elevated stress, such as plyometrics or additional loading, should be applied only when the athlete has achieved a full, pain-free range of motion, strength, and dynamic stability.

Exercises

The two main groups of upper extremity stabilization exercises can be differentiated: (1) closed kinetic chain exercises and (2) open kinetic chain exercises. During closed kinetic chain exercises, coactivation of glenohumeral muscles is high, enabling good stability in dynamic exercises.

WEIGHT TRANSFER FROM HAND TO HAND

The athlete may be supported by a wall, a bench (*a*), or the floor. The athlete steps each hand inward (*b*), shifting body weight from one arm to the other, then back out. The exercise may also be performed from a standing position. As the athlete progresses to a horizontal body position, the strain increases. To add additional stress, small exercise balls can be used or destabilizing movements can be initiated by a partner.

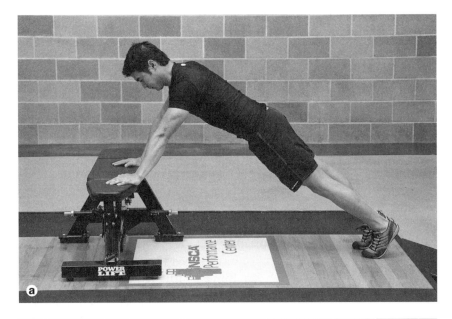

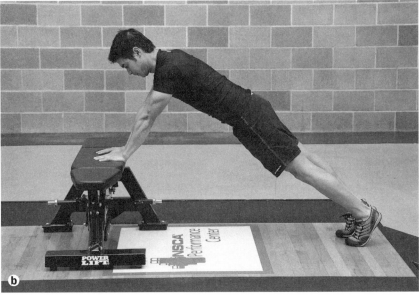

The use of elastic tubes enables movement in two-dimensional space. Since these exercises demand good stability of the upper body and lower limbs, they also influence torso stability. The same principle that is used in torso stability training should be followed, stressing preactivation of the abdominal muscles. The shoulders should also be positioned down and back (adduction and depression of the scapulae).

ELASTIC-BAR OSCILLATION
IN ABDUCTION AND ADDUCTION

The elbow should stay in a slightly flexed position during oscillation (*a-b*).

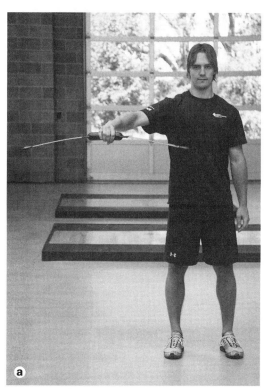
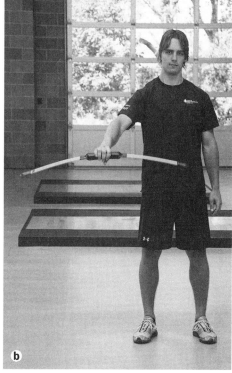

ELASTIC-BAR OSCILLATION IN MEDIOLATERAL SHOULDER ROTATION

Shoulder rotations can be performed during adduction, flexion in the sagittal plane, or abduction in the scapular plane. The difficulty increases with each respective position. In adduction, a small towel roll can be placed between the upper arm and the torso to relieve the subacromial space.

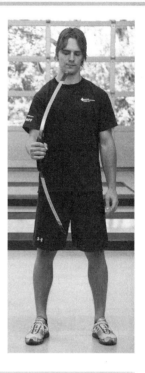

RHYTHMIC SHOULDER STABILIZATION WITH A PARTNER

The frequency and amplitude of perturbations can be varied.

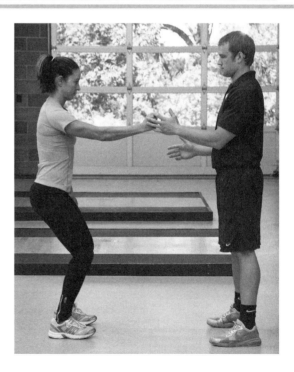

SUMMARY POINTS

- The positive effects of sensorimotor training have been widely accepted in rehabilitation and sports. An extensive body of literature and practical experience stresses the positive effects of sensorimotor training on compromised neuromuscular function after sport-induced injuries of the locomotor system.

- Practice and research also show a decreased number of sport-induced injuries after systematic implementation of sensorimotor training in standard training protocols of noninjured athletes at different quality levels. As such, sensorimotor training is an efficient tool for upgrading other training modalities and supporting athletes on their journey to reaching perfection in sports.

- When designing a training protocol in sports or rehabilitation, many aspects should be taken into consideration. As such, periodization presents the base for planning and decision making about which selection of training or rehabilitation modalities should be used.

- Strength and conditioning professionals and therapists should be acquainted with the specifics of their sport discipline, the involvement of different body parts, and the stresses placed on them. According to these basic directions, preventive measures can be taken to consider fatigue development and counteract negative effects of long-term and intensive training.

- Important joint complexes to consider when evaluating balance and stability are the torso (or core), knee, ankle and foot, and shoulder.

- Because core stabilizing movements are required for most athletes, core training should be a part of balance training for all athletes, even if it is not the location of injury or other joint instability.

Training Integration and Periodization

G. Gregory Haff, PhD, ASCC, CSCS*D, FNSCA

Erin E. Haff, MA

One of the primary concepts associated with the development and integration of training is *periodization*. Although periodization is widely accepted as a fundamental component of the training process, it is often misunderstood and misapplied. Contributing to this confusion is a misinterpretation of the classic literature on the topic and a common trend toward compartmentalizing the individual components of a training plan without considering how they are sequenced and integrated. These issues are best illustrated in the contemporary literature on resistance training, where periodization is incorrectly defined as the manipulation of sets, repetitions, or resistance (18, 47). Little or no attention is paid to how resistance training programs are affected by or integrated with other training factors, such as aerobic endurance, speed and agility, plyometric, technical, and tactical training. In reality, periodization is a much more inclusive theoretical and practical construct in which the management of workloads from all training factors are considered in relation to periods of restitution in order to direct training adaptations and, ultimately, elevate performance at appropriate times (38, 59, 64, 80).

The multifactorial nature of periodization is clearly demonstrated in the classic literature, where planned variation is considered in the context of appropriate sequencing and integration of multiple training factors (58, 59). For example, Nádori (57) and Nádori and Granek (58) suggest that periodization is the theoretical and methodological basis of training and planning. Here, predetermined training goals are accomplished through appropriate sequencing, integration, and variation of training factors in order to produce very specific physiological and performance adaptations at appropriate times. Central to this concept is the idea that interdependence exists between the various phases of training (38, 59). The aftereffects of one training phase exert a very powerful influence on subsequent training periods (40) and on the ability to direct the training process toward the desired outcomes (43, 44). Therefore, periodization should be defined as the logical, integrative, sequential manipulation of training factors (i.e., volume, intensity, training density, training frequency, training focus, and exercise selection) in order to optimize training outcomes at predetermined time points.

Ultimately, several distinct goals are targeted by a periodized training plan: (1) optimizing an athlete's performance at predetermined points or maintaining performance capacity for sports with a specific season, (2) structuring precise training interventions to target the development of specific physiological and performance outcomes, (3) managing the training stressors to reduce the potential for overtraining, and (4) promoting the athlete's long-term development (71, 80). The ability of a periodized training plan to achieve these specific goals largely depends on a multidimensional application of sequenced training variation. Although variation of training factors is a central component of an appropriately designed training plan, random or excessive variation should be avoided, since performance gains will be muted (80). It is essential that the training variation is applied in a logical, systematic fashion to modulate the training responses while decreasing fatigue and elevating performance at appropriate times.

General Principles of Periodization

When exploring the classic literature, it is clear that periodization is a method for employing sequential or phasic alterations in the workload, training focus, and training tasks contained within the microcycle, mesocycle, and annual training plan. The approach depends on the goals established for the specified training period (38, 52, 58). A periodized training plan that is properly designed provides a framework for appropriately sequencing training so that training tasks, content, and workloads are varied at a multitude of levels in a logical, phasic pattern in order to ensure the development of specific physiological and performance outcomes at predetermined time points.

In order for specific physiological responses and performance outcomes to develop, an appropriately sequenced and structured periodized training plan allows for the management of the recovery and adaptation processes (12, 18, 52, 64, 80). Since peak performance can only be maintained for brief periods of time (8-14 days) (9, 45, 55), the actual sequential structure of the periodized training plan is an essential consideration (64, 80, 85). Generally, the average intensity of the factors addressed by the training plan is inversely related to the average time that peak performance can be maintained and the overall magnitude of the performance peak (17, 38, 80).

For example, if the average intensity of all the training factors is high, the performance will elevate rapidly, but it will only be maintained for very brief periods. If, however, a more logical sequential modulation of training intensity is used, the period of peak performance can be extended. The magnitude of performance gain can also be significantly greater. Three basic mechanistic theories provide a foundational understanding for how periodization manages the recovery and adaptive responses: the general adaptive syndrome (GAS) (80, 88), stimulus-fatigue-recovery-adaptation theory (68, 80), and the fitness-fatigue theory (80, 88).

General Adaptive Syndrome

The general adaptive syndrome (GAS) is one of the foundational theories from which the concept of periodization of training was developed (78, 85). First conceptualized in 1956 by Hans Selye, the GAS describes the body's specific response to stress, either physical or emotional (68). These physiological responses appear to be similar regardless of what stimulates the stress. While the GAS does not explain all the responses to stress, it does offer a potential model that explains the adaptive responses to a training stimulus (figure 11.1) (27, 78).

When a training stress is introduced, the initial response, or *alarm phase*, reduces performance capacity as a result of accumulated fatigue, soreness, stiffness, and a reduction in energy stores (78). The *alarm phase* initiates

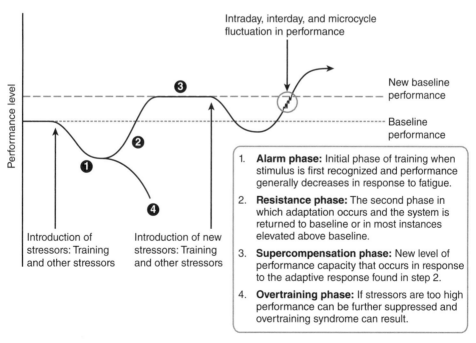

FIGURE 11.1   The general adaptive syndrome and its application to periodization.

Adapted from Fry et al. (36), Stone et al. (73), and Stone, Stone, and Sands (80).

the adaptive responses that are central to the *resistance phase* of the GAS. If the training stressors are not excessive and are planned appropriately, the adaptive responses will occur during the *resistance phase*. Performance will be either returned to baseline or elevated to new higher levels (supercompensation). Conversely, if the training stress is excessive, performance will be further reduced in response to the athlete's inability to adapt to the training stress, resulting in what is considered to be an overtraining response (20). From the standpoint of training response, it is important to realize that all stressors are additive and that factors external to the training program (e.g., interpersonal relationships, nutrition, and career stress) can affect the athlete's ability to adapt to the stressors introduced by the training program.

Stimulus-Fatigue-Recovery-Adaptation Theory

Whenever a training stimulus is applied, there is a general response that has been termed the *stimulus-fatigue-recovery-adaptation theory* (figure 11.2) (80). The initial response to a training stressor is an accumulation of fatigue, which results in a reduction in both preparedness and performance. The amount of accumulated fatigue and the corresponding reduction in preparedness and performance is proportional to the magnitude and duration of the workload encountered. As fatigue is dissipated and the recovery process is initiated, both preparedness and performance increase. If no new training stimulus is encountered after recovery and adaptation are completed, then preparedness and performance capacity will eventually decline. This is generally considered to be a state of involution.

When closely examining the general response to a training stimulus, it appears that the magnitude of the stimulus plays an integral role in deter-

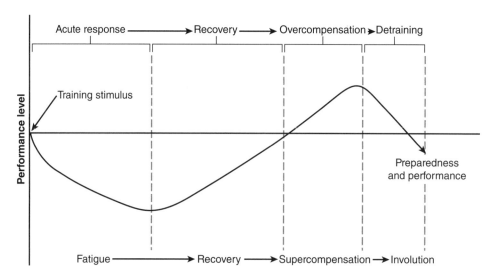

FIGURE 11.2   The stimulus-fatigue-recovery-adaptation theory.

Adapted from Verkishansky (81), Rowbottom (66), Yakovlev (87), and Stone, Stone, and Sands (80).

mining the time course of the recovery-adaptation portion of the process. For example, if the magnitude of the training load is substantial, a larger amount of fatigue will be generated, lengthening the time frame necessary for recovery and adaptation (66, 80). Conversely, if the training load is reduced, less fatigue will accumulate and the recovery-adaptation process will occur at a more rapid rate. This phenomenon is often referred to as the *delayed training effect*, in which the magnitude and duration of loading dictate the length of time necessary for recovery and adaptation. The modulation of the time course of the recovery-adaptation process through the appropriate variation and sequencing of workloads is a central theme of periodization.

In order to effectively develop periodized training plans, it is important to realize that the general pattern of response to a training stimulus can occur as a result of a single exercise, training session, training day, microcycle, meso-cycle, or macrocycle. It is important to note that it is not necessary to have complete recovery prior to initiating a subsequent training stimulus (58). In fact, it may be more prudent to modulate training intensities or workloads with the use of heavy or light days of training in order to facilitate recovery (19) while attempting to continue to develop fitness. Ultimately, the ability to appropriately sequence training stimuli is based on the manipulation of training factors in order to take advantage of the recovery-adaptation process. In fact, this process serves as a foundation for several sequential models of training presented in the periodization literature (64, 83, 84).

One sequential model that is largely based on the stimulus-fatigue-recovery-adaptation theory is the *concentrated loading* or *conjugated sequencing* model presented by several authors in the literature (figure 11.3) (64, 80, 83, 84). In this scenario, a concentrated training load (64, 80), or accumulation

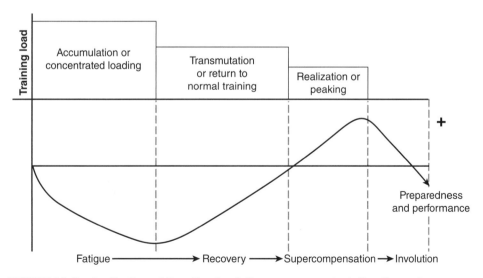

FIGURE 11.3 Application of the stimulus-fatigue-recovery-adaptation theory to sequential training.

Adapted from Verkishansky (81), Rowbottom (66), and Stone, Stone, and Sands (80).

load (43, 44, 88), is applied for a specific period of time (80). After this application of intentionally high training loads, there is a significant reduction in the training load, and training is returned to normal levels. This is often referred to as the *transmutation phase*, where preparedness and performance are elevated (69, 83-85). The final phase of this loading paradigm involves a further reduction in training load. This is sometimes referred to as a *peak*, *taper*, or *realization phase* (43, 44, 55, 84, 85, 88). During this phase, preparedness and performance generally supercompensate in response to the further reduction in fatigue that is stimulated by the reduction in training load (55). If, however, this phase is extended for too long (>14 days), *involution*, or a reduction in preparedness or performance, will occur.

Through the manipulation of training variables, an appropriately sequenced and integrated periodized training plan allows for the management of the accumulated fatigue and the process of recovery and adaptation. It also directs the training responses toward the targeted outcomes. If training loads are haphazardly applied and inappropriately sequenced, achieving performance goals becomes less likely as a result of the mismanagement of fatigue and or recovery.

Fitness-Fatigue Theory

The fitness-fatigue paradigm partially explains the relationships among fitness, fatigue, and preparedness (80, 88). It also gives a more complete picture of the physiological responses to a training stimulus (11). In this paradigm, the two aftereffects of training, fatigue and fitness, summate and exert an influence on the preparedness of the athlete (11, 88). The classic depiction of the fitness-fatigue theory presents the cumulative effects of training as one fatigue and one fitness curve (figure 11.4) (11, 80). In reality, multiple fitness and fatigue aftereffects likely exist in response to training that are interdependent and exert a cumulative effect (figure 11.5) (11).

The possibility of multiple fitness and fatigue aftereffects offers a partial explanation as to why there are individual response differences to variations in training (11, 80). Conceptually, the aftereffects of training are considered as residual training effects. They serve as the basis for sequential training (43, 44, 82, 85). Sequential training suggests that the rate of decay for a residual training effect can be modulated with either minimal training stimulus or through the periodic dosing of the specified training factor. Additionally, the residual effects of one training period can phase, potentiate, or elevate the level of preparedness of the subsequent periods, depending on the loading paradigms employed.

When the GAS, stimulus-fatigue-recovery-adaptation theory, and the fitness-fatigue theory are examined collectively, it is very clear that the ability to balance the development of various levels of fitness while facilitating the decay of fatigue is essential in modulating the adaptive responses to a training plan. An essential concept that allows for the appropriate

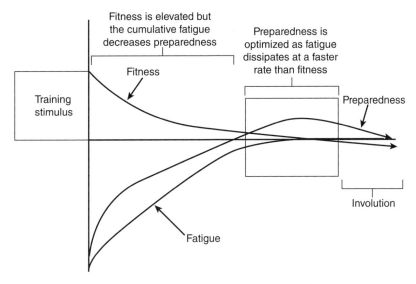

FIGURE 11.4 The fitness-fatigue paradigm.

Adapted from Stone, Stone, and Sands (80) and Zatsiorsky (88).

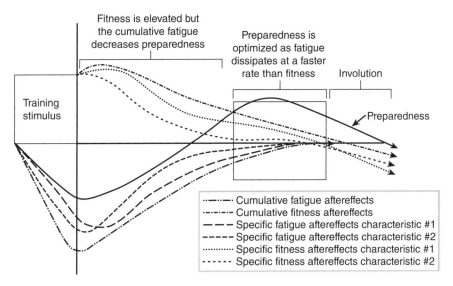

FIGURE 11.5 Modified fitness-fatigue paradigm depicting multiple training aftereffects.

Adapted from Stone, Stone, and Sands (80) and Chiu and Barnes (11).

modulation of training factors relates to sequencing training interventions to facilitate the management of fatigue and fitness while controlling the athlete's preparedness (64). Therefore, it is crucial when designing training interventions that the actual sequential pattern be considered in the context of how the training intervention is structured. This allows for the management of fatigue while maximizing the recovery adaptation process.

Ultimately, it results in the optimization of specific fitness parameters at key points so that preparedness and performance are elevated at the appropriate times.

Training Periods

Several distinct, interrelated levels of planning must be considered when constructing a training plan (table 11.1). Each of these levels must be considered in the context of the training goals established for the athlete. Once the training and performance goals are established, these periods are systematically structured, sequenced, and interrelated so that the athlete will be able to progress toward the training and performance outcomes specified by the training plan. The training periods are generally subdivided into various levels of planning, spanning from global or long-term structures, such as the multiyear training plan, to individual workouts that are contained during a specified training day (figure 11.6) (6, 16, 64, 67, 80, 88).

TABLE 11.1   Training Periods

Period	Duration	Description
Multiyear preparation	2-4 years	Also termed a *quadrennial plan*
Annual training plan	1 year	The overall training plan can contain a single or multiple macrocycles. It can be subdivided into preparatory, competitive, and transitional phases of training.
Macrocycle	Several months to a year	Some authors refer to this as an *annual plan*. It contains preparatory, competitive, and transitional phases of training.
Mesocycle	2-6 weeks	This medium-sized training cycle is sometimes called a *macrocycle* or a block of training. It consists of microcycles that are linked together.
Microcycle	Several days to 2 weeks	This small-sized training cycle can range from several days to 2 weeks in duration. It is comprised of multiple workouts.
Training day	1 day	One training day can contain multiple sessions. Is designed in the context of the microcycle in which it is contained.
Training session	Several hours	It generally consists of several hours of training. If the session has >30 min of rest between bouts of training, it should be considered as having multiple workouts.

Based on Bompa and Haff (6), Issurin (43, 44), Siff (70), and Stone et al. (78).

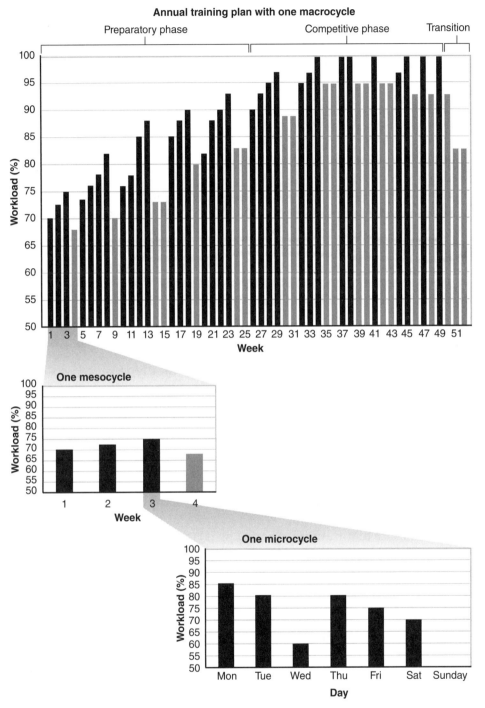

FIGURE 11.6 Breakdown of an annual training plan. The black bars represent a period of loading where workload (%) is increasing, while the gray bars represent a recovery microcycle where workload is markedly decreased. Conceptually, workload (%) is a composite of all the training factors undertaken during each period of training.

Adapted from Fry et al. (24) and Nádori and Granek (57).

From a hierarchical standpoint, the periodized training plan can be subdivided into seven periods: (1) multiyear training plan, (2) annual training plan, (3) macrocycle, (4) mesocycle, (5) microcycle, (6) training day, and (7) training session.

Multiyear Training Plan

The multiyear training plan is comprised of a series of annual training plans that are linked together to direct the athlete's training toward specific developmental and performance outcomes (6, 46, 58, 59, 67, 88). The quadrennial training plan (12, 24, 43, 46, 52, 66, 88) is commonly used by strength and conditioning professionals to develop training programs for athletes preparing for consecutive Olympic Games (12, 24, 43, 46, 52, 66, 88). This type of training has also been suggested to be a useful method for the development of high school and collegiate athletes (46, 61).

As a whole, multiyear training plans present the fundamental training tasks, main objectives, and directions of training that are to be targeted within each annual training plan in its structure (12). This is accomplished by establishing sequential training goals that develop the specific physiological, psychological, and performance outcomes necessary to realize the training goals established by the multiyear training plan (46). Sequencing is central to the successful application of the multiyear training plan, so that the adaptations established in one annual training plan serve as the foundation for subsequent annual plans. If the annual training plans contained within the multiyear training plan are structured and sequenced appropriately, optimal performance will occur at the appropriate time points.

Annual Training Plan

The annual training plan, sometimes called a *macrocycle* (12, 52), describes the overall training structures within a specific training year (12, 59, 66). The actual structure of the annual training plan largely depends on the athlete's developmental status (6, 43, 44, 59), the training objectives set forth by the multiyear training plan (12, 46, 59), and the competitive schedule of the athlete or team (6). In the classic literature, the annual training plan typically contains one macrocycle (52) (figure 11.7). However, an alternative training approach is to break the training year into two or three macrocycles in order to address multiple competitive seasons or the needs of athletes who participate in multiple sports (6, 44) (figure 11.8).

Regardless of the number of macrocycles in the annual training plan, the basic loading progression is from higher volumes of training toward higher intensity, lower volume training that is more technique oriented (31). Additionally, as the training load changes across the annual plan, the focus of training will be altered. These changes in focus can be easily seen in the three major subdivisions contained within the annual training plan: the (1) preparatory, (2) competitive, and (3) transitional phases (5, 6, 52, 66).

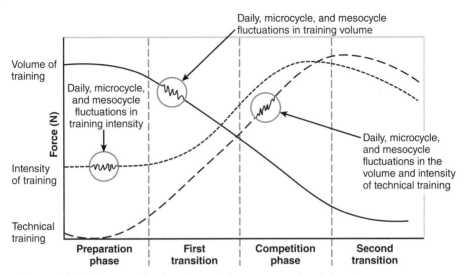

FIGURE 11.7 Matveyev's classic model of an annual training plan.

Reprinted from *Weight Training: A Scientific Approach 2nd edition*, by Michael H. Stone and Harold S. O'Bryant, copyright © 1987 by Burgess International Publishing. Reprinted by permission of Pearson Learning Solutions, A Pearson Education Company.

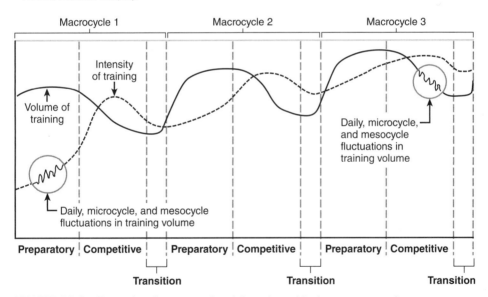

FIGURE 11.8 Example of an annual training plan with three macrocycles.

Adapted, by permission, from V. Issurin, 2008, *Block periodization: Breakthrough in sports training*, edited by M. Yessis (Ultimate Athlete Concepts), 213.

Preparatory Phase

The preparatory phase of the annual training plan induces physiological, psychological, and technical adaptations that serve as a foundation for the competitive phase (6). Depending on the athlete's level of development and the individual sport's requirements, the amount of time spent in the preparatory phase will range between three and six months (6). Conceptually, younger or less developed athletes should spend more time engaged in the general preparatory phase (6), while more advanced athletes can spend less time in this phase of training as a result of the training base already established. The total time spent in the preparatory phase will be divided among the macrocycles contained in the annual training plan. For example, in American football, a two-macrocycle annual training plan is generally used, with a three- to four-month preparatory phase in the early spring and a three-month preparatory phase before the fall season.

Regardless of the length and number of preparatory phases contained in the annual training plan, the classic literature on periodization breaks this phase into two broad subpreparatory categories: the (1) general and (2) specific preparatory phases (6, 44).

General Preparatory Phase   The general preparatory subphase is typically contained in the early part of the preparatory phase. It is designed to target the development of a general physical training base (6). This part of the preparatory phase is marked by high volumes of training, lower training intensities, and a large variety of training means that target the development of general motor abilities and skills (43, 52).

Specific Preparatory Phase   The specific preparatory subphase focuses on sport-specific motor and technical abilities in order to elevate sport-performance preparedness (12). This subphase generally contains higher training loads coupled with bursts of high-intensity training. A greater focus on sport-specific training is also included in order to build on the training base established during the general preparatory phase. Conceptually, this subphase strengthens the training base while preparing the athlete to transition into the competitive phase of the annual training plan.

Although the classic literature alters training focus by sequencing these subpreparatory phases, another model of training suggests that these two subphases should run concurrently with varying levels of focus (figure 11.9) (7, 12). This alternative model of sequencing so that the general and specific subphases run concurrently is based on the concept that the length of the preparatory phase is determined by the time necessary to achieve sporting form, not by the narrow structure of an annual training plan that contains between one and three macrocycles (7).

Competitive Phase

The primary goal of the competitive phase is to maintain or slightly improve the physiological and sport-specific skills acquired in the preparatory phase of development (58), while elevating preparedness and performance at the appropriate time points (6). These goals can be met by focusing on sport-specific activities, such as skill-based conditioning exercises (26), with a minor focus on general physical preparation activities (6). The use of skill-based conditioning activities also allows for the continued development of both technical and tactical skill sets, which are necessary for competitive success.

<table>
<tr><th colspan="2"></th><th colspan="12">Annual training plan</th></tr>
<tr><th colspan="2">Month</th><th>10</th><th>11</th><th>12</th><th>1</th><th>2</th><th>3</th><th>4</th><th>5</th><th>6</th><th>7</th><th>8</th><th>9</th></tr>
<tr><th>Model</th><th>Variant</th><th colspan="12"></th></tr>
<tr><td rowspan="10">Classic</td><td rowspan="2">1</td><td colspan="4">Preparatory phase</td><td rowspan="2">Competitive phase</td><td colspan="4">Preparatory phase</td><td colspan="3" rowspan="2">Competitive phase</td></tr>
<tr><td colspan="2">General prep.</td><td colspan="2">Specific prep.</td><td colspan="2">General prep.</td><td colspan="2">Specific prep.</td></tr>
<tr><td rowspan="2">2</td><td colspan="4">Preparatory phase</td><td colspan="4">Preparatory phase</td><td colspan="3" rowspan="2">Competitive phase</td><td rowspan="2">Transition</td></tr>
<tr><td colspan="2">General prep.</td><td colspan="2">Specific prep.</td><td colspan="2">General prep.</td><td colspan="2">Specific prep.</td></tr>
<tr><td rowspan="2">5</td><td colspan="4">Preparatory phase</td><td rowspan="2">Competitive phase</td><td colspan="4">Preparatory phase</td><td colspan="2" rowspan="2">Competitive phase</td><td rowspan="2">Transition</td></tr>
<tr><td colspan="2">General prep.</td><td colspan="2">Specific prep.</td><td colspan="2">General prep.</td><td colspan="2">Specific prep.</td></tr>
<tr><td rowspan="2">8</td><td rowspan="2">Transition</td><td colspan="6">Preparatory phase</td><td colspan="5" rowspan="2">Competitive phase</td></tr>
<tr><td colspan="3">General prep.</td><td colspan="3">Specific prep.</td></tr>
<tr><td rowspan="2">12</td><td rowspan="2">Transition</td><td colspan="8">Preparatory phase</td><td colspan="3" rowspan="2">Competitive phase</td></tr>
<tr><td colspan="4">General prep.</td><td colspan="4">Specific prep.</td></tr>
<tr><td rowspan="14">Alternative</td><td>3</td><td>Transition</td><td colspan="2">Preparatory phase</td><td>Transition</td><td colspan="2">Preparatory phase</td><td colspan="6">Competitive phase</td></tr>
<tr><td>4</td><td>Transition</td><td colspan="2">Preparatory phase</td><td colspan="4">Preparatory phase</td><td colspan="5">Competitive phase</td></tr>
<tr><td>6</td><td>Transition</td><td colspan="2">Preparatory phase</td><td>Competitive phase</td><td>Transition</td><td colspan="2">Preparatory phase</td><td colspan="5">Competitive phase</td></tr>
<tr><td>7</td><td>Transition</td><td colspan="2">Preparatory phase</td><td colspan="2">Competitive phase</td><td colspan="4">Preparatory phase</td><td colspan="3">Competitive phase</td></tr>
<tr><td>9</td><td>Transition</td><td colspan="3">Preparatory phase</td><td>Transition</td><td colspan="3">Preparatory phase</td><td colspan="4">Competitive phase</td></tr>
<tr><td>10</td><td>Transition</td><td colspan="3">Preparatory phase</td><td colspan="5">Preparatory phase</td><td colspan="3">Competitive phase</td></tr>
<tr><td>11</td><td>Transition</td><td colspan="3">Preparatory phase</td><td>Transition</td><td colspan="4">Preparatory phase</td><td colspan="3">Competitive phase</td></tr>
<tr><td>13</td><td>Transition</td><td colspan="4">Preparatory phase</td><td colspan="6">Preparatory phase</td><td>Competitive phase</td></tr>
<tr><td>14</td><td colspan="4">Preparatory phase</td><td>Transition</td><td colspan="4">Preparatory phase</td><td colspan="2">Competitive phase</td><td>Transition</td></tr>
<tr><td>15</td><td>Transition</td><td colspan="5">Preparatory phase</td><td colspan="6">Competitive phase</td></tr>
<tr><td>16</td><td>Transition</td><td colspan="6">Preparatory phase</td><td colspan="5">Competitive phase</td></tr>
<tr><td>17</td><td>Transition</td><td colspan="7">Preparatory phase</td><td colspan="4">Competitive phase</td></tr>
<tr><td>18</td><td>Transition</td><td colspan="8">Preparatory phase</td><td colspan="3">Competitive phase</td></tr>
</table>

FIGURE 11.9 Example of sequences for an annual training plan based on classic and alternative models.

Adapted from A. Bondarchuk, 1986, Periodization of sports training, *Legkaya Atletika* 12:8-9.

Generally, the volume of training is decreased across the competitive phase, while the intensity is increased. When following this basic loading pattern, it is important to realize that fluctuations in both volume and intensity occur throughout the competitive phase as a result of the competition schedule. Classic periodization literature often suggests that the competitive phase be divided into the precompetitive and main competitive subphases.

Precompetitive Subphase   The precompetitive subphase should be considered a link between the preparatory and main competitive subphases. A central component of this phase is the scheduling of unofficial competitions, such as exhibition games. It is important to note that the main objective of this phase is not to achieve the highest levels of performance, but to simply use competitions as training tools or as a means of preparation. Conceptually, these competitions serve as testing sessions that gauge the athlete's progress toward the main competitive goals (6).

Main Competitive Subphase   The main emphasis of this subphase is maximizing the athlete's preparedness and optimizing performance. A major factor in dictating the length of the main competitive subphase is the actual competitive schedule, which is often dictated by sport-governing bodies, such as the NCAA. As the athlete moves through this subphase, it is important that the training stimulus is modulated in order to allow for maintenance or continued elevation of the sport-specific fitness and skills attained in the previous phases. Generally, the primary competition is contained at the end of this subphase (i.e., conference championship track meet). A structured taper is employed for 8 to 14 days prior to this competition (6).

Transitional Phase

The transitional phase should be considered as an important bridge between either two annual training plans or two macrocycles(6, 58, 66). As a general rule, the transitional phase should consist of a significantly reduced training load, with a primary focus on general training activities that are used to maintain fitness levels (6, 58). Additionally, there should be a minimal emphasis on sport-specific skills in order to maintain technical proficiency (58). This important phase of the annual training plan typically lasts between two and four weeks, but if the annual training plan is particularly stressful, it can be extended to six weeks (6, 16, 49).

In some instances, a complete cessation of training during a portion of the transition phase may be warranted (i.e, if the athlete is recovering from an injury) (58). However, if training ceases for a significant time period, there will be a large reduction in the athlete's physical capacity (6), causing a significant planning problem. This scenario would require the next preparation phase to focus on reestablishing the baseline fitness levels achieved in the previous annual training plan, instead of elevating the athlete's capacity, as would normally be expected (6). Generally, the transition phase should be used to refresh the athlete both physically and mentally (58), while allowing him to exercise at a significantly reduced training load.

Macrocycle

Traditionally, the macrocycle has been considered as a single season (69) or annual training plan (6). However, it is likely that for many sports, multiple seasons will be contained within the annual training plan (i.e., distance runners often compete in cross-country running, indoor track, and outdoor track) and multiple macrocycles (2 or 3) will be needed in order to direct the training activities (59). Multiple macrocycle structures are typically seen, for example, in track and field, which has indoor and outdoor seasons, as well as in collegiate soccer, which has spring and fall seasons. Although the spring season in this example should not contain a true peak, since practice is the focus, some strength and conditioning professionals may place an emphasis on competition during this time frame when making decisions about their team structures. Theoretically, the macrocycle should be considered a training plan targeting specific training and competitive objectives (15, 16) that meet the overall goals set forth by the annual training plan. These objectives are met by manipulating specific training activities at both the mesocycle and microcycle levels.

The overall structure of the macrocycle is very similar to that of the annual training plan in that it contains preparatory, competitive, and transitional phases (6, 52, 66). As with the annual training plan, the general format of progression for each macrocycle is from higher volumes of training with lower intensities toward sport-specific training of higher intensity and lower volume (31). Each macrocycle is then linked by a transitional phase (figure 11.8). It is important to note with each successive macrocycle, the intensity of training and the focus on technical, tactical, and sport-specific training will be elevated. Overall, each macrocycle will be structured in the context of the annual training plan's overall goals and objectives. Typically, the last macrocycle of the annual training plan will be used to target the most important competitions contained in the training plan.

Mesocycle

In the traditional sense, the mesocycle is considered as a medium-duration training plan. It is generally comprised of two to six interlinked microcycles (43, 44, 59, 80, 83, 88). Typically, mesocycles are also considered to be blocks of training (43, 44), or summated microcycles (64, 78). When examining both the classic and contemporary literature on mesocycle structures, it is commonly noted that mesocycles generally last around four weeks (64, 86, 88). It appears that after about four weeks of a specific mesocycle, asymptotic training effects (i.e., a reduction in the adaptive responses to the training stimulus) begin to occur. These effects are most likely related to a state of involution in which physiological and performance gains either stagnate or begin to decline (86). It appears that if the training stimulus is altered at about four weeks, these reductions in fitness or performance can be avoided, and continued progress toward the targeted goals can occur. From a structural standpoint, four-week mesocycle blocks allow for delayed training effects to be superimposed, (43, 44, 80, 88) thus providing for the exploitation of cumulative training effects (80).

There are 8 to 10 potential classifications of mesocycles, which can be established based on their targeted objectives (table 11.2) (12, 39, 44, 52, 88). By sequencing and interlinking a series of specific mesocycles, the basic training plan can be established. Proponents of block mesocycle structures suggest a simplified mesocycle classification system, in which three basic blocks are designed: accumulation, transmutation, and realization (table 11.3) (8, 43, 44, 85, 88).

Accumulation Mesocycles

The main focus of an accumulation (43, 44), or concentrated loading (31, 64, 80), mesocycle is the development of the athlete's overall conditioning through the use of substantial workloads that target basic athletic abilities, such as muscular strength, anaerobic endurance, or aerobic endurance (44, 88). The length of accumulation mesocycles generally ranges between two and four weeks and depends on the time necessary to attain the targeted training effect, the rate of involution (i.e., performance decline), and the competitive schedule.

From a sequencing standpoint, the length of this mesocycle is proportional to the stability of the training effect (80, 88) and the time course of the involution of the residual training effects (64, 80). Longer accumulation mesocycles result in longer training residuals (43, 44) and substantially greater delay of training effects (64, 80). If structured correctly, this mesocycle establishes the training base on which subsequent mesocycles are based. Ultimately, this mesocycle should be considered a foundational training period that prepares the athlete for mesocycles that contain more intensive training and elevate performance.

Transmutation Mesocycles

After the completion of an accumulation mesocycle, the transmutation (43, 44, 88), or phase potentiating, mesocycle (64, 80) is undertaken. The central goal of this mesocycle is to elevate the athlete's overall level of preparedness by enhancing the abilities developed during the accumulation mesocycle (88). The goals of this mesocycle are met by targeting sport-specific training methods that focus on the competitive activity and utilize higher intensities that create a large amount of fatigue (43). For example, if the accumulation phase undertaken by the athlete targets strength-endurance, the transmutation

TABLE 11.2 Traditional Mesocycle Classifications

Type	Average duration (weeks)	Characteristics
Basic sport specific	6	Designed to elevate sport-specific fitness where performance in specific skills are targeted
Build-up	3	This more general form of training and conditioning is used to enhance foundational skills or fitness. It may be used after a period of specific or high-load training.
Competition	2-6	A mesocycle that specifically targets a competition during that mesocycle is used in the competitive phase of the annual training plan.
Competitive build-up	3	A period of increasing training loads that occurs during a long competitive phase and is used to reestablish foundational skills or fitness.
General	Any duration	This basic or general education and training targets the development of basic fitness. It generally occurs in the preparatory phase of the annual training plan.
Immediate preparatory	2	This training period occurs prior to a competition and targets peaking and restoration. It may be considered a taper and may proceed a testing period.
Precompetitive	6	Maximization of preparedness and performance for a specific competition or series of competitions. Marked by sport specific training. Designed to peak fitness, performance, and preparedness
Preparatory	6	Designed to develop a base necessary for competitive performance. Training moves from extensive to intensive. Fitness is established and utilized to develop skills
Recovery	1-4	Has a specific goal of inducing restoration. May follow a series of competitions. Serves to prepare athlete for subsequent training
Stabilization	4	Training used to perfect technique and fitness base. Technical errors are targeted as well as fitness deficits. Used to develop sport-specific fitness and skills base

Adapted from Harre (38) and Stone, Stone, and Sands (80).

TABLE 11.3   Simplified Sequential Mesocycle Structures

Phase	Alternative names	Duration	Methods	Characteristics
Accumulation	Concentrated loading	2-6 weeks	General physical development: General endurance, muscular strength, and basic technique	Tends to have the longest training residuals
				Creates the greatest amount of fatigue
				Increases general fitness the most
Transmutation	Normal training	2-4 weeks	Sport-specific abilities: Anaerobic conditioning (mixed), muscular endurance, technotactical preparedness	Shortened training residuals
				Increased preparedness
				Fatigue can become an issue
Realization	Peaking or tapering	7-14 days	Competition modeling: Maximal speed work, active recovery	Reduced training loads
				Increased preparedness
				Recovery

Adapted from Issurin (43, 44).

mesocycle may target the maximization of muscular strength, based on the foundation set forth in the previous mesocycle. The rate of involution (rate of decay) of training residuals from the accumulation mesocycle, the amount of fatigue generated during the current mesocycle, and the time course for the occurrence of asymptotic training effects all serve as the basis for the two- to four-week duration typically used in transmutation mesocycles. If the duration of this mesocycle is extended (>4 weeks), it is likely that the involution of residual training effects from the accumulation block will be maximized. If this occurs, the basic fitness necessary to perform during the realization (43, 44) or precompetitive mesocycle (85) will not be present and performance and preparedness will be muted.

Realization Mesocycles

The realization mesocycle is the final structure before a major competition that maximizes the athlete's level of preparedness (9, 45, 55, 56). This mesocycle is very similar to the taper typically seen in the classic literature in that it generally has the same goals and lasts between 8 and 14 days (43, 44). Similar to the classic taper, this mesocycle utilizes reductions in training load that maximize preparedness and performance while decreasing accumulated fatigue. Ultimately, the realization mesocycle attempts to create a situation in which the training residuals generated by the accumulation and transmutation mesocycles converge to elevate preparedness, maximize specifically trained abilities, and create a situation that maximizes performance (43, 44, 88).

The three main structural mesocycles serve as a foundation for the concept of sequential training. These mesocycles should be considered as interchangeable planning structures that can be used repetitively in order to direct the athlete's training toward targeted goals (80). The basic pattern for sequencing the three basic mesocycle structures is depicted as follows:

Accumulation → Transmutation → Realization

Ultimately, the actual sequencing and duration aspects of these planning structures are dictated by the objectives established by both the macrocycle and the annual training plan.

Microcycle

The microcycle is the smallest and most basic training structure, and it contains very specific training objectives (64, 80). The basic length of a microcycle is largely dictated by the phase of the overall training plan. It can last from several days to two weeks (31, 43, 44, 80). Microcycles contained in the preparatory phase generally last seven days, while those that are contained in the competitive phase vary in length depending on the actual competitive schedule (31, 43, 44 , 80). For example, during the general preparatory phase, the microcycle will be seven days long. In contrast, during the competitive phase, there may be two competitions during a week. This may require that two microcycles be created: one three days long and one four days long. The actual structure of the microcycle is largely predicated by its place within the overall planning structures (mesocycle, macrocycle, and annual training plans), the specific requirements of the sport or athlete, the athlete's ability to tolerate training stress, and the time allotted for training activities (49).

The general preparatory and sport-specific preparatory phases are the two main categories of microcycles (49, 80). During the early portion of the preparatory phase, training targets the development of general fitness with the use of what has been termed *general preparatory microcycles* (80). In the later stages of the preparatory phase, sport-specific preparatory microcycles will be used to develop sport-specific fitness and skills (49, 80). These two microcycle types can be further subdivided into the ordinary, shock, precompetitive, competitive, and recovery microcycles (49, 69, 80).

- *Ordinary microcycles.* This microcycle structure is comprised of lower training loads performed at submaximal intensities. With this type of microcycle, the training load is gradually and uniformly increased with successive microcycles (49, 69).

- *Shock microcycles.* A sudden increase in training load while maintaining a high volume of training is seen in a shock, (49, 52, 69, 80) or a concentrated loading, microcycle (64). Shock microcycles are widely used during both the preparatory and competitive phases of training by advanced athletes who have developed a substantial training base. This allows them to handle brief periods of intentionally high loading (49). If sequenced correctly within the mesocycle structure, the shock microcycle can be a very powerful tool for inducing significant physiological and performance adaptations (49, 64, 69, 80). Typically, after a shock microcycle, ordinary or recovery microcycles are employed, depending on the training status of the athlete and the overall goals of the program. However, in very unique situations, some elite athletes may employ two sequential shock microcycles. This has been termed a *double-shock microcycle* (69). Shock microcycles are commonplace in the training plans of elite athletes, but they should be avoided with beginner or novice athletes (49, 64). When considering the use of shock microcycles, it is important to note that their implementation should never place the athlete in danger of being injured. They should always employ logical and realistic loadings and should contain steps to monitor athletes' overall health status. For example, an illogical application of a shock microcycle would be to employ it with a collegiate football player after a winter-break transitional period, at the beginning of the general preparatory phase before an appropriate fitness base is established. This approach may increase the athlete's injury risk and the potential for overtraining, and may induce traumatic maladaptive responses, such as rhabdomyolysis. In this example, a better approach would be to undertake a period of base training that uses less aggressive loading schemes in order to elevate base fitness before attempting to employ shock microcycles.

- *Precompetitive microcycles.* The precompetitive (49), or introductory (69), microcycle prepares the athlete for the competitive microcycle. This microcycle may be considered an early portion of the precompetitive taper. It is marked by reduced training volumes, but it also emphasizes sport-specific training activities that elevate performance (49).

- *Competitive microcycle.* The competitive microcycle occurs immediately prior to a competition. It maximizes performance and preparedness (49, 69, 80). This microcycle should be considered an extension of the precompetitive microcycle. It contains the latter portion of the taper leading into the competition. Typically, this microcycle contains the immediate training preparation, travel to the competition, site preparation, warm-up, the actual competition, and the recovery activities undertaken after the competition (49, 80).

- *Recovery microcycle.* This microcycle is a training structure that contains a reduced training load in order to induce recovery by allowing the athlete to rest, heal, and prepare for upcoming training blocks (49, 69, 80).

The basic microcycle structures can be thought of as interchangeable building blocks from which the mesocycle training plan can be constructed. Depending on the targeted outcomes of the mesocycle, specific microcycle types can be selected and sequenced. For example, if athletes are in a realization mesocycle, they may perform the following sequential microcycles:

Precompetitive microcycle (7 days) → Competitive microcycle (7 days)

In comparison, an accumulation mesocycle can have a different targeted outcome. Thus, it would contain a different sequential approach of microcycles:

Ordinary (7 days) → Ordinary (7 days) → Ordinary (7 days) → Recovery (7 days)

Alternatively, if the mesocycle structure called for a concentrated load to be employed on week 1, the sequence of microcyles might be as follows:

Shock (7 days) → Ordinary (7 days) → Ordinary (7 days) → Recovery (7 days)

Ultimately, the various microcycle structures allow for various training sequences to be constructed, based on the needs of the athlete, the phase of training, and the goals of the mesocycle, macrocycle, and annual training plan.

Training Day

A training day is one of the smallest training units in a periodized training plan. Typically, a training day contains one or more interconnected training sessions (69) that are constructed in accordance with the objectives established by the microcycle plan. The density of training sessions in a training day largely depends on the athlete's level of development, the time allotted for training, and the phase of training. Generally, spacing multiple training sessions throughout the training day is recommended by many authors (28, 80, 82). By placing smaller periods of training throughout the day, it is believed that greater physiological adaptations may occur, which ultimately result in greater performance gains. Support for this contention can be found in the scientific literature, where studies have shown that greater neuromuscular and hypertrophic adaptations occur from training twice a day compared to a single training session, even when volume is held constant (36). Ultimately, by altering the density of training contained in a single day, an additional level of planning variation can be established.

Training Session

A training session or workout (43, 88) is the basic structural unit in a periodized training plan. Typically, multiple training sessions are performed each day in order to target several training factors (88). The organization of training during the day can either contain multiple sessions spaced periodically throughout the day or training sessions that contain short periods of rest (<40 min) (34-36). Based on these organizational strategies, one training session is traditionally defined having any rest interval less than 40 minutes (43, 44, 88).

Sequencing and Integration of the Training Process

The idea that periodized training programs should be sequenced and integrated is not new (7, 38, 50-53, 58, 60, 64, 83, 84). In fact, this concept can be seen in Matveyev's (52) seminal text, where he states that there is "a definite sequence of different links of the training process" and "a rational order of the interaction of various aspects of an athlete's training." Even though these concepts are echoed in other classic writings on periodization (3, 4, 7, 8, 38, 51-53, 57, 58), it appears that many contemporary coaches, especially strength and conditioning professionals, do not understand the importance of sequencing and integrating the training process (2, 10, 29, 61).

This lack of sequencing and integration of training can be seen in training programs where many or all training factors are addressed or emphasized at one time. This practice creates a scenario that generates high levels of fatigue and makes it virtually impossible to optimize performance at the appropriate times (30). It is likely that these high levels of fatigue increase the risk of overtraining (75) and potential for injury (26). Generally, an appropriately periodized training plan minimizes both these risks by manipulating various training factors, including intensity, volume, density, and training focus, in a sequential and integrative fashion (76, 77). Additionally, sequencing and integrating training factors exploit the physiological adaptations that occur in response to specific training interventions. When crafted correctly, these result in better management of training stressors and an increased ability to direct training toward specific performance goals.

As stated previously, the GAS, stimulus-fatigue-recovery-adaptation, and fitness-fatigue theories all provide a basis for sequential and integrative training (43, 44, 64, 78, 82, 84, 85). From a sequential standpoint, the residual (delayed) training effects developed in response to one mesocycle are used to potentiate the physiological and performance effects developed in subsequent mesocycles (80). Since the various residual effects, or physiological and performance adaptations, induced by a training intervention exhibit varying durations of stability and express different rates of involution, every training factor need not be trained in each stage of the periodized training plan (43, 44, 64). As a result of the various levels of involution that exist for the various training factors, a sequential training approach can be crafted in which complimentary training factors (table 11.4) are emphasized at specific time points across multiple mesocycles. This maximizes specific physiological or performance outcomes.

TABLE 11.4 Compatible Training Factors

Dominant (primary) training emphasis	Compatible training factors
Aerobic endurance	Strength-endurance training
	Maximal strength training
	Anaerobic endurance training
	Technical and tactical training (if done first)
Anaerobic endurance	Strength-endurance training
	Aerobic–anaerobic mixed endurance training
	Power endurance training
	Sprint (agility) training
	Explosive strength training / muscular power
	Muscular strength training
	Technical and tactical training (if done first)
Sprint ability	Maximal strength training
	Plyometric training
	Explosive strength training / muscular power
	Agility training
	Technical and tactical training (if done first)
Maximal strength	Sprint training
	Agility training
	Explosive strength training / muscular power
	Anaerobic endurance training
	Technical and tactical training (if done first)
Explosive strength/ muscular power	Sprint training
	Agility training
	Maximal strength training
	Plyometric training
	Technical and tactical training (if done first)
Technical training	Any emphasis as long as it is performed before other training factors
Tactical training	Any emphasis as long as it is performed before the other training factors

Adapted from Issurin (43, 44).

The success of a sequenced training plan is related to ordering successive mesocycles in accordance with mechanical specificity (64, 69, 79, 83), metabolic specificity (63, 80), and the time course of the stability and involution of residual training effects (43, 44, 69, 86, 88). Additionally, emphasis on actual training factors and the compatibility among factors are important considerations when attempting to sequence the mesocycle within a training plan. From a methodological standpoint, infinite sequencing possibilities can be employed when constructing a training plan. Three of the more commonly used methods are the (1) traditional or classic model, (2) summated microcycle model, and (3) conjugated sequencing model (64, 80).

Traditional or Classic Model

The traditional or classic model of periodization utilizes training structures that contain relatively limited variations in training methods and means. (64, 80) These are structured to create gradual wavelike increases in workload (figure 11.7) (50-52), which are sequenced into large multilateral training periods that uniformly distribute training loads across a predetermined training structure (12). Careful examination of the classic model reveals that the general training load is expressed as a ratio of volume to intensity of training (figure 11.7) (50). In the initial stages of training, the load is increased primarily by elevating the volume of work, while only marginally increasing intensity (12). As training progresses, the intensity will increase and training volume will subsequently decrease.

Matveyev's (50, 52) original depiction of the classic model was meant only as a graphical illustration of the central concepts (figure 11.7). It was not meant to be rigidly applied. The graphical depiction of the wavelike increases in workload presented by the model has been referred to as a *linear model of periodization* (1, 18, 47, 48, 65). However, a critical analysis of Matveyev's (50, 52) seminal text on the topic reveals that his model is, in fact, nonlinear. It contains several degrees of variation in volume, intensity, and training mode at the microcycle, mesocycle, and macrocycle levels.

A central component of the classic model is a complex system that employs the parallel development of physical abilities (12, 69, 82). Early research on this model suggested that it results in a simultaneous development of divergent physiological functions that are necessary for a variety of sports (69). However, careful inspection of this literature reveals that it was collected many decades ago from novice or beginner athletes (69, 82). Therefore, it may not optimize the physiological and performance adaptations of intermediate and advanced athletes (12, 82). There are several reasons why the rigid application of the classic model may not be advantageous for advanced athletes:

1. Advanced athletes already have a high level of special physical preparedness. They require a significant training stimulus that targets a

very finite emphasis to induce appropriate adaptations (69, 81). As a whole, the classic model produces a very small window of time where a novel stimulus is available to induce adaptation. This is followed by periods of monotonous training that are disadvantageous to advanced athletes. Conversely, with beginner or novice athletes, this model allows for stabilization of technical skills and other training factors (80, 83).

2. The classic model, mainly because of its reliance on a multifaceted training method that requires the simultaneous development of several training factors, cannot produce the highly specific physical preparedness that advanced athletes need (83). Conceptually, the multifaceted training approach results in an overall balanced development that does not stimulate an optimization of any specific training factor and may result in a muting of training adaptations and a smaller magnitude of performance gain.

3. The classic model relies on long periods of basic and sport-specific preparation (43, 44). These may be beneficial for novice athletes, but are considered a disadvantage for advanced athletes because of insufficient training variation (80). However, recent research indicates that the classic model may be advantageous in trained athletes when employed with college players of American football for relatively short-duration (e.g. 15 weeks), off-season training programs (42).

4. Elite competition requires a high level of technical competency. Developing technical competencies while simultaneously establishing special physical preparedness accumulates a large amount of fatigue. High levels of fatigue generally create a scenario where technical skills deteriorate, thus impeding the elite athlete's overall development (69, 81).

5. The modern athletic calendar often contains many competitions that the classic (traditional) periodization model cannot address (43, 44).

Based on these main points, it has generally been suggested that the classic model of periodization is best suited for beginner or novice athletes (12, 43, 44, 64, 80, 82). In contrast, complex sequential models, such as the summated microcycle or conjugated sequencing model, are more appropriate for intermediate and advanced athletes (43, 44, 64, 80, 82).

Summated Microcycle Model

The summated microcycle model increases training variation with an integrated, sequenced training structure. Typically utilized with intermediate to advanced athletes, this model introduces complementary training factors in a cyclical pattern that allows for a lower rate and magnitude of residual decay, or involution (64, 80). The typical structure of a summated microcycle is based on a four-week block of training, or mesocycle, that progresses from an extensive to an intensive workload, followed by a brief restitution period (43, 44). The basic four-week structure is often selected because this duration is associated with the time point at which asymptotic training effects arise and the involution (decay) of training residuals begins to occur (43, 44, 78, 86, 88).

In comparison to classic periodization models, the summated microcycle model uses a whole block of training, or mesocycle, to emphasize a very specific training factor, while other complementary training factors receive a minimal emphasis (64, 80). By structuring training in this fashion, a greater level of intermesocycle variation can be created (25, 52, 66, 80). At the same time, the training focus is better sequenced and integrated across the various training phases (43, 44, 69). If crafted correctly, this type of sequential model can minimize overtraining potential and decrease the involution of training aftereffects, while allowing for multiple training aftereffects to converge so that performance and preparedness are elevated at appropriate time points (80).

Central to the effective application of the summated microcycle model is the loading pattern and training-factor integration that is contained within each of the four interlinked microcycles that comprise the mesocycle block. Another important point is how each block of training is interrelated and sequenced. From a loading perspective, the basic summated model utilizes a loading structure that progresses from extensive-to-intensive workloads across three successive microcycles, followed by a recovery microcycle (figure 11.10, blocks 1-3) (64, 80). This general loading structure is traditionally referred to as a 3:1 loading paradigm (67, 71). Here, the first three microcycles increase in training volume, intensity, density, or some combination of each factor, followed by one recovery or unloading microcycle (32, 64). It is important to note that at the end of the third microcycle, the highest levels of fatigue are developed and performance capacity can be significantly impaired (80). Therefore, the recovery microcycle (where overall workload is reduced by manipulating training volume, intensity, or density) should be considered an extremely important component of the summated microcycle model because it reduces fatigue and potential for overtraining, elevates preparedness (31, 32), and facilitates the physiological adaptations necessary for the next block of training (80).

A second method of loading that is often used in conjunction with the summated microcycle model employs a concentrated loading (69, 84, 85), or planned overreaching, microcycle (14, 21-23, 37, 73). This method of loading is often used to initiate the block with a microcycle that contains an intentionally high workload, followed by a return to normal training loads (figure 11.10, blocks 4-5) (80). During the first microcycle, fatigue will be significantly elevated, while preparedness and performance markers (muscular strength, power, and endurance) will be reduced (13, 23). Ultimately, the degree of the reduction in preparedness and performance

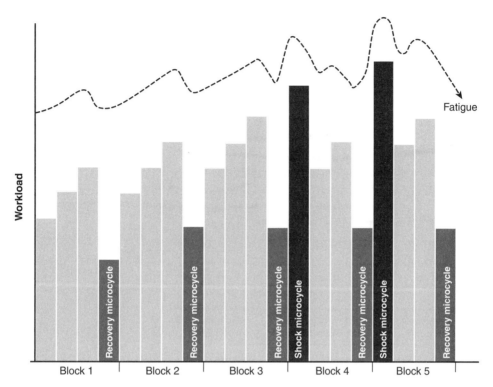

FIGURE 11.10   Example of a loading sequence for two variants of the summated micro-cycle model. Each block is four weeks in duration and each bar represents one microcycle.

Adapted from Stone, Stone, and Sands (80) and Plisk and Stone (64).

stimulated by the concentrated loading microcycle is directly proportional to the magnitude of loading (69). However, the greater the loading during this phase, the greater the potential performance elevation that can be stimulated once fatigue is dissipated (81). The dissipation of fatigue is accomplished in this model by sequencing the mesocycle so that after the concentrated loading microcycle ends, training workload is reduced to normal levels for two microcycles. Next, training loads are reduced further in a one-week recovery microcycle. If sequenced correctly, a supercompensation effect will occur at the end of the block in response to the convergence of the delayed training effects (69, 74, 80), or training residuals (43, 44).

The effectiveness of a summated microcycle model can be enhanced by employing intramicrocycle variation tactics. For example, the intensity of training can be altered across the microcycle, allowing for heavy and light days to be performed in the context of the microcycle's goal (80). An ath-lete may do resistance training on Monday and Friday, but the workload on Friday should be 40% less of that utilized on Monday. The inclusion of submaximal (light) days can exert a significant influence on the potential for positive adaptations, while minimizing the possibility of overtraining (19). Other intramicrocycle variations tactics, such as competitive-trial, interval, or repetition methods, may also be used to modulate the effectiveness of the summated microcycle (80). Ultimately, many methods can be used to introduce intramicrocycle variations or to modify the loading patterns utilized in the summated microcycle model.

Conjugated Sequencing Model

The conjugated sequencing model, or *coupled successive system*, as it was originally termed (64, 83), is a system for sequencing and integrating training factors typically employed with advanced athletes (41, 44, 64, 69, 71, 74, 78, 80, 86, 88). Central to this model is the sequencing of accumulation (64, 81, 84) (concentrated loading) (64, 80), transmutation (43, 44, 88), and realization (43, 44) or recovery (64, 80) mesocycles in order to take advantage of residual (delayed) training effects (figure 11.11). Theoretically, the annual training plan can be constructed by sequencing these three basic mesocycle structures and designing the training interventions in the context of the phases (i.e., preparatory or competitive) contained in the annual plan (figure 11.12).

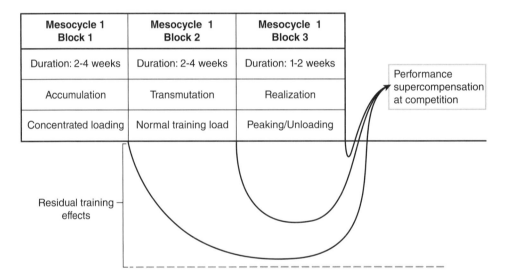

Mesocycle 1 Block 1	Mesocycle 1 Block 2	Mesocycle 1 Block 3
Duration: 2-4 weeks	Duration: 2-4 weeks	Duration: 1-2 weeks
Accumulation	Transmutation	Realization
Concentrated loading	Normal training load	Peaking/Unloading

Performance supercompensation at competition

Residual training effects

FIGURE 11.11 Basic conjugated sequencing structure.
Adapted from Issurin (43, 44).

Central to the effectiveness of the conjugated sequencing model is the use of *concentrated loading blocks*, which are considered as the primary component of the accumulation block. Typically, the accumulation block lasts between two and four weeks, during which either performance or preparedness is decreased in response to an elevated level of accumulative fatigue (64). Conceptually, the concentrated loading block saturates the system with one major training emphasis, while complimentary training factors are addressed with a smaller emphasis (figure 11.13). For example, when sequencing training for speed development, the primary emphasis in the *accumulation block* would target maximal strength development,

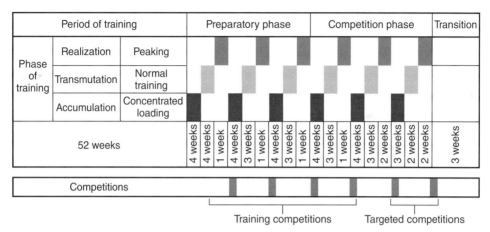

FIGURE 11.12 Example of an annual training plan containing a sequential application of accumulation, transmutation, and realization mesocycles.

Adapted by Issurin (43, 44).

while the secondary emphasis would focus on muscular power, and the tertiary emphasis would be on speed and agility (6, 62). As training shifts into the second block, or the *transmutation block*, the emphasis changes and the workloads are redistributed. In the example presented in figure 11.13, the primary emphasis of the transmutation block is muscular power, while

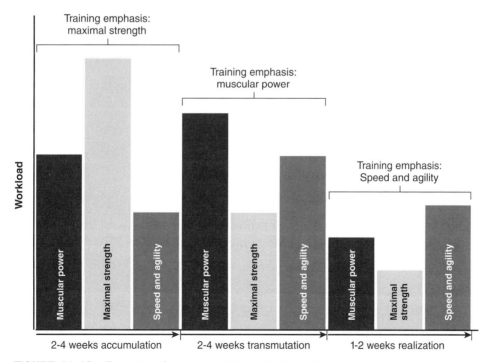

FIGURE 11.13 Example of a sequential application of accumulation, transmutation, and realization blocks for developing speed.

the secondary emphasis is speed and agility, and the tertiary emphasis is maximal strength.

The selection of these training factors is based on the relationships among maximal strength, power development, and the expression of speed. Typically, strength must be increased before power can be developed and then expressed as speed. The reorientation of the training emphasis facilitates recovery and takes advantage of the delayed training effects (residuals) developed by the accumulation block.

After completing two to four weeks of the transmutation block (43, 44), a *realization* or *restitution block*, which lasts between one and two weeks, will be performed (6). The realization block of the sequential plan results in continued dissipation of fatigue and a significant increase in preparedness and performance, which occurs in response to changes in training focus and a reduction in training load. For example, in figure 11.13, the realization block contains a primary emphasis on speed and agility, a secondary emphasis on muscle power, and a tertiary emphasis on maximal strength, while reducing workloads in order to maximize preparedness and performance.

When constructing a training plan, several blocks of accumulation, transmutation, and realization can be linked together in order to direct training toward specific physiological and performance outcomes. If sequenced appropriately, the athlete's level of preparedness and performance will increase across the sequentially linked blocks of training and in response to the realization block (figures 11.14-11.16). Figure 11.14 presents an example of a conjugated sequencing model in which a systematic overlapping of accumulation, transmutation, and realization blocks is used to direct preparedness for speed-strength performance.

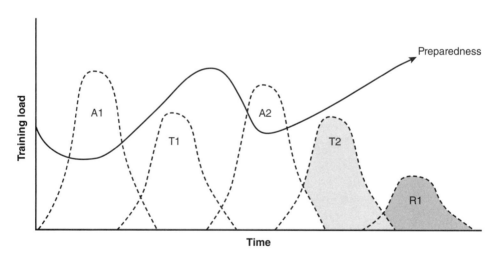

FIGURE 11.14   Sequencing of accumulation, transmutation, and restitution blocks of training for speed strength development.

Adapted from Siff (69), Siff and Verkoshansky (70), and Stone, Stone, and Sands (80).

In this example, two accumulation blocks (A1 and A2) contain high-volume, low-intensity strength training. During this time, performance is expected to decrease in response to accumulative fatigue (80). During the transmutation blocks (T1 and T2), the training focus shifts toward high-intensity speed work coupled with technical training. The reduction in training load and the shift in training emphasis results in a dissipation of accumulated fatigue and stimulates a corresponding elevation in preparedness. After the second transmutation phase (T2), a realization (R1) block is planned. In this block, training load will be further reduced and performance will supercompensate in response to a further reduction in accumulated fatigue (69, 80, 88).

Figure 11.14 represents a basic conjugated sequencing model, but more complex training structures can be created (figures 11.15 and 11.16). For example, in figure 11.15, the sequencing of training factors is more complex. In this example, the targeted performance outcome is, again, speed and strength. It presents a more complex illustration for a sequential ordering of the accumulation, transmutation, and realization blocks of training. The accumulation block is contained in the first half of the training structure. This block depicts an early emphasis that centers on strength-endurance and anaerobic conditioning, followed by a shift toward maximal strength and an increasing emphasis on technical (i.e., skill) training and speed training. In the second half of the this plan, the early portion represents the transmutation block, which shifts the emphasis toward the development of strength and power while continuing to focus on technical and speed training. Anaerobic conditioning is maintained. The final portion of the presented structure depicts the realization block, where technical and speed training are the primary focus and minimal emphasis

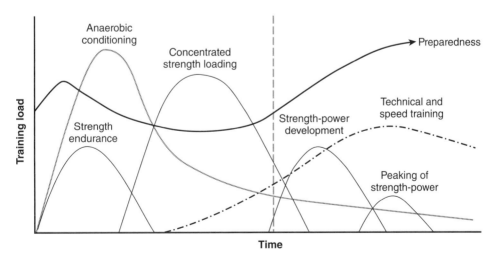

FIGURE 11.15 Sample sequencing of training that targets speed-strength development.

Adapted from Siff (69) and Siff and Verkoshansky (70).

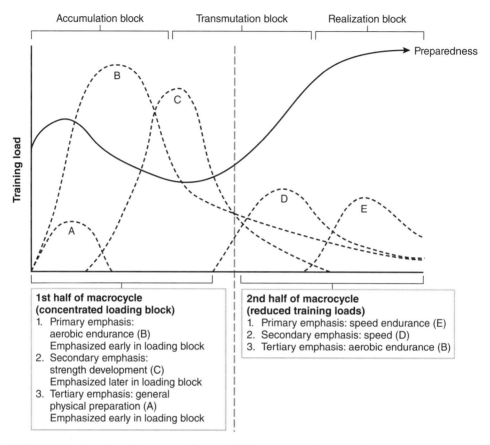

FIGURE 11.16 Sample sequencing model for a sport that requires medium-duration endurance.

Adapted from Issurin (43, 44), Plisk (62), and Bompa and Haff (6).

is placed on anaerobic conditioning. Here, strength/power capabilities peak.

Another example of a conjugated sequencing model is presented in figure 11.16. In this model, the targeted outcome is medium-duration endurance. Aerobic endurance, general physical preparation, strength development, and speed-endurance are all sequentially manipulated in order to direct preparedness.

Ultimately, if the blocks of training are sequenced and integrated appropriately with the conjugated sequencing model, the athlete's preparedness will be increased and performance will be supercompensated at the appropriate time points (69, 80, 88). When compared with a traditional, multidimensional training approach, the conjugated sequencing model has the potential to produce superior performance gains (33, 40, 54, 64, 76, 80). It appears that this model is particularly useful when targeting the development of power and speed, as compared to training heavy resistance or speed strength exclusively (33, 76).

Practical Guidelines

Periodization, as a whole, is a planning process that can be used to organize the training process of any athlete, regardless of developmental level or the sport being trained for. A simplified process that contains seven interrelated steps is presented in table 11.5.

TABLE 11.5 Basic Steps in the Planning Process

Step	Objective
1	1. Determine the athlete's long-term goals in order to develop a multiyear plan. Typically, this is accomplished with a quadrennial plan. 2. Outline the basic structure for the multiyear plan.
2	1. Prioritize the major objectives to be targeted by the annual training plan. 2. Evaluate the previous year's training plan, including competitive and performance results, and consult with the athlete or team about the training plan. 3. Create a working structure for the next annual training plan based on the competitive requirements of the athlete or team. 4. Determine the number of macrocycles contained in the annual training plan. 5. Establish the macrocycle lengths in the context of the structure established for the annual training plan.
3	1. Break the annual training plan into preparatory, competitive, and transitional phases based on the schedule of the athlete or team. 2. Divide the preparatory phases into general and specific subdivisions. 3. Create precompetitive and main competitive phases within the competitive phases of the annual training plan. 4. Insert testing days into the annual training plan at key time points.
4	1. Determine the lengths of the individual mesocycles. 2. Select and sequence the various structures of the mesocycles into the annual training plan. 3. Prioritize the focus of training factors for each mesocycle, considering how the factors are sequenced across each phase of training in the annual plan. 4. Establish the loading patterns in each mesocycle and determine how loading will progress across the macrocycles in the annual plan.
5	1. Construct each microcycle. 2. Divide the microcycle into training and recovery days according to the athlete's level of development and overall goals. 3. Establish which factors will be trained on each training day and how many training sessions will be contained during each day. 4. Create the loading structures used throughout the microcycle.
6	1. Design the individual training sessions. 2. Determine the loading structures for the training session. 3. Select the activities for the training plan.
7	1. Implement the training plan. 2. Continually monitor and evaluate the training plan and process.

When initiating the process by which a periodized training plan is developed, the first step is to establish a basic multiyear training plan. For example, with high-school athletes, Jeffreys (46) suggests year 1 (freshman year) is a foundational time that develops the requisite motor patterns and fitness characteristics that are essential for subsequent years of training. During year 2 of the training plan (sophomore year), the training plan builds on the foundation laid in year 1 through the continued development of sport-specific fitness and technical proficiency. In years 1 and 2, the emphasis should be not on competitive performance, but on the development of requisite skills needed for future competitive success. Competitive performance becomes more important during year 3 (junior year) of the multiyear training plan. During this annual plan, more emphasis is placed on the competitive phases and the actual optimization of sport performance. Finally, during year 4 (senior year), the major goal of the annual plan is to achieve the highest competitive performance. Although the example presented by Jeffreys (46) for a high-school athlete is excellent, it should be realized that a multitude of possible multiyear training structures can be developed, depending on the individual athlete's needs.

After establishing the multiyear training plan, the next step in the periodization process is to create the annual training plan for the next training year. Typically, it is best to structure the annual training plan during the transitional phase, which typically occurs at the end of the previous training year (6). At this time, the strength and conditioning professional can evaluate the training process of the previous year, examine competitive and performance test results, and consult with the athlete about the overall training plan. To facilitate the planning process, the strength and conditioning professional can develop a template for the annual training plan. An example of a possible planning template is available online at www.HumanKinetics.com/products/all-products/NSCAs-Guide-to-Program-Design, but professionals should create forms for individual athletes or teams based on their unique planning needs.

After careful thought and reflection about the previous training year, the strength and conditioning professional can then begin the next year's annual plan. The first step when compiling the annual training plan is to place all planned competitions and their locations on the planning sheet. Once this is completed, the competitions should be prioritized to determine where peak performance is needed and to allow the strength and conditioning professional to decide how many macrocycles will be contained in the annual training plan.

Once the macrocycles have been determined, the annual training plan should be further subdivided into preparatory, competitive, and transitional phases. The length of the competitive phase largely depends on the competition schedule established. After dividing the macrocycles into these major phases, the training plan is further divided into general preparatory, specific preparatory, precompetitive, and competitive subphases.

Based on these structural decisions, the strength and conditioning professional can then determine where peak performance is needed. This is indicated with the peaking index. The peaking index is demonstrated on a scale of 1 to 5, where 1 is the highest level of preparedness and 5 is the lowest level of preparedness (6). Conceptually, the higher the volume of work or training stressors, the higher the peaking index number. The decisions made about the peaking index will aid the decision-making process when establishing the mesocycle and microcycle structures.

Figure 11.17 on page 250 is an example of what a annual training planning sheet for a Division I women's soccer team will look like after completing steps 2 and 3 of the planning process presented in table 11.5. In this example, the first macrocycle, which is comprised of the spring season, runs from January 4 to May 9, with an 11-week preparatory phase (January 4-March 21) and a 5-week competitive phase (March 22-April 24). After completing competitive phase 1, the athletes will undergo a 3-week transitional phase prior to initiating macrocycle 2. It is important to note that competitive performance is not a major priority at this point in the annual training plan; therefore, the athletes are not taken to a true peak as indicated by the peaking index.

The second macrocycle (figure 11.17) is the most important macrocycle contained in the annual training plan. It begins on May 10 and runs until December 26. Since the sample team is one of the top teams in their conference, typically qualifying for the NCAA tournament, the major peak should occur for the tournament. As with the first macrocycle of the annual training plan, the second macrocycle is subdivided into preparatory, competitive, and transitional phases. The early part of the summer, May 10 to July 17, contains the general preparation subphase, while the specific preparatory subphase runs from July 18 to August 22. As noted on the planning chart, an exhibition game is scheduled for August 22 that serves as an evaluative tool. Therefore, decisions about tactical or technical skills need to be addressed in the competitive phase of the annual plan.

The early part of competitive phase 2 (August 23-September 12) is delineated as the precompetitive phase. This subphase progressively elevates the competitive capacity of the athletes and culminates with a minor peak (or unloading) for the September 11 competition. After completing the precompetitive subphase, the main competitive phase is initiated. A relatively long competitive phase is planned as a result of the nature of the sport. A minor peak is planned for the conference tournament that occurs in microcycles 44 and 45, while the major peak will occur during the NCAA tournament.

The next planning step is to determine the mesocycle lengths contained in each macrocycle. In this example, the annual training plan is broken into 14 mesocycles, with 5 mesocycles contained in macrocycle 1 and 9 contained in macrocycle 2. Once the macrocycles are established, the strength and conditioning professional can begin sequencing and integrating the various training factors. Figure 11.18 on pages 252-257 is an expansion of figure 11.17, where these steps are integrated into the planning for a Division I women's soccer team. In this example, the strength training is sequenced and integrated with the other training factors in order to better manage fatigue and training stressors. In this step, the strength and conditioning professional should consider which training factors are of primary emphasis, and then integrate the training factors by indicating if they are a high, moderate, or low emphasis. Figure 11.18 should be viewed as just one example of how this might be done for a women's soccer team.

The next step of the planning process is to determine the loading patterns contained in each mesocycle and macrocycle in the annual training plan. Note that this is merely an estimation of the workload. Additionally, the graphical representation is a summation of each of the training factors. It is important to remember that each bar represented in figure 11.18 is a summation of all the individual training factors. For example, in microcycle 3, the workload represents the integration of the resistance training (strength endurance and basic strength work), aerobic endurance training, sprint and agility training, and technical or tactical work.

After completing steps 1 through 4 of the planning process, the strength and conditioning professional can then begin to construct the individual microcycles, paying particular attention to the emphasis placed on each training factor (step 5, table 11.5). When undergoing this process, the strength and conditioning professional must consider the athlete's daily schedule, the need for recovery days, and the overall context of the mesocycle and macrocycle for which the microcycle is designed. Once the microcycle has been outlined, the strength and conditioning professional can then undertake step 6 of the planning process and design the individual training sessions.

To see larger versions of figures 11.17 and 11.18, visit www.HumanKinetics. com/products/all-products/NSCAs-Guide-to-Program-Design.

SUMMARY POINTS

- Periodization of training is an essential component of the athlete's long-term development. It should be considered a logical, integrative, and sequential manipulation of training factors in order to optimize training outcomes at predetermined time points.

- Periodization is a theoretical and practical paradigm that is well established in the scientific literature as a superior method of developing athletes, especially over the long term.

- Periodization is a planning process that allows the strength and conditioning professional to structure training that targets specific physiological and performance outcomes, while managing the training and life stressors that the athlete is exposed to.

- Training periods that should be considered and structured when designing an athlete's program include the multiyear training plan, annual training plan, macrocycle, mesocycle, microcycle, and training day and session.

- Although the classic model of periodization is helpful for novice or beginner athletes, advanced athletes require sequential models of periodization that are more complex. These include the summated microcycle model and the conjugated sequencing model.

Dates	Month	January				February				March			March		April					May	
	Week ending	10	17	24	31	7	14	21	28	7	14	21	28		4	11	18	24	25	2	9
Competitions	Away match					C							C	C							
	Home match														C	C	C	C			
	Competition name					2/28-Penn State							3/28-Tennessee	3/28-Georgia	4/4-Pitt.	4/5-Team Ontario	4/18-Purdue	4/25-Ohio State			
Periodization	Training phase	Preparatory phase 1											Competitive 1						Transition 1		
	Training subphase	General preparatory							Specific prep				Precompetitive			Competitive			Transition		
	Macrocycle	Macrocycle 1																			
	Mesocycle																				
	Microcycle	1	2	3	4	5	6	7	8	9	10	11	12		13	14	15	16	17	18	19
	Peaking index	5	5	5	5	4	4	4	4	5	5	5	4		3	3	3	2	5	5	5
	Testing dates	T																	T		
	Recovery weeks																				

Competition key
P = major peak
p = minor peak
c = competition

Abbreviations
R = recovery week
Specific prep = specific preparatory
T = testing

Peaking index
1 = highest level of preparedness
2
3
4
5 = lowest level of preparedness

FIGURE 11.17 Example of steps 2-3 of the planning process for a Division 1 women's soccer team

FIGURE 11.17 (continued)

Category		May			June				July				August					September			
	Month	May	May	May	June	June	June	June	July	July	July	July	August	August	August	August	August	September	September	September	September
	Week ending	16	23	30	6	13	20	27	4	11	18	25	1	8	15	22	29	5	12	19	26
Dates																					
Competitions	Away match																C	C	p	C	C
	Home match															C	C	C	C	C	C
	Competition name															8/16-Exhibition Maryland	8/23-Ohio State; 8/29-Penn State	8/31-BYU; 9/3-Duquesne	9/6-Boston; 9/11-Virginia	9/13-Dartmouth; 9/18-Pitt.	9/20-Tennessee; 9/24-Marquette
Periodization	Training phase	Preparatory phase 2															Competitive 2				
	Training subphase	General preparatory										Specific prep					Precompetitive		Competitive		
	Macrocycle	Macrocycle 2															Macrocycle 2				
	Mesocycle																				
	Microcycle	20	21	22	23	24	25	26	27	28	29	30	31	32	33	34	35	36	37	38	39
	Peaking index	5	5	5	5	5	5	5	5	5	4	4	4	4	5	5	4	3	2	3	3
	Testing dates										T								T		
	Recovery weeks																				

251

FIGURE 11.17 (continued)

Dates / Competitions

Competition name	Away match	Home match
9/27-USF	C	
10/2-Notre Dame	p	
10/4-DePaul		C
10/9-Syracuse		C
10/11-St. Johns		C
10/16-Villanova	C	
10/18-Georgetown	C	
10/23-Connecticut	C	
10/25-Providence	C	
Big East Tournament (Storrs, Conn.)	p	
11/13-NCAA First Round	p	
11/15-NCAA Second Round	p	
11/20-11/22: NCAA Championships	p	
11/21, 11/22, or 11/23-NCAA Third Round	p	
12/4-NCAA Semifinals	p	p
12/6-NCAA Finals	p	p

Periodization

Training phase: Competitive 2 | Transition 2
Training subphase: Competitive | Transition
Macrocycle: Macrocycle 2

Month	Week ending	Microcycle	Peaking index	Testing dates	Recovery weeks
October	3	40	2		
October	10	41	3		
October	17	42	3		
October	24	43	2		
October	31	44	1		
November	7	45	1		
November	14	46	2		
November	21	47	2		
November	28	48	2		
December	5	49	1	T	
December	12	50	5		R
December	19	51	5		R
December	26	52	5		R

252

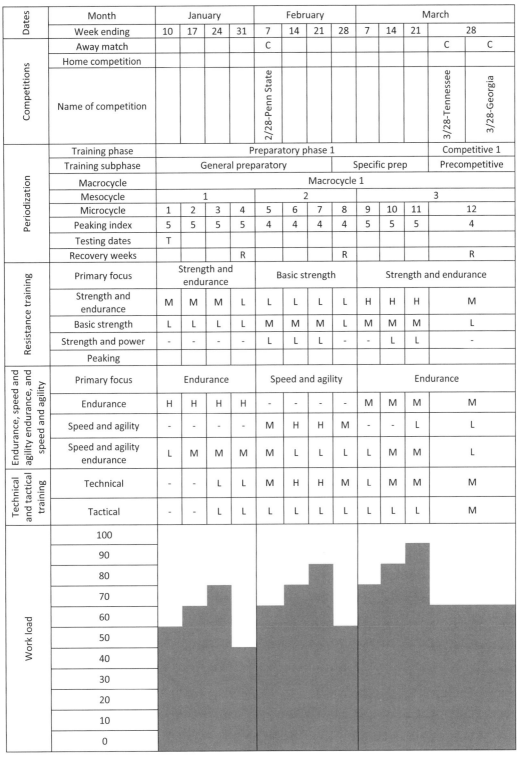

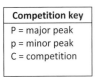

FIGURE 11.18 Example of step 4 of the planning process for a Division 1 women's soccer team.

Dates		4	11	18	24	25	2	9	16	23	30	6
Month		April					May					June
	Week ending	4	11	18	24	25	2	9	16	23	30	6
Competitions	Away match											
	Home competition	C	C	C	C							
	Name of competition	4/4-Pitt.	4/5-Team Ontario	4/18-Purdue	4/25-Ohio State							
Periodization	Training phase	Competitive 1					Transition 1		Preparatory phase 2			
	Training subphase	PreC	Competitive				Transition		General preparatory			
	Macrocycle	Macrocycle 1							Macrocycle 2			
	Mesocycle	4					5		6			
	Microcycle	13	14	15	16	17	18	19	20	21	22	23
	Peaking index	3	3	3	2	5	5	5	5	5	5	5
	Testing dates					T						
	Recovery weeks				U	R	R	R				R
Resistance training	Primary focus	Strength and power					Recovery		Strength and endurance			
	Strength and endurance	M	M	L	-	-	-	-	M	H	H	M
	Basic strength	H	H	M	L	-	-	-	L	L	L	L
	Strength and power	M	M	H	M	-	-	-	-	-	-	-
	Peaking				H							
Endurance, speed and agility	Primary focus	Speed and agility				Recovery			Endurance			
	Endurance	-	-	-	-	-			M	M	M	M
	Speed and agility	M	H	H	L	-			-	-	L	L
	Speed and agility endurance	M	L	L	L	-			L	M	M	M
Technical and tactical training	Technical	M	M	L	L	-			L	L	L	L
	Tactical	M	M	H	H	-			L	L	L	L

Work load (y-axis): 100, 90, 80, 70, 60, 50, 40, 30, 20, 10, 0

FIGURE 11.18 (continued)

254

	Month	June			July				August			
Dates	Week ending	13	20	27	4	11	18	25	1	8	15	22
Competitions	Away match											
	Home competition											C
	Name of competition											8/16-Exhibition Maryland
Periodization	Training phase	Preparatory phase 2										
	Training subphase	General				Specific prep						
	Macrocycle	Macrocycle 2										
	Mesocycle	7				8			9			10
	Microcycle	24	25	26	27	28	29	30	31	32	33	34
	Peaking index	5	5	5	5	5	4	4	4	4	5	5
	Testing dates					T						
	Recovery weeks				R			R				R
Resistance training	Primary focus	Basic strength				Strength and endurance			Basic strength			
	Strength and endurance	L	L	L	L	M	H	H	L	L	L	L
	Basic strength	M	H	H	M	L	M	M	M	M	M	M
	Strength and power	L	L	M	L	-	-	L	M	M	M	M
	Peaking											
Endurance, speed and agility, agility endurance, and speed and agility	Primary focus	Speed and agility				Speed and agility endurance						
	Endurance	L	L	L	L	H	M	M	L	L	L	L
	Speed and agility	M	M	M	M	-	M	M	M	H	H	M
	Speed and agility endurance	L	L	L	L	M	L	L	M	M	M	H
Technical and tactical training	Technical	M	M	M	M	L	L	L	M	M	L	L
	Tactical	L	L	L	L	L	L	L	H	H	H	H

Work load (scale 100, 90, 80, 70, 60, 50, 40, 30, 20, 10, 0) — shown as a bar graph.

FIGURE 11.18 *(continued)*

	Aug 8/23-Ohio State	8/29-Penn State	8/31-BYU	9/3-Duguense	9/6-Boston	9/11-Virginia	9/13-Dartmouth	9/18-Pitt.	9/20-Tennessee	9/24-Marquette	9/27-USF	10/2-Notre Dame
Dates — Month	August	August	September	September	September	September	September	September	September	September	October	October
Week ending	29	29	5	5	12	12	19	19	26	26	3	3
Competitions — Away match		C	C			p	C	C			C	
Home competition	C			C	C				C	C		p
Name of competition	8/23-Ohio State	8/29-Penn State	8/31-BYU	9/3-Duguense	9/6-Boston	9/11-Virginia	9/13-Dartmouth	9/18-Pitt.	9/20-Tennessee	9/24-Marquette	9/27-USF	10/2-Notre Dame
Periodization — Training phase	Competitive 2											
Training subphase	Precompetitive						Competitive					
Macrocycle	Macrocycle 2											
Mesocycle	10						11					
Microcycle	35	35	36	36	37	37	38	38	39	39	40	40
Peaking index	4	4	3	3	2	2	3	3	3	3	2	2
Testing dates					T							
Recovery weeks					U				U			
Resistance training — Primary focus	Strength and power						Strength and power					
Strength and endurance	-		-		-		L		-		-	
Basic strength	M		M		L		M		L		L	
Strength and power	H		M		L		M		M		L	
Peaking					H						H	
Endurance, speed and agility endurance, and speed and agility — Primary focus	Tactics and maintenance											
Endurance	L		L		L		M		L		L	
Speed and agility	L		L		L		L		L		L	
Speed and agility endurance	L		L		L		M		L		L	
Technical and tactical training — Technical	L		L		L		L		L		L	
Tactical	H		H		H		H		H		H	
Work load (scale: 100, 90, 80, 70, 60, 50, 40, 30, 20, 10, 0)	bar graph											

FIGURE 11.18 (continued)

Dates	Month	October									November
	Week ending	10		17		24		31			7
Competitions	Away match				C	C	C	C	p		p
	Home competition	C	C	C							
	Name of competition	10/4-DePaul	10/9-Syracuse	10/11-St. Johns	10/16-Villanova	10/18-Georgetown	10/23-Connecticut	10/25-Providence			Conference Tournament (Storrs, Conn.)

Periodization						
	Training phase	Competitive 2				
	Training subphase	Competitive				
	Macrocycle	Macrocycle 2				
	Mesocycle	12				
	Microcycle	41	42	43	44	45
	Peaking index	3	3	2	1	1
	Testing dates					
	Recovery weeks	U			U	U

Resistance training						
	Primary focus	Strength and power				
	Strength and endurance	L	-	-	-	-
	Basic strength	M	L	L	L	L
	Strength and power	M	M	M	L	L
	Peaking				H	H

Endurance, speed and agility, and speed and agility endurance						
	Primary focus	Tactics and maintenance				
	Endurance	M	L	L	L	L
	Speed and agility	L	L	L	L	L
	Speed and agility endurance	M	L	L	L	L

Technical and tactical training						
	Technical	L	L	L	L	L
	Tactical	H	H	H	H	H

Work load: 100, 90, 80, 70, 60, 50, 40, 30, 20, 10, 0

FIGURE 11.18 *(continued)*

Dates	Month		November				December		
	Week ending		14		21	28	5	12	19	26

Competitions		14 (11/13)	14 (11/15)	21	28	5	12	19	26
	Away match	P	P	P	P	P	P		
	Home competition								
	Name of competition	11/13-NCAA First Round	11/15-NCAA Second Round	11/20-11/22: NCAA Championships	11/21, 11/22, or 11/23-NCAA Third Round	12/4-NCAA Semifinals	12/6-NCAA Finals		

Periodization		14	21	28	5	12	19	26
	Training phase	Competitive 2					Transition 2		
	Training subphase	Competitive					Transition		
	Macrocycle	Macrocycle 2							
	Mesocycle	13				14			
	Microcycle	46	47	48	49	50	51	52
	Peaking index	2	2	2	1	5	5	5
	Testing dates				T			
	Recovery weeks				U	R	R	R

Resistance training		14	21	28	5	12
	Primary focus	Strength and power				Recovery
	Strength and endurance	L	-	-	-	-
	Basic strength	M	L	L	-	-
	Strength and power	M	L	L	L	-
	Peaking				H	-

Endurance, speed and agility endurance, and speed and agility		14	21	28	5	12
	Primary focus	Tactics and maintenance				-
	Endurance	M	L	L	L	-
	Speed and agility	L	L	L	L	-
	Speed and agility endurance	M	L	L	L	-

Technical and tactical training		14	21	28	5	12
	Technical	L	L	L	L	-
	Tactical	H	H	H	H	-

Work load	
	100
	90
	80
	70
	60
	50
	40
	30
	20
	10
	0

FIGURE 11.18 *(continued)*

12

Training Program Implementation

Jay R. Hoffman, PhD, CSCS*D, FNSCA
Lee E. Brown, EdD, CSCS*D, FACSM, FNSCA
Abbie E. Smith, PhD, CSCS*D, CISSN

Often, the most complicated aspect of strength and conditioning is putting the entire program together. The previous chapters detail methodologies used to improve specific fitness components involved in athletic performance. However, strength and conditioning professionals must incorporate all of the information and create a yearly training plan that maximizes performance at the appropriate time and minimizes the risk for overtraining. Much of the theory for developing a periodized training program is covered in chapter 11. This chapter focuses on the practical aspects of developing a training program. Examples of specific training programs are used to emphasize important aspects of the discussion.

For all sample resistance training programs in this chapter, the range of repetitions assumes that the last repetition is a maximal effort. The resistance should be adjusted so that the athlete's RM falls into the range given. See pages 84-86 for more on load selection based on the RM.

It is important to note that the yearly training program is specific for each sport. The take-home message from this chapter should be the examples that provide insight on how to build a program and the various influences that may affect program progression. Although no single method has universal acceptance regarding the development of a training program (it is quite specific to the individual sport and athlete), it is understood that for a training program to be effective, it needs to be based on sound science. The various training methods that exist simply give the strength and conditioning professional tools that need to be used at the appropriate times in the yearly training cycle. Many of the examples in this chapter have been used with collegiate basketball and American football programs. Other sports have specific nuances that need to be considered for integration in the yearly training program.

Workout Sessions

Before the onset of any workout, the strength and conditioning professional must lead or direct a structured warm-up routine to prepare athletes for the subsequent workout. Proper warm-up routines can also reduce the risk for injury during training sessions. Whether the use of static stretching exercises should be incorporated into the warm-up is questionable (see chapter 3 for a more detailed discussion). A dynamic warm-up that utilizes exercise-specific movement patterns likely provides the greatest benefit in preparing for the workout. It is important to note that the warm-up should not fatigue athletes for subsequent performance. An example of a dynamic warm-up is shown in the following sidebar.

Sample Dynamic Warm-Up

All exercises are performed for 30 yards (27 m).

1. Lunge walk with reach
2. Lateral step (switch side every 10 yards, or 9 m)
3. Tin soldier (Opposite foot to opposite hand, knee to chest)
4. High-knee walk, followed by glute kick (heel of foot to butt)
5. Side shuffle (switch sides every 10 yards)
6. Carioca
7. Speed skip into skip taps
8. Backward run (reach long)
9. Backward run (shorter steps)
10. Resistive run
11. Two to four bounds that accelerate into a run for 30 yards

As athletes move from one training phase to another, it is imperative that they be physically ready for each proceeding step. The variables of intensity, volume, and exercise selection should progress to provide physical challenges in each subsequent training phase. Emphasis on proper technique should always be a priority. Load should not be emphasized until athletes have demonstrated successful technique in the exercise. The order of exercises within a training session is another variable that can be manipulated for better training results. Refer to chapter 4 for more specific guidelines on the development of the resistance training program, including guidelines for exercise order.

Off-Season Training

The goals of the off-season training program should be specific for each athlete. The key is to find the most effective way to accomplish the goals. For an experienced strength/power athlete, ballistic exercises (e.g., squat jump or bench press throws) may be more effective than for the novice athlete. The strength and conditioning professional needs to examine which training component has the greatest window of adaptation (or the most potential for improvement). This is identified through careful evaluation of the testing results (see chapter 2).

Although high levels of performance ability need to be maintained, the focus of the training prescription should be in the area that has the greatest room for adaptation. The focus of the early part of the off-season training program is primarily on developing hypertrophy, strength, power, and speed, but athletes should maintain a minimal level of conditioning. When possible, they should practice their sport skill. For example, basketball players often accomplished this by participating in pick-up games. For football players, this is more challenging. Still, regardless of sport, athletes should be encouraged to maintain their athleticism and competitiveness by participating in off-season sports, such as basketball and racquet sports.

The basic goal of all off-season training programs is to enhance the performance capability of the athlete. This generally involves training programs that increase power, speed, and strength. Other off-season training goals include altering body composition by increasing lean muscle mass and decreasing fat mass.

As the off-season program begins, the focus should be primarily in the weight room. Every athlete can benefit from being stronger or more powerful. As chapters 4 and 11 discuss, the resistance training program generally begins with a paradigm of high-volume (greater number of repetitions performed per set) and low-intensity (loads with a low percentage of the athlete's 1RM) exercises. The purpose for this is to prepare athletes for the higher intensity lifting that they will perform during the latter stages of the training program, and to focus on the hypertrophy phase of the periodized training program. The duration of time spent at this stage will depend on the athlete's training goals. If the athlete is focused on increasing muscle size (may be common among younger athletes), more time may be spent at this phase of training. If the athlete's primary goal is to increase strength and power, then this phase will be used to prepare for more complicated exercises of higher intensity that will be incorporated into the latter phases of the training program.

Figure 12.1*a* and *b* provide examples of off-season training programs for a strength/power athlete who plays a fall sport. This can be adjusted to meet other athletes' needs using the approximate time frames for each phase. Two examples are provided. One uses a longer duration for each training phase and assumes that no sport-specific practices, such as spring football, will interrupt

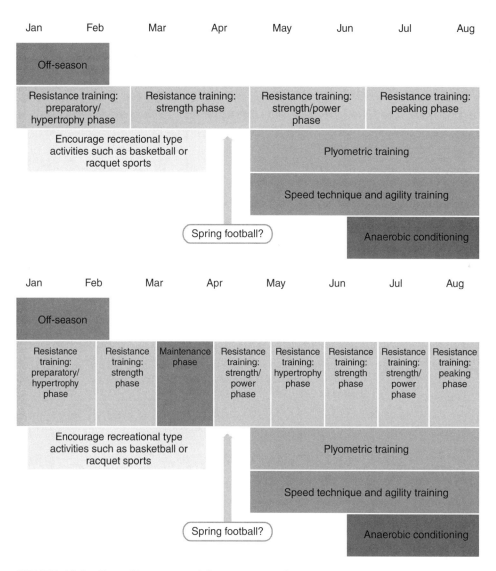

FIGURE 12.1 Two off-season training programs for a strength/power sport, such as American football: (*a*) Does not allow for interruptions in the training program, but (*b*) makes allowances for spring competition.

the training program. The other example repeats the various training cycles and accounts for spring football. In addition, it may be prudent to use an off-loading period (one week) between each training phase for recovery.

Although many examples in this chapter show programs for strength/ power athletes, keep in mind that a well-designed resistance training program can benefit athletes in a wide range of sports. Table 12.1 depicts a 15-week resistance training program for tennis, which is not considered to be a strength/power sport. However, tennis athletes can benefit tremendously from resistance training.

TABLE 12.1 15-Week Tennis Program (Training Three Days per Week)

Exercise	Sets × repetitions, weeks 1-5	Sets × repetitions, weeks 6-10	Sets × repetitions, weeks 11-15
Monday			
Hang clean	3 × 4-6	4 × 3-5	5 × 2-4
Back squat	3 × 10-12	3 × 8-10	3 × 6-8
Bench press	3 × 10-12	3 × 8-10	3 × 6-8
Lunge	3 × 8-10		
Lateral dumbbell raise	3 × 10-12		
Trunk rotation	3 × 25		
Internal/external rotations	3 × 10		
Wednesday			
Leg press	4 × 8-10	4 × 6-8	4 × 4-6
Stiff-leg deadlift	3 × 10-12	3 × 8-10	3 × 6-8
Front pulldown	3 × 10-12	3 × 8-10	3 × 6-8
Calf raise	3 × 10-12		
Reverse fly	3 × 10-12		
Russian twist	3 × 25-30		
Ulnar/radial deviation	2 × 10		
Scapula stabilizer circuit	2 × 10		
Friday			
Hang snatch	3 × 4-6	4 × 3-5	5 × 2-4
Front squat	3 × 10-12	3 × 8-10	3 × 6-8
Seated row	3 × 10-12	3 × 8-10	3 × 6-8
Inclined dumbbell press	3 × 10-12	3 × 8-10	3 × 6-8
Wrist/reverse curl	3 × 10-12		
Internal/external rotations	3 × 10-12		
Abdominal crunch	3 × 25-30		

Intensity: 60% to 85% of 1RM periodized

Rest intervals: 2-3 min for core exercises, 1-2 min for assistance exercises, 30-60 s for abdominal exercises

Preparatory Phase

The initial training phase, as mentioned previously, is the preparatory/hypertrophy phase. Table 12.2 provides an example of the resistance training program used for a strength/power athlete during this time. This program is generally four to eight weeks in length, depending on the athlete's goals. During this phase of training, the athlete may also perform recreational activities (e.g., basketball, racquet sports), but the primary focus will be on the resistance exercise program.

If losing body fat is an important part of the off-season training goals, then appropriate adjustments must be made to account for a greater aerobic endurance aspect of the training program. However, good evidence indicates that high-intensity training is an effective stimulus for increasing fat oxidation (11). It must be acknowledged that for the resistance trained athlete, a greater emphasis on aerobic endurance activity will likely have a negative effect on maximum strength and power gains (1, 10). Considering the potential beneficial effects of high-intensity training on fat oxidation, a combination between these two forms of training (resistance and high-intensity running) may be more accommodating to the desired training outcomes.

TABLE 12.2 Example of a Split-Routine Resistance Training Program (4 Days per Week): Preparatory/Hypertrophy Phase for a Strength/Power Athlete

Exercise	Sets × repetitions	Exercise	Sets × repetitions
Days 1 and 3		**Days 2 and 4**	
Squat	1*, 4 × 8-12	Bench press	1*, 4 × 8-12
Leg extension	3 × 8-12	Inclined bench press	3 × 8-12
Leg curl	3 × 8-12	Inclined fly	3 × 8-12
Standing calf raise	3 × 8-12	Seated shoulder press	1*, 4 × 8-12
Lat pulldown	1*, 4 × 8-12	Upright row	3 × 8-12
Seated row	1*, 4 × 8-12	Lateral raise	3 × 8-12
Dumbbell biceps curl	3 × 8-12	Triceps pushdown	3 × 8-12
Barbell biceps curl	3 × 8-12	Triceps extension	3 × 8-12
Hyperextension	3 × 8-12	Sit-up	3 × 20
Crunch	3 × 20		

Rest: 1 min between each set, 72 hours between days 1 and 3 and between days 2 and 4. Days 1 and 2 and days 3 and 4 can be performed consecutively. For instance, this split-routine training program can be performed on Monday, Tuesday, Thursday, and Friday (4 days per week).

*Indicates at least one warm-up set.

The training program depicted in table 12.2, is a four-day split routine, in which each body part is trained twice per week. The athlete is required to use the same relative intensity during each resistance training session. However, some variability to training volume is to be expected, since the number of repetitions per training session may differ to account for recovery from the preceding training session. In following with the progressive overload principle, once the athlete can achieve the desired training goal (e.g., maximum number of repetitions per session), the resistance can be elevated during the next training session. Although the relative intensity remains the same, training volume actually increases (load × number of repetitions). This is often called a *traditional* or *classic periodization program* and has been referred to in recent sport-science literature as *linear periodization*. However, chapter 11 discusses, there is a very good debate regarding the appropriateness of the *linear* term.

An alternative method of training uses a different loading scheme for each workout. This has been referred to as an *undulating* or *nonlinear periodization program* (9). Table 12.3 provides an example of a three-day nonlinear

TABLE 12.3 Undulating Program for Competitive Strength/Power Athletes

Exercise	Sets × reps	Exercise	Sets × reps	Exercise	Sets × reps
Monday		**Wednesday**		**Friday**	
Squat	1*, 4 × 3-5	Front squat	1*, 4 × 6-8	Dumbbell lunges	3 × 10-12
Bench press	1*, 4 × 3-5	Inclined bench press	1*, 4 × 6-8	Dumbbell bench press	3 × 10-12
Push press	1*, 4 × 3-5	Seated dumbbell shoulder press	1*, 4 × 6-8	Seated shoulder press	3 × 10-12
High pull	3 × 3-5	Dumbbell upright row	3 × 6-8	Compound set: Shrugs and lateral raises	3 × 10-12 × 2
Lat pulldown	3 × 3-5	Seated row	3 × 6-8	Dumbbell bent-over rows	3 × 10-12
Triceps pushdown	3 × 6-8	Triceps extension	3 × 6-8	Weighted dips	3 × 10-12
Standing biceps curl	3 × 3-5	Dumbbell seated biceps curl	3 × 6-8	Dumbbell hammer curls	3 × 10-12
Sit-up	3 × 20	Crunches	3 × 20	Back extensions	3 × 8-10

*Indicates at least one warm-up set.

training program that may be considered for athletes in the off-season. However, it is important to note that recent research has suggested that the traditional periodized training model may be more effective during short-term (~15 weeks), off-season training programs for collegiate strength/power athletes (8). An additional concern for strength and conditioning professionals developing off-season training programs is the experience level of their athletes. For the more experienced resistance-trained athlete, it appears that the inclusion of assistance exercises (e.g., inclined bench press, inclined fly) is important for providing the necessary training stimulus (7).

Strength

The next training cycle during the off-season generally focuses on strength development. The intensity during this training phase increases as compared to the preparatory/hypertrophy phase, resulting in fewer repetitions being performed per set. As a result, the total volume of training (expressed as sets × number of repetitions) is decreased. During this training phase, the strength and conditioning professional may incorporate additional exercises (primarily multiple-joint, structural movement exercises) into the training program to increase the training stimulus. An example of this training program can be viewed in table 12.4. In comparison to the train-

TABLE 12.4 Example of a Split-Routine Resistance Training Program: Strength Phase for Strength/Power Athletes (4 Days per Week)

Exercise	Sets × reps	Exercise	Sets × reps
Days 1 and 3		**Days 2 and 4**	
Squat	1*, 4 × 6-8	High pulls	1*, 4 × 6-8
Dead lifts	3 × 6-8	Bench press	1*, 4 × 6-8
Leg curls	3 × 6-8	Inclined bench press	3 × 6-8
Standing calf raise	3 × 6-8	Inclined fly	3 × 6-8
Lat pulldown	1*, 4 × 6-8	Seated shoulder press	1*, 4 × 6-8
Seated row	1*, 4 × 6-8	Front/lateral raise	3 × 6-8
Dumbbell biceps curl	3 × 6-8	Triceps pushdown	3 × 6-8
Barbell biceps curl	3 × 6-8	Triceps extension	3 × 6-8
Hyperextension	3 × 8-12	Sit-up	3 × 20
Crunch	3 × 20		

Rest: 3 min between each set, 72 hours between days 1 and 3 and between days 2 and 4. Days 1 and 2 and days 3 and 4 can be performed consecutively. For instance, this split-routine training program can be performed on Monday, Tuesday, Thursday, and Friday (4 days per week).

*Indicates at least one warm-up set.

ing program for the preparatory/hypertrophy phase seen in table 12.2, this program begins to incorporate Olympic-style lifting movements (e.g., high pulls). These exercises could also appear during the initial phase of training, but inexperienced or novice athletes may benefit from developing a strength base and proper technique with traditional power lifting exercises. In addition, the incorporation of these exercises in the latter phases of training provides a degree of variation to the training program that prevents monotony. This training phase can also last between four and six weeks.

In some programs, strength and conditioning professionals may begin to incorporate additional modes of training. For instance, plyometric exercises or speed and agility drills can be incorporated into the training schedule. During the off-season conditioning program for American football, plyometric exercises can be incorporated into the strength mesocyle. The incorporation of plyometric exercises should also move progressively from low-intensity to high-intensity exercises. Table 12.5 provides a list of plyometric exercises that are separated by level of intensity.

Typically, exercises of low intensity incorporate two-leg jumps from ground level. Single-leg jumps, bounds, jumps from height (depth jumps), and repeated jumps onto boxes increase the intensity of training. An important aspect of program design is the decision whether to include or to limit the volume of plyometric training. Consider the type of sport. For instance, basketball and volleyball athletes can be expected to play pick-up games during the off-season. The jumps that the athletes perform during this recreational play need to be considered, since they will still contribute to overall fatigue. Adding plyometric exercises to the training programs of these athletes without accounting for their recreational participation can increase the risk for overtraining syndrome.

In general, the ideal training program has athletes perform plyometric exercises on the days for upper body resistance training. If upper body plyometric exercises are to be included, they should be performed on days for lower body resistance training. A sample training program for integrating both strength and plyometric training can be seen in table 12.6. It is also possible to include several lower body plyometric exercises as part of the lower body resistance training program. However, the strength and conditioning professional should be careful to not fatigue the athlete. As different modes of exercise are added, to reduce the incidence of overreaching, it would be prudent to reduce the volume of training for other exercises. For instance, if a few plyometric exercises are included on days for a lower body lifting routine, a few of the lower body assistance exercises should be removed. Using the training program described in table 12.4, the strength and conditioning professional can substitute box jumps for deadlifts on one of the lower body lifting days to avoid overtraining the athlete.

TABLE 12.5 Examples of Plyometric Exercises

Drill	Intensity	Starting position	Action
Standing long jump	Low	Stand in a semisquat position with feet shoulder-width apart.	With a big arm swing and a counter-movement with the legs, jump as far forward as possible.
Squat jump	Low	Stand in squat position with thighs parallel with floor and with fingers interlocked and hands behind head.	Jump to maximum height without moving hands. On landing, return to starting position.
Skipping	Low	Stand comfortably.	Lift one leg with knee bent to 90° while lifting the opposite arm (elbow also bent to 90°). Alternate between both sides. For added difficulty, push off ground for more upward extension.
Power skipping	Low	Stand comfortably.	With a double-arm action, move forward in a skipping motion, bringing the lead leg as high as possible in an attempt to touch the hands. Try to get as much height as possible when pushing off with the back leg. Each repetition should be performed with alternate leg.
Front cone hop	Low	Stand with feet shoulder-width apart in front of a line of cones.	Keeping feet shoulder-width apart, jump over each cone, landing on both feet at the same time. Use a double-arm swing and attempt to stay on the ground for as little time as possible.
Single-leg push-off with box	Low	Stand on ground in front of box 6-12 in. (15-30 cm) high. Place heel of one foot on the box near the closest edge.	Push off the top foot to gain as much height as possible by extending through entire leg and foot. Use a double-arm swing to gain height and maintain balance.
Medicine ball throw	Low	Stand and hold a medicine ball overhead.	Step forward and throw the ball with both arms to a partner or for a specified distance. This drill can also be performed as a chest pass, either sitting or standing.
Front box jump	Low-Moderate	Stand in front of box 12-42 in. (30-107 cm) high (depending on ability), with feet shoulder-width apart and hands behind head.	Jump up and land with both feet on the box, and then step down. For a more advanced exercise, hop down and immediately hop back on top. Use a variety of box heights.
Tuck jump with knees up	Moderate	Stand with knees slightly bent and feet shoulder-width apart.	Jump vertically as high as possible, bringing the knees to the chest and grasping them with the hands before returning to the floor. Land in a standing vertical position.

Drill	Intensity	Starting position	Action
Lateral cone hop	Moderate	Stand with knees slightly bent and feet shoulder-width apart to the side of a row of cones.	Jump sideways down the row of cones, landing on both feet. When the row is completed, begin to jump back to starting position. This drill should be performed with 3-5 cones placed 2-3 ft (60-90 cm) apart.
Standing triple jump	Moderate	Stand with feet shoulder-width apart and bend at knee with a slight forward lean.	With a countermovement, jump as far up and forward as possible with both feet, as in the long jump. On landing, make contact with only one foot. Immediately jump off, using the same foot. Get maximal distance and land with the opposite foot, then take off again. Land from this jump is with both feet.
Multiple box-to-box jumps	Moderate	Stand in front of 3-5 boxes 12-42 in. high (depending on ability), with feet shoulder-width apart.	Jump onto the first box then off of it. Jump onto the next box and continue to the end of the line, using a double-arm action for gaining height and maintaining balance.
Depth jump to prescribed height	Moderate	Stand on a box 12-42 in. high (the higher the box, the greater the intensity of the exercise) in front of a box of similar height, with toes close to edge and feet shoulder-width apart.	Step from the box and drop to the ground with both feet. As soon as foot contact is made, jump explosively as high as possible onto the second box. Try to make as little contact with the ground as possible.
Alternate-leg bounding	Moderate	Begin with one foot slightly in front of the other and arms at the side. Use a rocker step or begin from a jog.	Push off with the front leg and drive the knee up and out. Try to get maximal horizontal and vertical distance with either an alternating or double-arm action. Try to hang in the air for as long as possible. On landing, repeat with opposite leg. The goal is to cover maximal distance with each jump. This is not designed to be a race or sprint.
Power drop with medicine ball	Moderate -High	Lie supine on the ground with arms outstretched next to a box 12-42 in. high. A partner stands on the box holding a medicine ball.	When the partner drops the ball, catch it and immediately throw it back.
Double-leg or single-leg zigzag hop	Moderate -High	Place about 6-10 cones about 1.5-2 ft (46-60 cm) apart in a zigzag pattern. Begin with feet shoulder-width apart and knees slightly bent.	Jump diagonally over the first cone. After landing, change directions and jump diagonally over each of the remaining cones. Jumping with a single leg is considered to be a high-intensity plyometric exercise.

(continued)

TABLE 12.5 *(continued)*

Drill	Intensity	Starting position	Action
Pike jump	Moderate-High	Stand with feet shoulder-width apart and knees slightly bent.	Jump up and bring the legs together in front of the body. Flexion should occur at only the hips. Attempt to touch the toes at the peak of the jump. Return to starting position.
Depth jump	High	Stand on a box 12-42 in. high (the higher the box, the greater the intensity of the exercise), with toes close to the edge and feet shoulder-width apart.	Step from the box and drop to the ground with both feet. As soon as the feet make contact, jump explosively as high as possible. Try to have as little contact with the ground as possible.
Split squat with cycle	High	Stand upright, with feet split front to back as far as possible. The front leg forms a 90° angle at the hip and 90° at the knee.	Perform a maximal vertical jump while switching leg position. As the legs switch, attempt to flex the knee so that the heel of the back foot comes close to the buttocks. Land in the split-squat position and jump again.
Single-leg hop	High	Place one foot slightly ahead of the other as in initiating a step. The arms are at the side.	Using a rocker step or jogging into the starting position, drive the knee of front leg up and out as far as possible. At the same time, using a double-arm action. Hold the nonjumping leg in a stationary position, with the knee flexed during the exercise. The goal is to hang in the air as long as possible. Land with the same leg and repeat.
Multiple box-to-box squat jump	High	Stand in front of 3-5 boxes that are 12-42 in. high (depending on ability). Assume a parallel squat position, with feet shoulder-width apart and hands behind head or on hips.	Jump onto the first box, maintaining squat position, then jump off. Jump onto the next box, and then continue to the end of the line. Keep the hands behind the head or at the hips.
Single-leg depth jump	High	Stand on a box 12-18 in. high, with toes close to the edge and feet shoulder-width apart.	Step from the box and drop to the ground, landing with one foot. As soon as the foot contacts the ground, jump explosively as high as possible with a single foot. Try to touch the ground as little as possible.
Single-leg bounding	High	Stand on one foot.	Bound from one foot as far forward as possible, using the other leg and arms to cycle in air for balance and increase forward momentum.

TABLE 12.6 Sample of Integrated Strength and Plyometric Training Program

Day	Resistance training	Plyometric training
Monday	High-intensity upper body exercises	Low-intensity lower body exercises
Tuesday	High-intensity lower body exercises	—
Wednesday	—	—
Thursday	Low-intensity upper body exercises	High-intensity lower body exercises
Friday	Low-intensity lower body exercises	—

Reprinted, by permission, from J.R. Hoffman, 2002, *Physiological aspects of sport training and performance* (Champaign, IL: Human Kinetics), 169-184.

Strength and Power

The next phase of training is the power or strength/power phase. During this training phase, the intensity of exercise is elevated further and training volume is reduced from the levels for the initial strength phase. For the collegiate football player, this phase may be interrupted by spring football. If this is the case, the athlete will likely enter a maintenance program for the duration of spring football. Next, the strength and conditioning professional can begin the resistance training program again from the hypertrophy phase and then proceed to the other training phases. The purpose of returning to the hypertrophy phase is to reduce the intensity of training and to help the athlete recover from spring football. However, this is often not a concern for other sports, so those athletes will continue to focus on their off-season training goals.

During the strength/power phase, a greater emphasis is placed on Olympic and ballistic exercises. Power performance is enhanced by using multiple-joint, compound structural movements that combine both speed of movement and high force output. Exercises such as the snatch, power clean, and push press are often added to the program. Some of the traditional power lifting exercises or assistance exercises are removed. Table 12.7 provides an example of a split-routine resistance training program performed four days per week that is used for the strength/power phase. Previous research has shown that Olympic exercises can enhance speed and power development in resistance trained athletes during their off-season training program to a greater extent than traditional power lifting exercises can (3). In addition, a speed and agility program is often included in this training phase. These exercises generally do not result in a change to the resistance training program.

TABLE 12.7   Example of a Split-Routine Resistance Training Program: Power Phase for Strength/Power Athletes (4 Days per Week)

Exercise	Sets × reps	Exercise	Sets × reps
Days 1 and 3		**Days 2 and 4**	
Squat	1*, 4 × 4-6	High pulls/power clean	1*, 4 × 4-6
Dead lifts/snatch	4 × 4-6	Bench press	1*, 4 × 4-6
Leg curl	3 × 4-6	Inclined bench press	3 × 4-6
Lat pulldown	1*, 4 × 4-6	Push press/push jerk	1*, 4 × 4-6
Seated row	1*, 4 × 4-6	Front/lateral raise	3 × 4-6
Dumbbell biceps curl	3 × 4-6	Triceps pushdown	3 × 4-6
Barbell biceps curl	3 × 4-6	Triceps extension	3 × 4-6
Hyperextension	3 × 8-12	Abdominal/core routine	3 × 20
Crunch	3 × 20		

Rest: 3 min between each set, 72 hours between days 1 and 3 and between days 2 and 4. Days 1 and 2 and days 3 and 4 can be performed consecutively. For instance, this split-routine training program can be performed on Monday, Tuesday, Thursday, and Friday (4 days per week).

*Indicates at least one warm-up set.

Speed and Agility

During the power phase of training, a speed and agility routine is often incorporated into the weekly routine. For team sports, one purpose of these exercises is often to get the team to work together. A more important goal is to enhance the athlete's performance in these movement variables. This routine is not designed for conditioning. As such, the work-to-rest interval is relatively longer than one would expect when goals include conditioning.

For example, the work-to-rest ratio for an exercise that enhances anaerobic capacity (see chapter 6) may be 1:4; however, when focusing on the quality per repetition, the work-to-rest ratio can elongate to 1:8. The focus during this training phase, as related to agility, speed, and plyometric exercises, is on the quality of work, not the quantity. As the athlete moves into the later stages of the off-season training program, the speed and agility work becomes more up-tempo to contribute to aspects of anaerobic conditioning. However, a longer work-to-rest ratio still requires 100% effort for each drill.

Examples of speed technique and agility drills for athletes participating in a strength/power phase are depicted in the sidebar. These drills are often performed in a circuit fashion twice per week. For example, circuit-format agility drills could include (in order) stations for the *T* drill, Edgren side step, pro-agility drill, *L* drill, and agility ladder drill. A circuit for plyometric drills might include stations for the standing long jump, front or side box jumps, single-leg hops, medicine ball throw, and depth jumps, in that order. These circuits are commonly used for American football, basketball, baseball, and other strength/power sports. These circuits would also be very beneficial for soccer, field hockey, and lacrosse athletes, since they require greater levels of cardiorespiratory endurance but would still benefit from power development.

Administratively, the team is divided into five groups of players. Players go through each drill for 3 minutes. For instance, 60 players are participating in these drills, each group would consist of 12 players. If the drill takes 5 seconds to complete, then each athlete would receive approximately 3 repetitions. Again, as mentioned earlier, the quality is much more important than the quantity. Thus, using the previous time example, each athlete

Sprinting Technique and Agility Drills

Sprinting technique drills:

- Heel ups (p. 172)
- Arm action (p. 173)
- Lean fall and run (p. 174)
- Drop and go (p. 175)
- Bound into run (p. 176)
- Jump and go (p. 176)
- Scramble and go (p. 177)
- Light sled pulls (p. 180)
- Cone jumps and sprint (p. 184)
- Sprint starts: first 4 steps out of the stance
- Sprint starts: first 8 steps out of the stance
- Two sprints of 30 yards (27 m)

Agility Drills:

- T test (p. 43)
- Pro-agility test (p. 44)
- Figure eights (p. 156)
- 40-yard lateral shuffle (p. 154)
- 15-yard turning drill (p. 154)
- Z-pattern run (p. 156)
- 20-yard square (p. 155)
- Agility ladder drills (pp. 157-160)

would perform approximately 15 repetitions. Athletes can be randomly assigned to each drill area (athletes of similar ability are recommended to be grouped together, perhaps separated by position). They should move from one drill to the next in a clockwise fashion.

The following sections describe sample agility training programs for basketball and field sports. Keep in mind that as agility drills are added to the training program, the volume of training in the resistance exercise program is generally reduced (fewer repetitions performed per workout). If the added training volume is not accounted for, the risk of overtraining may increase.

Basketball Agility Program

Table 12.8 provides an example of a simple basketball agility program. The drills included contain similar movement patterns to those a basketball player would encounter in a game situation (e.g., figure eight). The training frequency is two or three times per week, since this has been demonstrated to be effective in previous training studies. Also, as previously discussed, agility drills should be performed at maximal or near-maximal intensity to elicit optimal adaptations. Volume will consist of two sets of 10 repetitions for each exercise.

TABLE 12.8 Basketball Agility Program

Exercise	Frequency	Intensity	Volume	Rest
20 yd shuttle	2-3	Max	2 sets of 10	2-3 min
20 yd square	2-3	Max	2 sets of 10	2-3 min
Figure eight	2-3	Max	2 sets of 10	2-3 min
Ladder: In-out	2-3	Max	2 sets of 10	2-3 min
Carioca	2-3	Max	2 sets of 10	2-3 min

For example, the athlete will perform 10 consecutive repetitions of the exercise. This constitutes one set. The very fast paced nature of basketball, which is evident in the offense-to-defense transitions required throughout the game, necessitates continuous change of direction. This is provided by the shuttle sprints at the prescribed volume assignments. The 2- or 3-minute recovery periods should be adequate between sets; however, this may be adjusted accordingly by the strength and conditioning professional, depending on factors like athlete fatigue.

Field Sports Agility Program: Fast Footwork, Close Quarters

This sample agility program (table 12.9) would be appropriate for many of the field sports, such as American football, soccer, lacrosse, and rugby. It emphasizes fast footwork and change of direction in enclosed or limited spaces. Since both teams in these particular sports can have multiple players on the field at once, it is very common to operate in tight spaces. For example, an attacking soccer player attempting to advance the ball toward the goal will have to maneuver through multiple opponents. As the opposing team closes in, fast footwork within the confined space will be crucial to maintain possession of the ball. For the defender, one-on-one situations will require the athlete to mirror the offensive player, using close-quarter footwork and change of direction to avoid getting beaten. Dead-ball situations, such as free kicks and corner kicks, also involve a substantial number of attacking and defending players in one area, severely limiting space availability. To obtain a more suitable position to put the ball in the back of the net, players on the attacking team will often try to lose their marks, using fast feet and quick changes of direction. This clearly demonstrates a need for agile movements in tight spaces.

TABLE 12.9   Agility Program for Field Sports: Fast Footwork, Close Quarters

Exercise	Frequency (per week)	Intensity	Volume	Rest
Hexagon	1-3	Max	3 sets of 3 (clockwise and counterclockwise)	1-2 min
Double-leg lateral hop	1-3	Max	5 sets of 1	1-2 min
Ladder: Ickey shuffle	1-3	Max	5 sets of 1	1-2 min
Ladder: Side right-in	1-3	Max	5 sets of 1	1-2 min
Ladder: Crossover shuffle	1-3	Max	5 sets of 1	1-2 min
Ladder: Snake jump	1-3	Max	5 sets of 1	1-2 min

The exercises listed in table 12.9 all consist of fast-footwork, change-of-direction drills in enclosed or limited spaces. The frequency is listed as one to three times per week depending on scheduling considerations. For instance, if this agility program is utilized in conjunction with other training programs (e.g., resistance training) or during the in-season phase, the lower end of the range might be more appropriate. If this program is used exclusively, three times per week may be more beneficial.

The volume and rest periods for most of the drills are listed as five sets of 1 minute or 1 to 2 minutes respectively, with the exception of the hexagon drill. The volume for the hexagon drill is prescribed as three sets of three for both directions, meaning three consecutive repetitions should be performed both clockwise and counterclockwise. The volume for the remainder of the drills has been established at five sets of one because it is assumed that teams will train together. Thus, instead of doing all five repetitions consecutively, everyone on the team will complete one repetition at a time and then wait for their teammates to perform the same drill before moving on the next set. Furthermore, as a result of going through the drill in turns, the time between repetitions should provide close to the 1 to 2 minutes of rest time prescribed.

Field Sports Agility Program: Change of Direction Over Varying Distances

In addition to close quarter agility needs, field-sport athletes also cover large amounts of ground with change-of-direction events interspersed throughout an event. This program (table 12.10) aims to integrate change-of-direction tasks with a variety of distances encountered throughout a game. The strength and conditioning professional may also want to consider adding sport specificity to these drills if desired. Examples include soccer athletes performing a shuttle sprint while dribbling and lacrosse athletes running with the stick. Training frequency is prescribed as one to three times per week for the same reasons described previously for the fast-footwork, close-quarters agility program. For example, this workout could be conducted once per week and the fast-footwork, close-quarters program could be conducted twice per week, or vice versa. As always, intensity should be maximum or near-maximum. Volume assignments decrease as the total distance covered in a given drill increases, such as in the 60- and 100-yard (55 and 91 m) shuttle sprints. Greater recovery periods are also provided for these drills, since they consist of more changes of direction and longer distances.

TABLE 12.10 Agility Program for Field Sports: Change of Direction Over Varying Distances

Exercise	Frequency (per week)	Intensity	Volume	Rest
15 yd turn drill	1-3	Max	5 sets of 1	1-2 min
20 yd square	1-3	Max	5 sets of 1	1-2 min
Z-pattern run	1-3	Max	5 sets of 1	1-2 min
40 yd lateral shuffle	1-3	Max	3 sets of 1	2-3 min
60 yd shuttle sprint	1-3	Max	3 sets of 1	3-5 min
100 yd shuttle sprint	1-3	Max	3 sets of 1	3-5 min

Peaking

The next phase of training is the peaking phase. During this phase of training, the intensity of training is at its highest, while the volume of training is reduced further. Here, the athlete begins to make final preparations for either the most important competition or the start of preseason training camp. The lower training volume also gives the athlete additional time to focus on anaerobic conditioning exercises. During the final two to three weeks of the strength/power phase and throughout the peaking phase, the athlete will focus on getting in anaerobic condition to play a competitive season. Table 12.11 provides an example of a resistance training program during the peaking phase, and table 12.12 depicts a 13-week anaerobic conditioning program for speed, technique, and agility for athletes preparing for a competitive season. Note that the conditioning phase begins approximately eight weeks prior to the onset of the preseason.

TABLE 12.11   Example of a Split-Routine Resistance Training Program: Peaking Phase for Strength/Power Athletes (4 Days per Week)

Exercise	Sets × reps	Exercise	Sets × reps
Monday		**Tuesday**	
Clean (floor)	5 × 1-3	Snatch (floor)	5 × 1-3
Push jerk	5 × 1-3	Clean pulls (above knee)	3 × 1-3
Squat	5 × 1-3	Bench press	5 × 1-3
Box jump	3 × 5	Push press	4 × 3
Core	4x	Core	4x
Thursday		**Friday**	
Snatch (floor)	5 × 1-3	Clean pull (waist)	4 × 1-3
Clean pulls (above knee)	3 × 1-3	Bench press	5 × 1-3
Bench press	5 × 1-3	Inclined bench press	3 × 5
Push press	4 × 3	Push jerk	4 × 1-3
Core	4x	Power shrug	4 × 3
Clean (above knee)	5 × 1-3	Core	4x

The daily goal is to achieve a 3 rep max with each lift. The athlete may fall short of 3 reps on your last sets (e.g., 1-2). Prior to reaching the workout session weight, the athlete may need to perform 2-3 warm-up sets. The rest period between sets should be 3-5 min.

Anaerobic Conditioning in the Peaking Phase

Anaerobic conditioning is comprised of short- and long-distance sprints, as well as interval training. Chapter 6 discusses the basis of this conditioning program. The volume of training for anaerobic conditioning will increase from week to week. Intensity is controlled by altering the work-to-rest ratio. As the athlete gets closer to preseason training, the time between each sprint should decrease. Toward the end of the training cycle, the work-to-rest ratio should simulate that typical of actual performance. At specific times

TABLE 12.12 Agility, Speed, and Conditioning Program

Week	Monday	Tuesday	Wednesday	Thursday	Friday	Saturday
1		Agility and form running		Agility and form running		
2		Agility and form running		Agility and form running		
3		Agility and form running		Agility and form running		
4		Agility and form running		Agility and form running		
5		Agility and form running		Agility and form running		
6		Agility and form running	2 × 200 yd, 5 × 60 yd sprints	Agility and form running	1 × line drill, 2 × intervals	
7		Agility and form running	4 × 200 yd, 6 × 60 yd sprints	Agility and form running	1 × line drill, 3 × intervals	
8	4 × starts, 3 × intervals	Agility and form running	4 × 200 yd, 6 × 60 yd sprints	Agility and form running	1 × line drill, 3 × intervals	4 × 200 yd, 4 × 100 yd, 4 × 40 yd sprints
9	6 × starts, 3 × intervals	Agility and form running	5 × 200 yd, 8 × 60 yd sprints	Agility and form running	2 × line drill, 3 × intervals	4 × 200 yd, 4 × 100 yd, 4 × 40 yd sprints
10	8 × starts, 4 × intervals	Agility and form running	6 × 200 yd, 8 × 60 yd sprints	Agility and form running	2 × line drill, 4 × intervals	5 × 200 yd, 5 × 100 yd, 5 × 40 yd sprints
11	10 × starts, 4 × intervals	Agility and form running	7 × 200 yd, 10 × 60 yd sprints	Agility and form running	3 × line drill, 4 × intervals	5 × 200 yd, 5 × 100 yd, 5 × 40 yd sprints
12	10 × starts, 5 × intervals	Agility and form running	8 × 200 yd, 10 × 60 yd sprints	Agility and form running	3 × line drill, 4 × intervals	6 × 200 yd, 6 × 100 yd, 6 × 40 yd sprints
13	10 × starts, 6 × intervals	3 × line drill	8 × 200 yd, 10 × 60 yd sprints	Agility and form running	Rest	Report to camp

(i.e., near the onset of the season), the work-to-rest ratio may exceed that seen during actual performance. This may be needed to provide an additional overload that can stimulate further physiological adaptations.

As discussed earlier in this chapter, many athletes continue to stay in condition during the off-season by playing their sports. These athletes will maintain a certain level of conditioning that has to be acknowledged. If not, a mistake could be made in the exercise prescription that can put these athletes at risk for overtraining. In general, strength and conditioning professionals should plan for six to eight weeks of anaerobic conditioning to prepare their athletes for competition.

Anaerobic athletes should not start preparing to be metabolically ready for a season of competition until two to four weeks before the preseason training program (4). Until this phase, the athlete's off-season conditioning program is primarily focused on resistance training, power development (plyometrics), and sport-specific skill development (including agility and speed development). Anaerobic conditioning is not emphasized until the preseason phase to prevent any possible overtraining syndrome from occurring during the season. However, athletes should be strongly encouraged to maintain some level of fitness throughout the off-season.

For many sports (both professional and collegiate), the preseason period is approximately six weeks in duration. The goal during this phase of training is to bring the athlete close to peak condition, but not necessarily all the way there. Although this last statement is quite ambiguous, there is a reason for it. For instance, in the off-season, the primary contact person for college athletes is the strength and conditioning professional. Once official practice begins, the team will begin practicing with the rest of the coaching staff. This time period before the competitive season begins is also referred to as the *preseason*. However, for the athlete, this will be *preseason II*. Depending on the specific situation involved, many strength and conditioning professionals devote much of this time to conditioning drills. During this phase of training, it may be prudent for strength and conditioning professionals to provide room for improvement. A problem of fatigue or overreaching may develop if athletes peak too soon. The ideal situation is for the strength and conditioning professional and the coaching staff of the athlete's sport to work together regarding the development of the yearly training program. Although this appears to be quite logical, many mistakes are made in exercise prescription that result from poor communication. A clear understanding of the goals of a practice session determines whether additional conditioning drills are needed or whether practice is sufficient in stimulating physiological adaptation.

Anaerobic Conditioning for Team Sports

An example of a preseason anaerobic conditioning program is presented in table 12.13. This program was developed for college basketball players and is performed four days per week with a progression in both intensity and volume. It is also important to notice how the intensity of the workouts is manipulated by changes in the work-to-rest ratio during the sprint training. The aim in reducing the work-to-rest ratio is to improve the recovery time between the bouts of high-intensity activity typically seen during a basketball game. In addition, as described previously, there is a great deal of variability in the movement patterns and intensity levels of these movements. To provide for a greater similarity to the game, it may be prudent to design the training program with exercises that simulate such changes. The use of interval or Fartlek training should become an integral part of the program. Considering the variation in intensity and length of sprints that these drills use, it gives the strength and conditioning professional a more effective way to simulate the changes that may occur in a game of basketball. Specific descriptions of these types of training exercises will be presented later.

TABLE 12.13   Example of an Anaerobic Conditioning Program for Basketball

	Day 1	Day 2	Day 3	Day 4
Weeks 1-2	Intervals 3-4 laps	Sprints (distance × reps) 400 m × 1 100 m × 2 30 m × 8 Work-to-rest ratio = 1:4	Intervals 3-4 laps	Sprints (distance × reps) 200 m × 4-5 Work-to-rest ratio = 1:4
Weeks 3-4	Intervals 4-5 laps	Sprints (distance × reps) 400 m × 1 100 m × 3-4 30 m × 8-10 Work-to-rest ratio = 1:4	Intervals 4-5 laps	Sprints (distance × reps) 200 m × 5-6 Work-to-rest ratio = 1:4
Weeks 5-6	Intervals 5-6 laps	Sprints (distance × reps) 400 m × 2 100 m × 4-5 30 m × 10-12 Work-to-rest ratio = 1:3	Intervals 5-6 laps	Sprints (distance × reps) 200 m × 6-7 Work-to-rest ratio = 1:3

Reprinted, by permission, from J. Hoffman, *Physiological Aspects of sport training and performance* (Champaign, IL: Human Kinetics), 93-108.

Anaerobic Conditioning for Individual Sports

As discussed in chapter 6, anaerobic training for individual sports, such as sprint-distance running events, should focus on decreasing fatigue rate over the course of a single sprint, rather than preparing the athlete for repeated high-intensity activity over a long time. Table 12.14 depicts the rest intervals recommended for enhancing speed-endurance for the 400 m sprinter. Notice the long rest intervals between sprints. Obviously, the goal for the 400 m sprinter is not to improve recovery time but to maximize the quality of each sprint.

TABLE 12.14   Speed-Endurance Training for 400 m Sprinters

Number of sprints	Distance of each sprint (m)	Recovery time between sprints (min)
10	100	5-10
6	150	5-10
5	200	10
4	300	10
3	350	10
2	450	10

The distance of each sprint can vary. However, the total distance run per workout should be approximately 2.5 times the distance of the athlete's event. Thus, if the athlete were a 400 m sprinter, then he should run 1,000 m in sprints per workout. The length of the rest period should ensure complete recovery.

Adapted from USA Track and Field (12).

Competitive Season

Once the preseason begins and as the athlete enters the competition, the primary focus will be actual sport performance. Although coaches may continue to condition their athletes during practice, the actual intensity of practice should be taken into consideration regarding the volume of conditioning drills. The duration and frequency of actual sprinting that occurs during practice sessions should also be calculated and taken into account to determine whether specific conditioning drills should be performed during practice or whether they would pose a greater risk for overtraining. However, strength and conditioning professionals may decide to provide additional conditioning exercises for team-sport players who are not in their regular playing rotation. This will provide them with the necessary physiological stimulus to maintain a high level of conditioning and to be ready if the need for an increase in playing time occurs.

The effort necessary to maintain the strength and power gains made during the off-season is extremely important. At times, it is overlooked by sport strength and conditioning professionals. Research has clearly shown that these strength and power gains can be maintained by a resistance training program performed two days per week (2, 5, 6). Typically, the volume and intensity utilized during the strength phase is incorporated, and only the core lifts are required (see table 12.15). The purpose is to use exercises that recruit the largest muscle mass and simulate sport performance. Interestingly, several studies have shown that strength improvements can also be seen during the maintenance phase in young athletes who have limited experience with resistance training (5, 6).

TABLE 12.15 In-Season Resistance-Training Maintenance Program

Exercise	Sets	Reps
Power clean	4	4-6
Squat	4	6-8
Bench press	4	6-8
Push press	4	4-6

Considerations for Endurance Athletes

Similar to that for strength/power athletes, the training program for athletes participating in an aerobic endurance sport is periodized to help them reach peak condition at the appropriate time of the year. One of the largest differences between these two types of athletes is that the majority of strength/power athletes participating in a team sport focus on a competitive season in which importance is placed on all contests. In contrast, aerobic endurance athletes, although participating in several meets during the season, are preparing to peak at a specific contest at the end of the competitive season. These athletes actually train through the earlier contests in order to reach peak performance for the more important contests that occur at the end of the season. Another difference between the two types of athletes is that aerobic endurance athletes generally do not perform speed or agility training. However, some may use resistance training to support specific goals (see chapter 4). The following sections discuss specific training strategies for aerobic endurance events. In addition, examples of training programs are provided.

Long Distance: Marathon

The marathon distance is becoming more and more popular for recreational runners. Once thought of as a race for only serious runners, the distance offers a challenge that is now appealing and, with proper training, feasible for many runners. Many websites offer free training plans for the marathon that allow athletes to modify volume and intensity based on current race time, number of weeks before the event, and current fitness level. If their goal is not just to finish a marathon, but rather to improve performance time, athletes might consider adding a tempo or hill workout each week. Table 12.16 shows a 16-week marathon training program for a beginner. A more advanced runner might use a program more like that shown in table 12.17.

Training for a half marathon calls for reduced volume, specifically by reducing the training day for long, slow distance (LSD) work, and perhaps by adding an additional speed session each week. Athletes may also increase the intensity of existing speed sessions. Training for an ultra-endurance run requires more volume and less intensity over a longer training period.

TABLE 12.16   Beginner Training Program for a Marathon

Monday	Tuesday	Wednesday	Thursday	Friday	Saturday	Sunday
Weeks 1-7						
Rest	3 miles	4 miles	Rest	3 miles 2-3 hill sprints	Rest	5 miles
Weeks 8-11						
Rest	6 miles	4 miles	5 miles	4 miles 5-6 hill sprints	Rest	12 miles
Weeks 12-15						
Rest	6 miles	7 miles	5 miles	4 × 1 mile @ 10K pace	Rest	20 miles
Week 16						
Rest	4 miles	Rest	3 miles	Rest	Easy run or rest	Race

TABLE 12.17   Intermediate Training Program for a Marathon

Monday	Tuesday	Wednesday	Thursday	Friday	Saturday	Sunday
Weeks 1-7						
Rest or easy run	3 miles	5 miles	Rest or easy run	4 miles 2-3 hill sprints	3 miles	8 miles
Weeks 8-11						
Rest	5 miles	4 × 1 mile @ 10K pace	8 miles	6 miles 5-6 hill sprints	8 miles	16 miles
Weeks 12-15						
Rest	8 miles	10 miles	6 miles	10 × 800 m @ 3K/5K pace	Rest	20 miles
Week 16						
Rest	6 miles	Rest or easy run	5 miles	Rest	2-3 miles easy	Race

Moderate Distance: Triathlon

Triathlon training can cross a wide spectrum of training areas, depending on the distance of competition. In all cases, training strategies include a variety of swim, bike, and running workouts that use all the concepts covered in this chapter: LSD, intervals, Fartlek training, and, of course, recovery. Several helpful websites are available to help establish specific programs. Table 12.18 provides a sample two-week triathlon training cycle.

TABLE 12.18   Example of a Two-Week Triathlon Training Cycle

Monday	Tuesday	Wednesday	Thursday	Friday	Saturday	Sunday
Week 1						
Day off	Swim: Speed-endurance 100 s Cycling: Tempo 90 min (60 min in zone)	Run: 60 min (30 min tempo)	Swim: Aerobic endurance (base)—intervals Cycling: Hill reps 60-75 min (5 × 3 min/6 reps)	Run: 30 min easy	Cycling: Aerobic endurance 90-120 min Run: Transition immediately after bike 15 min	Swim: 30-45 min technique Run: Aerobic endurance 80 min
Week 2						
Day off	Swim: Speed-endurance 25 s/50 s Cycling: Tempo 90 min (60 min in zone)	Run: 60 min (40 min tempo)	Swim: Aerobic endurance (base) 400s/200s/100s Cycling: Hill reps 75 min (5 × 3 min/6 reps)	Day off	Swim: 1,500 m time trial Cycling: Aerobic endurance 120 min Run: Transition immediately after bike 20 min	Run: Aerobic endurance 90 min Cycling: Easy 30 min

Shorter Endurance Events

A benefit of the 5K distance is that almost anyone, at any fitness level, can train to run a 5K in as little as six to eight weeks. Training for a 5K consists of less volume and more intensity than that required for longer aerobic endurance events. Table 12.19 is a sample 5K training plan for an intermediate runner.

Training for a 10K requires more volume than the 5K because of the increased length of the race. Intermediate runners should perform one

TABLE 12.19   Three-Week 5K Training Plan for Intermediate Runners

Monday	Tuesday	Wednesday	Thursday	Friday	Saturday	Sunday
Rest/easy run	2 miles 4 × 100 m strides	3 miles	Rest/easy run	3 miles 2-3 hill sprints	2 miles	4 miles
Rest/easy run	2 miles 6 × 200 m @ 5K pace	4 miles	Rest/easy run	3 miles 4-5 hill sprints	2 miles	6 miles
Rest/easy run	2 miles 6 × 400 m @ 5K pace	4 miles	Rest/easy run	3 miles 5-7 hill sprints	3 miles	8 miles

or two training runs per week that are longer than the race distance. For beginners, longer training runs may not be as necessary if their primary goal is just to finish the race. When completing speed workouts geared towards a specific distance, the goal should be to have the distance of the speed workout eventually equal the race distance (e.g., when training for a 5K, 12 × 400 m nearly equals a 5K). It's important to gradually work up to this volume of speed work to avoid injury.

Swim Training

For either an advanced swimmer or a novice, designing daily workouts can be a challenge. Variation, technique, and speed are elements that are important and are often overlooked. Table 12.20 provides example days of a swimming training plan.

Rowing

Rowing can also be considered an aerobic endurance sport, depending on the length of competition and fitness goals. It may also serve as a great method of cross-training for various aerobic endurance athletes. Unfamiliarity is a common roadblock when looking for other avenues to improve fitness. Table 12.21 shows a sample rowing workout.

Program Evaluation

An integral part in the development of athletes' training program and the evaluation of the effectiveness of the training program is the continual monitoring and evaluation of the fitness and performance levels of the athletes. The ability to properly assess athletes provides strength and conditioning professionals with a greater understanding of how to maximize their players' athletic performance and, as a result, maximize the effort placed in developing optimal training programs. As discussed in chapter 2, this type of testing provides a thorough analysis of all the components comprising athletic performance (i.e., strength, anaerobic power, speed, agility, maximal aerobic capacity and endurance, flexibility, and body composition). Results from testing can help determine the relevance and importance of each fitness component to a particular sport. They also permit appropriate emphasis to be placed on that variable in the athletic training program. Athletes and strength and conditioning professionals alike can use these standards as a motivational tool when establishing personal training goals by comparing their results to normative data from similar athletic populations. Performance testing can also be used to provide baseline data for prescribing individual exercise programs, giving feedback in the evaluation of a training program, and providing information concerning the extent of recovery following injury.

TABLE 12.20 Example Days for Swim Training Plan

EXAMPLE DAY 1			EXAMPLE DAY 2		
Duration	45-60 min		Duration	30-45 min	
Distance	2,800 yd		Distance	2,000 yd	
Pool length	25 yd		Pool length	25 yd	
Stroke	**Sets × reps**	**Notes**	**Stroke**	**Sets × reps**	**Notes**
Warm-up					
Any stroke (even pace)	4 × 100 yd	Rest 0:15 / 100 yd (Swim your choice of stroke at a steady pace)	Any stroke (even pace)	4 × 50 yd	Rest 0:15 / 50 yd
Build-up (repeat 6 times day 1, 4 times day 2)					
Front scull and kick	1 × 50 yd	Rest 0:15 / 50 yd (Streamline body position with straight arms and kicking)	Streamline kicking	1 × 50 yd	Rest 0:15 / 50 yd
Freestyle push and glide	1 × 50 yd	Rest 0:15 / 50 yd (Freestyle swim, pausing at the end of every stroke with arms outstretched, one held out from, the other loosely against the body)	Freestyle push and glide	1 × 50 yd	Rest 0:15 / 50 yd
Core					
Freestyle swim	2 × 200 yd	Leave on 4:10 / 200 yd	Freestyle swim	6 × 50 yd	Target time 00:56 / 50 yd Rest 0:20 / 50 yd
Freestyle swim	4 × 100 yd	Leave on 2:10 / 100 yd	Freestyle swim	6 × 50 yd	Target time 00:56 / 50 yd Rest 0:15 / 50 yd
Freestyle swim	2 × 200 yd	Leave on 4:10 / 200 yd	Freestyle swim	6 × 50 yd	Target time 00:56 / 50 yd Rest 0:20 / 50 yd
Freestyle swim	80 × 50 yd	Leave on 1:05 / 50 yd	Freestyle swim	6 × 50 yd	Target time 00:56 / 50 yd Rest 0:10 / 50 yd
Cool-down					
Freestyle easy	2 × 50 yd	Rest 0:15 / 50 yd	Freestyle easy	2 × 50 yd	Rest 0:15 / 50 yd
Backstroke easy	2 × 50 yd	Rest 0:15 / 50 yd	Backstroke easy	2 × 50 yd	Rest 0:15 / 50 yd

TABLE 12.21   Sample Workouts From a Rowing Training Plan

COMPETITION TRAINING		
Duration	45 min	
Difficulty	Intermediate	
Action	**Time**	**Intensity**
Warm-up		
10 stroke bursts	5 min	Increasing
Core		
5 rowing intervals	1 min hard, 30 s easy	Moderate
5 rowing intervals	1 min hard, 30 s easy	Fast
5 rowing intervals	1 min hard, 30 s easy	Moderate
5 rowing intervals	1 min hard, 30 s easy	Very fast
Cool-down		
Active recovery	10 min	Easy
GENERAL FITNESS		
Duration	45 min (including warm-up and cool-down)	
Difficulty	Beginner	
Stroke rate	**Time**	**Pace**
22	Row 16 min Rest 3 min	Easy, conversational
26	Row 16 min	Slightly faster

SUMMARY POINTS

- The key to successfully developing the training regimen for athletes is to base the program on sound scientific evidence. The information that is presented in this book is based on evidence found in sport science literature. This allows strength and conditioning professionals to defend the program and to provide the best techniques to train their athletes.
- Individual workout sessions should always include a proper dynamic warm-up. Workouts should emphasize proper technique before increasing load.
- The basic goal of off-season training is to enhance athletes' capabilities. The basic phases of most off-season training programs are the preparatory phase, strength phase, strength/power phase, and peaking phase.
- Off-season training goals should be specific to the needs of the athlete.

In many programs, plyometric training and speed-agility training can be introduced during the strength and strength/power phases.

- During the season, the goal is to maintain gains made in the off-season. For strength/power gains, this goal can be accomplished with a program that runs two days per week.

- Although this book provides examples of various training routines, as discussed in chapter 1, the individual responses to the same training program will be quite varied. This is due to a host of reasons that include training experience and genetic potential. Strength and conditioning professionals need to evaluate their programs based on the response of the athletes.

References

Chapter 1

1. Alentorn-Geli E, Myer GD, Silvers HJ, et al. Prevention of non-contact anterior cruciate ligament injuries in soccer players. Part 2: A review of prevention programs aimed to modify risk factors and to reduce injury rates. *Knee Surgery, Sports Traumatology, Arthroscopy.* 2009; 17: 859-879.

2. Andrews JR, Harrelson GL, Wilk KE. *Physical Rehabilitation of the Injured Athlete.* 3rd ed. Philadelphia, PA: Saunders; 2004.

3. Baker D, Wilson G, Carlyon R. Periodization: The effect on strength of manipulating volume and intensity. *Journal of Strength and Conditioning Research.* 1994; 8: 235-242.

4. Bloomer RJ, Ives JC. Varying neural and hypertrophy influences in a strength program. *Strength and Conditioning Journal.* 2000; 22: 30-35.

5. Bloomfield J, Polman R, O'Donoghue P, McNaughton L. Effective speed and agility conditioning methodology for random intermittent dynamic type sport. *Journal of Strength and Conditioning Research.* 2007; 21: 1093-1100.

6. Borghuis J, Hof AL, Lemmink KA. The importance of sensory-motor control in providing core stability: Implications for measurement and training. *Sports Medicine.* 2008; 38: 893-916.

7. Campos GE, Luecke TJ, Wendeln HK, et al. Muscular adaptations in response to three different resistance-training regimens: Specificity of repetition maximum training zones. *European Journal of Applied Physiology.* 2002; 88: 50-60.

8. Dudley GA, Djamil R. Incompatibility of endurance- and strength-training modes of exercise. *Journal of Applied Physiology.* 1985; 59: 1446-1451.

9. Fleck SJ, Kraemer WJ. *Designing Resistance Training Programs.* 3rd ed. Champaign, IL: Human Kinetics; 2004.

10. Folland JP, Williams AG. The adaptations to strength training: Morphological and neurological contributions to increased strength. *Sports Medicine.* 2007; 37: 145-168.

11. Fry AC, Kraemer WJ. Resistance exercise overtraining and overreaching. Neuroendocrine responses. *Sports Medicine.* 1997; 23: 106-129.

12. Fry RW, Morton AR, Keast D. Overtraining in athletes. An update. *Sports Medicine.* 1991; 12: 32-65.

13. Giza E, Micheli LJ. Soccer injuries. *Medicine and Sport Science.* 2005; 49: 140-169.

14. Halson SL, Jeukendrup AE. Does overtraining exist? An analysis of overreaching and overtraining research. *Sports Medicine.* 2004; 34: 967-981.

15. Hreljac A. Impact and overuse injuries in runners. *Medicine and Science in Sports and Exercise.* 2004; 36: 845-849.

16. Kerssemakers SP, Fotiadous AN, deJonge MC, Karantanas AH, Mass M. Sport injuries in the paediatric and adolescent patient: A growing problem. *Pediatric Radiology.* 2009; 39: 471-484.

17. Knobloch K, Jagodzinski M, Haasper C, Zeichen J, Krettek C. Gymnastic school injuries—Aspects of preventive measures. *Sportverltz Sportsschaden.* 2006; 20: 81-85.

18. Kraemer WJ. Exercise prescription in weight training: A needs analysis. *National Strength and Conditioning Association Journal.* 1983; 5: 64-65.

19. Kraemer WJ. Exercise prescription: Needs analysis. *National Strength and Conditioning Association Journal.* 1984; 6: 47.

20. Kraemer WJ. A series of studies: The physiological basis for strength training in American football: Fact over philosophy. *Journal of Strength and Conditioning Research.* 1997; 11: 131-142.

21. Kraemer WJ, Fleck SJ. *Optimizing Resistance Training Programs.* Champaign, IL: Human Kinetics; 2007.

22. Kraemer WJ, Nindl BA. Factors involved with overtraining for strength and power. In: Kreider RF, O'Toole AM, eds. *Overtraining in Sport.* Champaign, IL: Human Kinetics; 1998: 69-86.

23. Kraemer WJ, Ratamess NA. Fundamentals of resistance training: Progression and exercise prescription. *Medicine and Science in Sports and Exercise.* 2004; 36: 674-688.

24. Kraemer WJ, Fry AC, Rubin MR, et al. Physiological and performance responses to tournament wrestling. *Medicine and Science in Sports and Exercise.* 2001; 33: 1367-1378.

25. Kraemer WJ, Patton JF, Gordon SE, et al. Compatibility of high-intensity strength and endurance training on hormonal and skeletal muscle adaptations. *Journal of Applied Physiology.* 1995; 78: 976-989.

26. Kraemer WJ, Noble BJ, Clark MJ, Culver BW. Physiological responses to heavy resistance exercise with very short rest periods. *International Journal of Sports Medicine.* 1987; 8: 247-252.

27. McArdle WD, Katch FI, Katch VL. *Exercise Physiology; Energy, Nutrition, and Human Performance.* 5th ed. Philadephia, PA: Lippincott Williams & Wilkins; 2001.

28. Myer GD, Ford KR, Palumbo JP, Hewett TE. Neuromuscular training improves performance and lower-extremity biomechanics in female athletes. *Journal of Strength and Conditioning Research.* 2005; 19: 51-60.

29. Paulsen G, Myklestad D, Raastad T. The influence of volume of exercise on early adaptations to strength training. *Journal of Strength and Conditioning Research.* 2003; 17: 115-120.

30. Pearce PZ. Prehabilitation: Preparing young athletes for sports. *Current Sports Medicine Reports.* 2006; 5: 155-160.

31. Ratamess NA, Kraemer WJ, Volek JS, et al. The effects of amino acid supplementation on muscular performance during resistance training overreaching. *Journal of Strength and Conditioning Research.* 2003; 17: 250-258.

32. Sale DG. Neural adaptation to resistance training. *Medicine and Science in Sports and Exercise.* 1985; 20: S135-S145.

33. Smith CE, Nyland J, Caudill P, Brosky J, Carbon DN. Dynamic trunk stabilization: A conceptual back injury prevention program for volleyball athletes. *Journal of Orthopaedic and Sports Physical Therapy.* 2008; 38: 703-720.

34. Smith LK, Weiss EL, Lehmkuhl LD. *Brunnstrom's Clinical Kinesiology.* 5th ed. Philadelphia, PA: FA Davis; 1996.

35. Taimela S, Kujala UM, Osterman K. Intrinsic risk factors and athletic injuries. *Sports Medicine.* 1990; 9: 205-215.

36. Woods K, Bishop P, Jones E. Warm-up and stretching in the prevention of muscular injury. *Sports Medicine.* 2007; 37: 1089-1099.

37. Zatsiorsky VM, Kraemer WJ. *Science and Practice of Strength Training,* 2nd ed. Champaign, IL: Human Kinetics; 2006.

Chapter 2

1. American College of Sports Medicine (ACSM). *Guidelines for Exercise Testing and Prescription*. Franklin BA, ed. Philadephia, PA: Lippincott Williams & Wilkins; 2000.

2. Anderson DE. Reliability of air displacement plethysmography. *Journal of Strength and Conditioning Research*. 2007; 21: 169-171.

3. Ayalon A, Inbar O, Bar-Or O. Relationships among measurements of explosive strength and anaerobic power. In: Nelson and Morehouse, eds. *International Series on Sport Sciences. Vol I Biomechanics IV*. Baltimore, MD: University Park Press; 1974: 527-532.

4. Ballard T.P., L. Fafara and M.D. Vukovich. Comparison of Bod Pod and DXA in female collegiate athletes. *Medicine and Science in Sports and Exercise*. 2004. 36: 731-735.

5. Bar-Or O. The Wingate anaerobic test: An update on methodology, reliability and validity. Sports Medicine. 1987; 4:381-394.

6. Bar-Or O, Dotan R, Inbar O, Rotstein A, Karlsson J, Tesch P. Anaerobic capacity and muscle fiber type distribution in man. International Journal of Sports Medicine. 1980; 1:89-92.

7. Bosco C, Mognoni P, Luhtanen P. Relationship between isokinetic performance and ballistic movement. European Journal of Applied Physiology. 1983; 51:357-364.

8. Brzycki M. Strength testing: Predicting a one-rep max from reps to fatigue. *Journal of Health, Physical Education, Recreation and Dance*. 1993. 64:88-90.

9. Cook EE, Gray VL, Savinar-Nogue E, Medeiros J. Shoulder antagonistic strength ratios: A comparison between college-level baseball pitchers and nonpitchers. *Journal of Orthopedic and Sports Physical Therapy*. 1987; 8:451-460.

10. Davis JA, Dorado S, Keays KA, Reigel KA, Valencia KS, Pham PH. Reliability and validity of the lung volume measurement made by the BOD POD body composition system. *Clinical Physiology Functional Imaging*. 2007; 27: 42-46.

11. Durnin JV, Womersley J. Body fat assessment from total body density and its estimation from skinfold thickness: Measurements on 481 men and women aged 16-72 years. *British Journal of Nutrition*. 1974; 32:77-97.

12. Ebbeling CB, Ward A, Puleo EM, Widrick J, Rippe JM. Development of a single-stage submaximal treadmill walking test. *Medicine and Science in Sports and Exercise*. 1991; 23:966-973.

13. Ellenbecker TS. A total arm strength isokinetic profile of highly skilled tennis players. *Isokinetic Exercise Science*. 1991; 1:9-21.

14. Epley B. Poundage chart. Lincoln, NE. *Boyd Epley Workout*. 1985.

15. Falk B, Weinstein Y, Dotan R, Abramson DR, Mann-Segal D, Hoffman JR. A treadmill test of sprint running. *Scandinavian Journal of Medicine and Science in Sports*. 1996; 6:259-264.

16. Fornetti WC, Pivarnik JM, Foley JM, Fliechtner JJ. Reliability and validity of body composition measures in female athletes. *Journal of Applied Physiology*. 1999; 87:1114-1122.

17. Gettman LR. Fitness testing. In: Durstine JL, King AC, Painter PL, Roitman JL, Zwiren LD, eds. *ACSM's Resource Manual for Guidelines for Exercise Testing and Prescription*. 2nd ed. Philadelphia, PA: Williams & Wilkins; 1993: 229-246.

18. Hakkinen K, Komi PV, Alen M, Kauhanen H. EMG, muscle fibre and force production characteristics during a 1 year training period in highly competitive weightlifters. *European Journal of Applied Physiology and Occupational Physiology*. 1987; 56:419-427.

19. Harman EA, Rosenstein MT, Frykman PN, Rosenstein RM, Kraemer WJ. Estimation of human power output from vertical jump. *Journal of Applied Sport Science Research*. 1991; 5:116-120.

20. Harris RC, Edwards RH, Hultman E, Nordesjo LO, Nylind B, Sahlin K. The time course of phosphorylcreatine resynthesis during recovery of the quadriceps muscle in man. *Pflugers Archives*. 1976; 367:137-142.

21. Heyward VH, Stolarczyk LM. *Applied Body Composition Assessment*. Champaign, IL: Human Kinetics; 1996.

22. Hoeger WW, Hopkins DR, Barette SL, Hale DF. Relationship between repetitions and selected percentages of one repetition maximum: A comparison between untrained and trained males and females. *Journal of Applied Sports Science Research*. 1990; 4:47-54.

23. Hoffman JR.. *Physiological Aspects of Sport Training and Performance*. Champaign, IL: Human Kinetics; 2002: 169-184.

24. Hoffman JR. *Norms for Fitness, Performance, and Health*. Champaign, IL: Human Kinetics; 2006: 3-115.

25. Hoffman JR, Fry AC, Howard R, Maresh CM, Kraemer WJ. Strength, speed and endurance changes during the course of a division I basketball season. *Journal of Applied Sport Science Research*. 1991; 5:144-149.

26. Hoffman JR, Kang J, Ratamess NA, Hoffman MW, Tranchina CP, Faigenbaum AD. Examination of a high energy, pre-exercise supplement on exercise performance. *Journal of the International Society of Sports Nutrition*. 2009; 6:2.

27. Hoffman JR, Kraemer WJ, Fry AC, Deschenes M, Kemp M. The effect of self-selection for frequency of training in a winter conditioning program for football. *Journal of Applied Sport Science Research*. 1990; 3:76-82.

28. Hoffman JR, Ratamess NA, Faigenbaum AD, Mangine GT, Kang J. Effects of maximal squat exercise testing on vertical jump performance in college football players. *Journal of Sports Science and Medicine*. 2007; 6:149-150.

29. Hoffman JR, Ratamess NA, Faigenbaum AD, Ross R, Kang J, Stout JR. Short duration β-alanine supplementation increases training volume and reduces subjective feelings of fatigue in college football players. *Nutrition Research*. 2008; 28:31-35.

30. Jackson AS, Pollock ML. Practical assessment of body composition. *Physician and Sports Medicine*. 1985; 13:76-90.

31. Katch V, Weltman A, Martin R, Gray L. *Optimal test characteristics for maximal anaerobic work on the bicycle ergometer*. Research Quarterly. *1977; 48:319-327.*

32. Knapik JJ, Bauman CL, Jones BH, Harris JM, Vaughan L. Preseason strength and flexibility imbalances associated with athletic injuries in female collegiate athletes. *American Journal of Sports Medicine*. 1991; 19:76-81.

33. Landers J. Maximum based on reps. *National Strength and Conditioning Association Journal*. 1985; 6: 60-61.

34. Leveritt M, Abernethy PJ. Acute effects of high-intensity endurance exercise on subsequent resistance activity. *Journal of Strength and Conditioning Research*. 1999; 13: 47-51.

35. Lohman TG. Skinfolds and body density and their relation to body fatness: A review. *Human Biology*. 1981; 53: 181-225.

36. Mayhew JL, Ball TE, Bowen JC. Prediction of bench press lifting ability from submaximal repetitions before and after training. *Sports Medicine, Training and Rehabilitation*. 1992; 3:195-201.

37. Mayhew JL, Ware JS, Bemben MG, et al. The NFL-225 test as a measure of bench press strength in college football players. *Journal of Strength and Conditioning Research*. 1999; 13:130-134.

38. O'Toole ML, Douglas PS, Hiller WD. Applied physiology of a triathlon. *Sports Medicine*. 1989; 8: 201-225.

39. Pineau JC, Guihard-Costa AM, Bocquet M. Validation of ultrasound techniques applied to body fat measurement. A comparison between ultrasound techniques, air

displacement plethysmography and bioelectrical impedance vs. dual-energy X-ray absorptiometry. *Annals of Nutrition and Metabolism*. 2007; 51: 421-427.

40. Pipes TV. Variable resistance versus constant resistance strength training in adult males. *European Journal of Applied Physiology and Occupational Physiology*. 1978; 17; 39(1): 27-35.

41. Radley D, Gately PJ, Cooke CB, Carroll S, Oldroyd B, Truscott JG. Estimates of percentage body fat in young adolescents: A comparison of dual-energy X-ray absorptiometry and air displacement plethysmography. *European Journal of Clinical Nutrition*. 2003; 57: 1402-1410.

42. Radley D, Cooke CB, Fuller NJ, Oldroyd B, Truscott JG, Coward WA, Wright A, Gately PJ. Validity of foot-to-foot bio-electrical impedance analysis body composition estimates in overweight and obese children. *International Journal of Body Composition Research*. 2009; 7: 15-20.

43. Ross RE, Ratamess NA, Hoffman JR, Faigenbaum AD, Kang J, Chilakos A. The effects of treadmill sprint training and resistance training on maximal running velocity and power. *Journal of Strength and Conditioning Research*. 2009; 23:385-394.

44. Sargeant AJ, Hoinville E, Young A. Maximum leg force and power output during short-term dynamic exercise. *Journal of Applied Physiology*. 1981; 26:188-194.

45. Visser M, Fuerst T, Lang T, Salamone L, Harris T. Validity of fan-beam dual-energy X-ray absorptiometry for measuring fat-free mass and leg muscle mass. *Journal of Applied Physiology*. 1999; 87: 1513-1520.

Chapter 3

1. American College of Sports Medicine. *ACSM's Guidelines for Exercise Testing and Prescription*. 8th ed. Baltimore, MD: Lippincott, Williams and Wilkins; 2010.

2. Asmussen E, Bonde-Peterson F, Jorgenson K. Mechano-elastic properties of human muscles at different temperatures. *Acta Physiologica Scandinavica*. 1976; 96: 86-93.

3. Behm D, Button D, Butt JC. Factors affecting force loss with prolonged stretching. *Canadian Journal of Applied Physiology*. 2001; 26: 262-272.

4. Behm DG, Bambury A, Cahill F, Power K. Effect of acute static stretching on force, balance, reaction time, and movement time. *Medicine and Science in Sports and Exercise*. August 2004; 36(8): 1397-1402.

5. Bergh U, Ekblom B. Influence of muscle temperature on maximal strength and power output in human muscle. *Acta Physiologica Scandinavica*. 1979; 107: 332-337.

6. Bradley P, Olsen P, Portas M. The effect of static, ballistic, and proprioceptive neuromuscular facilitation stretching on vertical jump performance. *Journal of Strength and Conditioning Research*. 2007; 21(1): 223-226.

7. Burkett LN, Phillips WT, Ziuraitis J. The best warm-up for the vertical jump in college-age athletic men. *Journal of Strength and Conditioning Research*. August 2005; 19(3): 673-676.

8. Chatzopoulos D, Michailidis C, Giannakos A, et al. Postactivation potentiation effects after heavy resistance exercise on running speed. *Journal of Strength and Conditioning Research*. 2007; 21(4): 1278-1281.

9. Cissik J, Barnes M. *Sport Speed and Agility*. Monterey, CA: Healthy Learning; 2004.

10. Cornwell A, Nelson A, Sidaway B. Acute effects of stretching on the neuromuscular properties of the triceps surae muscle complex. *European Journal of Applied Physiology*. 2002; 86: 428-434.

11. Cornwell A, Nelson AG, Heise GD, Sidaway B. Acute effects of passive muscle stretching on vertical jump performance. *Journal of Human Movement Studies*. 2001; 40: 307-324.

12. de Villarreal SS, Gonzalez-Badillo JJ, Izquierdo M. Optimal warm-up stimuli of muscle activation to enhance short and long-term acute jumping performance. *European Journal of Applied Physiology.* July 2007; 100(4): 393-401.

13. Devore P, Hagerman P. A pre-game soccer warm-up. *Strength and Conditioning Journal.* 2006; 28(1): 14-18.

14. Faigenbaum A, Kang J, McFarland J. Acute effects of different warm-up protocols on anaerobic performance in teenage athletes. *Pediatric Exercise Science.* 2006; 17: 64-75.

15. Faigenbaum A, McFarland J. Guidelines for implementing a dynamic warm-up for physical education. *Journal of Physical Education Recreation and Dance.* 2007; 78: 25-28.

16. Faigenbaum A, Westcott W. *Youth Strength Training: Programs for Health, Fitness and Sport.* Champaign, IL: Human Kinetics; 2009.

17. Faigenbaum AD, Mcfarland JE, Kelly N, Ratamess NA, Kang J, Hoffman JR. Influence of recovery time on warm-up effects in adolescent athletes. *Pediatric Exercise Science.* 2010; 22: 266-77.

18. Faigenbaum AD, McFarland JE, Schwerdtman JA, Ratamess NA, Kang J, Hoffman JR. Dynamic warm-up protocols, with and without a weighted vest, and fitness performance in high school female athletes. *Journal of Athletic Training.* Oct-Dec 2006; 41(4): 357-363.

19. Fletcher IM, Jones B. The effect of different warm-up stretch protocols on 20 meter sprint performance in trained rugby union players. *Journal of Strength and Conditioning Research.* 2004; 18(4): 885-888.

20. Fowles J, Sale D, MacDougall J. Reduced stretch after passive stretch of the human plantarflexors. *Journal of Applied Physiology.* 2000; 89: 1179-1188.

21. Fradkin AJ, Gabbe BJ, Cameron PA. Does warming up prevent injury in sport? The evidence from randomized controlled trials. *Journal of Science and Medicine in Sport.* 2006; 9(3): 214-220.

22. Gullich A, Schmidleicher D. MVC-induced short term potentiation of explosive force. *New Studies in Athletics.* 1996; 11: 67-81.

23. Hayes P, Walker A. Pre-exercise stretching does not impact upon running economy. *Journal of Strength and Conditioning Research.* 2007; 21(4): 1227-1232.

24. Hedrick A. Dynamic flexibility training. *Strength and Conditioning.* 2000; 22(5): 33-38.

25. Herman SL, Smith D. Four-week dynamic stretching warm-up intervention elicits longer-term performance benefits. *Journal of Strength and Conditioning Research.* 2008; 22(4): 1286-1297.

26. Hoffman JR. *Physiological Aspects of Sports Training and Performance.* Champaign, IL: Human Kinetics; 2002.

27. Jeffreys I. *Total Soccer Fitness.* Monterey, CA: Healthy Learning; 2007.

28. Jeffreys I. Warm-up and stretching. In: Baechle T, Earle R, eds. *Essentials of Strength and Conditioning.* 3rd ed. Champaign, IL: Human Kinetics; 2008: 296-324.

29. Jones J. Warming up for intermittent endurance sports. *Strength and Conditioning Journal.* 2007; 29(6): 70-77.

30. Judge L, Craig BW, Baudendistal S, Bodey K. An examination of the stretching practices of Division I and Division III college football programs in the midwestern United States. *Journal of Strength and Conditioning Research.* 2009; 23(4): 1091-1096.

31. Kilduff L, Bevan H, Kingsley M, et al. Postactivation potentiation in professional rugby players: Optimal recovery. *Journal of Strength and Conditioning Research.* 2007; 21(4): 1134-1138.

32. Knudson D. Current issues in flexibility fitness. *Presidents Council on Physical Fitness and Sport.* 2000; 3(1): 1-6.

33. Knudson D, Noffal G, Bahamonde R, Bauer JA, Blackwell J. Stretching has no effect on tennis serve performance. *Journal of Strength and Conditioning Research.* 2004; 18(3): 654-656.

34. Kokkonen J, Nelson A, Cornwell A. Acute muscle stretching inhibits maximal strength performance. *Research Quarterly for Exercise and Sport.* 1998; 69: 411-415.

35. Kokkonen J, Nelson A, Eldredge C, Winchester JB. Chronic static stretching improves exercise performance. *Medicine and Science in Sports and Exercise.* 2007; 39(10): 1825-1831.

36. Martens R. *Successful Coaching.* 3rd ed. Champaign, IL: Human Kinetics; 2004.

37. Masamoto N, Larson R, Gates T, Faigenbaum A. Acute effects of plyometric exercise on maximum squat performance in male athletes. *Journal of Strength and Conditioning Research.* 2003; 17(1): 68-71.

38. McMillian DJ, Moore JH, Hatler BS, Taylor DC. Dynamic vs. static-stretching warm up: The effect on power and agility performance. *Journal of Strength and Conditioning Research.* August 2006; 20(3): 492-499.

39. Nelson A, Kokkonen J. Acute ballistic msucle stretching inhibits maximal stretch performance. *Research Quarterly for Exercise and Sport.* 2001; 72(4): 415-419.

40. Nelson A, Kokkonen J, Arnall DA. Acute muscle stretching inhibits muscle strength endurance performance. *Journal of Strength and Conditioning Research.* 2005; 19(2): 338-343.

41. Nelson A, Kokkonen J, Eldredge C. Strength inhibition following an acute stretch is not limited to novice stretchers. *Research Quarterly for Exercise and Sport.* 2005; 76(4): 500-506.

42. Pearce AJ, Kidgell DJ, Zois J, Carlson JS. Effects of secondary warm up following stretching. *European Journal of Applied Physiology.* January 2009; 105(2): 175-183.

43. Rassier D, MacIntosh B. Coexistence of potentiation and fatigue in skeletal muscle. *Brazilian Journal of Medical and Biological Research.* 2000; 33: 499-508.

44. Sale D. Postactivation potentiation: Role in human performance. *Exercise and Sport Sciences Reviews.* 2002; 30: 138-143.

45. Sargeant A, Hoinville E, Young A. Maximum leg force and power output during short term dynamic exercise. *Journal of Applied Physiology.* 1981; 26: 188-194.

46. Shehab R, Mirabelli M, Gorenflo D, Fetters M. Pre-exercise stretching and sports related injuries: Knowledge, attitudes and practices. *Clinical Journal of Sports Medicine.* 2006; 16(3): 228-231.

47. Shrier I. Stretching before exercise does not reduce the risk of local muscle injury: A critical review of the clinical and bsic science literature. *Clinical Journal of Sports Medicine.* 1999; 9(4): 221-227.

48. Shrier I. Does stretching improve performance? *Clinical Journal of Sports Medicine.* 2004; 14(5): 267-273.

49. Shrier I. When and whom to stretch? *Physician and Sports Medicine.* 2005; 33(3): 22-26.

50. Small K, Naughton L, Matthews M. A systematic review into the efficacy of static stretching as part of a warm-up for the prevention of exercise-related injury. *Research in Sports Medicine.* 2008; 16(3): 213-231.

51. Smith L, Brunetz M, Chenier M, et al. The effects of static stretching and ballistic stretching on delayed onset muscle soreness and creatine kinase. *Research Quarterly for Exercise and Sport.* 1993; 64(1): 103-107.

52. Stone M, O'Bryant HS, Ayers C, Sands W. Stretching: Acute and chronic? The potential consequences. *Strength and Conditioning Journal.* 2006; 28(6): 66-74.

53. Thacker S, Gilchrist D, Stroup C, Kimsey C. The impact of static stretching on sports injury risk: A systematic review of the literature. *Medicine and Science in Sports and Exercise.* 2004; 36: 371-378.

54. Tillin N, Bishop D. Factors modulating post-activation potentiation and its effect on performance of subsequent explosive activities. *Sports Medicine.* 2009; 39(2): 147-166.

55. Verstegen M, Williams P. *Core Performance.* New York: Rodale; 2004.

56. Wilcox J, Larson R, Brochu K, Faigenbaum A. Acute explosive-force movements enhance bench press performance in athletic men. *International Journal of Sports Physiology and Performance.* 2006; 1: 261-269.

57. Winchester JB, Nelson A, Landin D, Young M, Schexnayder IC. Static stretching impairs sprint performance in collegiate track and field athletes. *Journal of Strength and Conditioning Research.* 2008; 22(1): 13-18.

58. Yamaguchi T, Ishii K. Effects of static stretching for 30 seconds and dynamic stretching on leg extension power. *Journal of Strength and Conditioning Research.* 2005; 19(3): 677-683.

59. Young WB, Behm DG. Should static stretching be used during a warm-up for strength and power activities? *Strength and Conditioning Journal.* 2002; 24(6): 33-37.

60. Young WB, Behm DG. Effects of running, static stretching and practice jumps on explosive force production and jumping performance. *Journal of Sports Medicine and Physical Fitness.* March 2003; 43(1): 21-27.

61. Young WB, Elliot S. Acute effects of static stretching, proprioceptive neuromuscular facilitation stretching and maximal voluntary contractions on explosive force production and jumping performance. *Research Quarterly for Exercise and Sport.* 2001; 72: 273-279.

Chapter 4

1. Augustsson J, Esko A, Thomee R, Svantesson U. Weight training of the thigh muscles using closed vs. open kinetic chain exercises: A comparison of performance enhancement. *Journal of Orthopaedic and Sports Physical Therapy.* 1998; 27: 3-8.

2. Baker D, Nance S, Moore M. The load that maximizes the average mechanical power output during explosive bench press throws in highly trained athletes. *Journal of Strength and Conditioning Research.* 2001; 15: 20-24.

3. Baker D, Nance S, Moore M. The load that maximizes the average mechanical power output during jump squats in power-trained athletes. *Journal of Strength and Conditioning Research.* 2001; 15: 92-97.

4. Blackburn JR, Morrissey MC. The relationship between open and closed kinetic chain strength of the lower limb and jumping performance. *Journal of Orthopaedic and Sports Physical Therapy.* 1998; 27: 430-435.

5. Borst SE, Dehoyos DV, Garzarella L, et al. Effects of resistance training on insulin-like growth factor-1 and IGF binding proteins. *Medicine and Science in Sports and Exercise.* 2001; 33, 648-653.

6. Boyer BT. A comparison of the effects of three strength training programs on women. *Journal of Applied Sport Science Research.* 1990; 4: 88-94.

7. Cormie P, McBride JM, McCaulley GO. Validation of power measurement techniques in dynamic lower body resistance exercises. *Journal of Applied Biomechanics.* 2007; 23: 103-118.

8. Cormie P, McCaulley GO, McBride JM. Power versus strength-power jump squat

training: Influence on the load-power relationship. *Medicine and Science in Sports and Exercise.* 2007; 39: 996-1003.

9. Fleck SJ, Kraemer WJ. *Designing Resistance Training Programs.* 2nd ed. Champaign, IL: Human Kinetics; 1997.

10. Graves JE, Pollock ML, Leggett SH, et al. Effect of reduced training frequency on muscular strength. *International Journal of Sports Medicine.* 1988; 9:316-319.

11. Hansen S, Kvorning T, Kjaer M, Szogaard G. The effect of short-term strength training on human skeletal muscle: The importance of physiologically elevated hormone levels. *Scandinavian Journal of Medicine and Science in Sports.* 2001; 11: 347-354.

12. Hoffman JR, Ratamess NA. *A Practical Guide to Developing Resistance Training Programs.* 2nd ed. Monterey, CA: Coaches Choice Books; 2008.

13. Hoffman JR, Kraemer WJ, Fry AC, Deschenes M, Kemp DM. The effect of self-selection for frequency of training in a winter conditioning program for football. *Journal of Applied Sport Science Research.* 1990; 3: 76-82.

14. Hunter GR. Changes in body composition, body build, and performance associated with different weight training frequencies in males and females. *NSCA Journal.* 1985; 7:26-28.

15. Jones K, Hunter G, Fleisig G, Escamilla R, Lemak L. The effects of compensatory acceleration on upper-body strength and power in collegiate football players. *Journal of Strength and Conditioning Research.* 1999; 13: 99-105.

16. Kawamori N, Crum AJ, Blumert PA, et al. Influence of different relative intensities on power output during the hang power clean: Identification of the optimal load. *Journal of Strength and Conditioning Research.* 2005; 19: 698-708.

17. Keeler LK, Finkelstein LH, Miller W, Fernhall B. Early-phase adaptations of traditional-speed vs. superslow resistance training on strength and aerobic capacity in sedentary individuals. *Journal of Strength and Conditioning Research.* 2001; 15: 309-314.

18. Kemmler WK, Lauber D, Engelke K, Weineck J. Effects of single- vs. multiple-set resistance training on maximum strength and body composition in trained postmenopausal women. *Journal of Strength and Conditioning Research.* 2004; 18: 689-694.

19. Keogh JW, Wilson GJ, Weatherby RP. A cross-sectional comparison of different resistance training techniques in the bench press. *Journal of Strength and Conditioning Research.* 1999; 13: 247-258.

20. Kraemer WJ. A series of studies—The physiological basis for strength training in American football: Fact over philosophy. *Journal of Strength and Conditioning Research.* 1997; 11: 131-142.

21. Kraemer WJ, Ratamess NA. Fundamentals of resistance training: Progression and exercise prescription. *Medicine and Science in Sports and Exercise.* 2004; 36: 674-678.

22. Kraemer WJ, Ratamess NA, Fry AC, et al. Influence of resistance training volume and periodization on physiological and performance adaptations in college women tennis players. *American Journal of Sports Medicine.* 2000; 28, 626-633.

23. McBride JM, Triplett-McBride T, Davie A, Newton RU. The effect of heavy- vs. light-load jump squats on the development of strength, power, and speed. *Journal of Strength and Conditioning Research.* 2002; 16: 75-82.

24. McCurdy KW, Langford GA, Doscher MW, Wiley LP, Mallard KG. The effects of short-term unilateral and bilateral lower-body resistance training on measures of strength and power. *Journal of Strength and Conditioning Research.* 2005; 19: 9-15.

25. McGuigan M, Ratamess NA. Strength. In: Ackland TR, Elliott BC, Bloomfield J, eds. *Applied Anatomy and Biomechanics in Sport.* 2nd ed. Champaign, IL: Human Kinetics; 2009: 119-154.

26. Mookerjee S, Ratamess NA. Comparison of strength differences and joint action durations between full and partial range-of-motion bench press exercise. *Journal of Strength and Conditioning Research.* 1999; 13: 76-81.

27. Morrissey MC, Harman EA, Frykman PN, Han KH. Early phase differential effects of slow and fast barbell squat training. *American Journal of Sports Medicine.* 1998; 26: 221-230.

28. Peterson MD, Rhea MR, Alvar BA. Maximizing strength development in athletes: A meta-analysis to determine the dose-response relationship. *Journal of Strength and Conditioning Research.* 2004; 18: 377-382.

29. Ratamess NA. Adaptations to anaerobic training programs. In: Baechle TR, Earle RW, eds. *Essentials of Strength Training and Conditioning.* 3rd ed. Champaign, IL: Human Kinetics; 2008: 93-119.

30. Ratamess, NA, Falvo MJ, Mangine GT, Hoffman JR, Faigenbaum AD, Kang J. The effect of rest interval length on metabolic responses to the bench press exercise. *European Journal of Applied Physiology.* 2007; 100: 1-17.

31. Ratamess NA, Alvar BA, Evetovich TK, et al. American College of Sports Medicine's position stand: Progression models in resistance training for healthy adults. *Medicine and Science in Sports and Exercise.* 2009; 41: 687-708.

32. Rhea MR, Alvar BA, Ball SD, Burkett LN. Three sets of weight training superior to 1 set with equal intensity for eliciting strength. *Journal of Strength and Conditioning Research.* 2002; 16: 525-529.

33. Schilling BK, Falvo MJ, Chiu LZ. Force-velocity, impulse-momentum relationships: Implications for efficacy of purposely slow resistance training. *Journal of Sports Science and Medicine.* 2008; 7: 299-304.

34. Siegel JA, Gilders RM, Staron RS, Hagerman FC. Human muscle power output during upper- and lower-body exercises. *Journal of Strength and Conditioning Research.* 2002; 16: 173-178.

35. Simao R, Farinatti PT, Polito MD, Maior AS, Fleck SJ. Influence of exercise order on the number of repetitions performed and perceived exertion during resistive exercises. *Journal of Strength and Conditioning Research.* 2005; 19: 152-156.

36. Simao R, Farinatti PT, Polito MD, Viveiros L, Fleck SJ. Influence of exercise order on the number of repetitions performed and perceived exertion during resistance exercise in women. *Journal of Strength and Conditioning Research.* 2007; 21: 23-28.

37. Starkey DB, Pollock ML, Ishida Y, et al. Effect of resistance training volume on strength and muscle thickness. *Medicine and Science in Sports and Exercise.* 1996; 28, 1311-1320.

38. Willoughby DS, Gillespie JW. A comparison of isotonic free weights and omnikinetic exercise machines on strength. *Journal of Human Movement Studies.* 1990; 19: 93-100.

39. Wilson GJ, Newton RU, Murphy AJ, Humphries BJ. The optimal training load for the development of dynamic athletic performance. *Medicine and Science in Sports and Exercise.* 1993; 25:1279-1286.

Chapter 5

1. Adams K, O'Shea JP, O'Shea KL, Climstein M. The effect of six weeks of squat, plyometric and squat-plyometric training on power production. *Journal of Applied Sport Science Research.* 1992; 6(1): 36-41.

2. Atha J. Strengthening muscle. *Exercise and Sport Sciences Review.* 1981; 9: 1-73.

3. Baker D. A series of studies on the training of high-intensity muscle power in rugby league football players. *Journal of Strength and Conditioning Research.* 2001; 15(2): 198-209.

4. Bauer T, Thayer RE, Baras G. Comparison of training modalities for power development in the lower extremity. *Journal of Applied Sport Science Research.* 1990; 4(4): 115-21.

5. Behm DG, Sale, DG. Intended rather than actual movement velocity determines velocity-specific training response. *Journal of Applied Physiology.* 1993; 74(1): 359-68.

6. Berger RA. Optimum repetitions for the development of strength. *Research Quarterly.* 1962; 33(3): 334-37.

7. Berger RA. Effects of dynamic and static training on vertical jumping ability. *Research Quarterly.* 1963; 34(4): 419-24.

8. Blazevich AJ, Gill ND, Bronks R, Newton RU. Training-specific muscle architecture adaptation after 5-week training in athletes. *Medicine and Science in Sports and Exercise.* 2003; 35(12): 2013-2022.

9. Bobbert MF, Van Soest AJ. Effects of muscle strengthening on vertical jump height: A simulation study. *Medicine and Science in Sports and Exercise.* 1994; 26(8): 1012-1020.

10. Bobbert MF, Gerritsen KG, Litjens MC, Van Soest AJ. Why is countermovement jump height greater than squat jump height? *Medicine and Science in Sports and Exercise.* 1996; 28(11): 1402-1412.

11. Bosco C, Komi PV. Potentiation of the mechanical behavior of the human skeletal muscle through prestretching. *Acta Physiologica Scandinavica.* 1979; 106(4): 467-472.

12. Bosco C, et al. Bosco C, Viitasalo JT, Komi PV, Luhtanen P. Combined effect of elastic energy and myoelectrical potentiation during stretch-shortening cycle exercise. *Acta Physiologica Scandinavica.* 1982; 114: 557-565.

13. Bottinelli R, Pellegrino MA, Canepari M, Rossi R, Reggiani C. Specific contributions of various muscle fibre types to human muscle performance: An in vitro study. *Journal of Electromyography and Kinesiology.* 1999; 9(2): 87-95.

14. Brown ME, Mayhew JL, Boleach LW. Effect of plyometric training on vertical jump performance in high school basketball players. *Journal of Sports Medicine and Physical Fitness.* 1986; 26(1): 1-4.

15. Caiozzo VJ, Perrine JJ, Edgerton VR. Training-induced alterations of the in vivo force-velocity relationship of human muscle. *Journal of Applied Physiology.* 1981; 51(3): 750-754.

16. Campos GE, Luecke TJ, Wendeln HK, et al. Muscular adaptations in response to three different resistance-training regimens: Specificity of repetition maximum training zones. *European Journal of Applied Physiology.* 2002; 88: 50-60.

17. Canavan PK, Garrett GE, Armstrong LE. Kinematic and kinetic relationships between an Olympic-style lift and the vertical jump. *Journal of Strength and Conditioning Research.* 1996; 10(2): 127-130.

18. Carlock JM, Smith SL, Hartman MJ, et al. The relationship between vertical jump power estimates and weightlifting ability: A field-test approach. *Journal of Strength and Conditioning Research.* 2004; 18(3): 534-539.

19. Chimera NJ, Swanik KA, Swanik CB, Straub SJ. Effects of plyometric training on muscle-activation strategies and performance in female athletes. *Journal of Athletic Training.* 2004; 39(1): 24-31.

20. Chu DA. *Jumping into Plyometrics.* Champaign, IL: Leisure Press; 1992.

21. Clutch D, Wilton M, McGown C, Bryce GR. The effect of depth jumps and weight training on leg strength and vertical jump. *Research Quarterly for Exercise and Sport.* 1983; 54(1): 5-10.

22. Cormie P. A series of investigations into the effect of strength level on muscular power in athletic movements. In *School of Exercise, Biomedical and Health Science.* Perth, WA: Edith Cowan University; 2009: 263.

23. Cormie P, McCaulley GO, McBride JM. Power versus strength-power jump squat training: Influence on the load-power relationship. *Medicine and Science in Sports and Exercise.* 2007; 39(6): 996-1003.

24. Cormie P, McBride JM, McCaulley GO. Power-time, force-time, and velocity-time curve analysis during the jump squat: Impact of load. *Journal of Applied Biomechanics.* 2008; 24(2): 112-120.

25. Cormie P, McCaulley GO, Triplett NT, McBride JM. Optimal loading for maximal power output during lower-body resistance exercises. *Medicine and Science in Sports and Exercise.* 2007; 39(2): 340-349.

26. Coyle EF, Feiring DC, Rotkis TC, et al. Specificity of power improvements through slow and fast isokinetic training. *Journal of Applied Physiology.* 1981; 51(6): 1437-1442.

27. de Haan A, Jones DA, Sargent AJ. Changes in velocity of shortening, power output and relaxation rate during fatigue of rat gastrocnemius muscle. *Pflugers Archive.* 1989; 412(4): 422-428.

28. de Villarreal ES, Kellis E, Kraemer WJ, Izquierdo M. Determining variables of plyometric training for improving vertical jump height performance: A meta-analysis. *Journal of Strength and Conditioning Research.* 2009; 23(2): 495-506.

29. Delbridge A, Bernard JR. *The Macquarie Concise Dictionary.* Sydney, Australia: Macquarie Library; 1988.

30. Desmedt JE, Godaux E. Ballistic contractions in man: Characteristic recruitment pattern of single motor units of the tibialis anterior muscle. *Journal of Physiology.* 1977; 264: 673-693.

31. Desmedt JE, Godaux E. Ballistic contractions in fast or slow human muscles: Discharge patterns of single motor units. *Journal of Physiology.* 1978; 285: 185-196.

32. Duchateau J, Hainaut K. Isometric or dynamic training: Differential effects on mechanical properties of human muscle. *Journal of Applied Physiology.* 1984; 56: 296-301.

33. Dugan EL, Doyle TL, Humphries B, Hasson CJ, Newton RU. Determining the optimal load for jump squats: A review of methods and calculations. *Journal of Strength and Conditioning Research.* 2004; 18(3): 668-674.

34. Ebben WP, Carroll RM, Simenz CJ. Strength and conditioning practices of national hockey league strength and conditioning coaches. *Journal of Strength and Conditioning Research.* 2004; 18(4): 889-897.

35. Ebben WP, Hintz MJ, Simenz CJ. Strength and conditioning practices of major league baseball strength and conditioning coaches. *Journal of Strength and Conditioning Research.* 2005; 19(3): 538-546.

36. Elliott BC, Wilson DJ, Kerr GK. A biomechanical analysis of the sticking region in the bench press. *Medicine and Science in Sports and Exercise.* 1989; 21: 450-462.

37. Ettema GJ, van Soest AJ, Huijing PA. The role of series elastic structures in prestretch-induced work enhancement during isotonic and isokinetic contractions. *Journal of Experimental Biology.* 1990; 154: 121-136.

38. Faulkner JA, Claflin DR, McCully KK. Power output of fast and slow fibers from human skeletal muscles. In: Jones NL, McCartney N, McComas AJ, eds. *Human Muscle Power.* Champaign, IL: Human Kinetics; 1986: 81-94.

39. Fielding RA, LeBrasseur NK, Cuoco A, Bean J, Mizer K, Fiatarone Singh MA. High-velocity resistance training increases skeletal muscle peak power in older women. *Journal of the American Geriatric Society.* 2002; 50(4): 655-662.

40. Garhammer J. A review of power output studies of Olympic and powerlifting: Method-

ology, performance prediction and evaluation tests. *Journal of Strength and Conditioning Research.* 1993; 7(2): 76-89.

41. Garhammer J, Gregor R. Propulsion forces as a function of intensity for weightlifting and vertical jumping. *Journal of Applied Sport Science Research.* 1992; 6(3): 129-134.

42. Gollhofer A, Kyrolainen H. Neuromuscular control of the human leg extensor muscles in jump exercises under various stretch-load conditions. *International Journal of Sports Medicine.* 1991; 12(1): 34-40.

43. Gollnick PD, Bayley WM. Biochemical training adaptations and maximal power. In: Jones NL, McCartney N, McComas AJ, eds. *Human Muscle Power.* Champaign, IL: Human Kinetics; 1986: 255-267.

44. Haff GG, Stone M, O'Bryant HS, et al. Force-time dependent characteristics of dynamic and isometric muscle actions. *Journal of Strength and Conditioning Research.* 1997; 11(4): 269-272.

45. Hakkinen K. Neuromuscular and hormonal adaptations during strength and power training. A review. *Journal of Sports Medicine and Physical Fitness.* 1989; 29(1): 9-26.

46. Häkkinen K, Alen M, Komi PV. Changes in isometric force- and relaxation-time, electromyographic and muscle fibre characteristics of human skeletal muscle during strength training and detraining. *Acta Physiologica Scandinavica.* 1985; 125(4): 573-85.

47. Häkkinen K, Komi PV, Alen M. Effect of explosive type strength training on isometric force- and relaxation-time, electromyographic and muscle fibre characteristics of leg extensor muscles. *Acta Physiologica Scandinavica.* 1985; 125(4): 587-600.

48. Häkkinen K, Komi PV, Tesch PA. Effect of combined concentric and eccentric strength training and detraining on force-time, muscle fibre and metabolic characteristics of leg extensor muscles. *Scandinavian Journal of Sport Science.* 1981; 3: 50-58.

49. Häkkinen K, Mero A, Kauhanen H. Specificity of endurance, sprint and strength training on physical performance capacity in young athletes. *Journal of Sports Medicine and Physical Fitness.* 1989; 29(1): 27-35.

50. Häkkinen K, Komi PV, Alén M, Kauhanen H. EMG, muscle fibre and force production characteristics during a 1 year training period in elite weight-lifters. *European Journal of Applied Physiology.* 1987; 56: 419-427.

51. Häkkinen K, Kallinen M, Izquierdo M, et al. Changes in agonist-antagonist EMG, muscle CSA, and force during strength training in middle-aged and older people. *Journal of Applied Physiology.* 1998; 84(4): 1341-1349.

52. Hannerz J. Discharge properties of motor units in relation to recruitment order in voluntary contraction. *Acta Physiologica Scandinavica.* 1974; 91(3): 374-385.

53. Harris GR, Stone MH, O'Bryant HS, Proulx CM, Johnson RL. Short-term performance effects of high power, high force, or combined weight-training methods. *Journal of Strength and Conditioning Research.* 2000; 14(1): 14-20.

54. Hatfield FC. *Power: A Scientific Approach.* Chicago, IL: Contemporary Books; 1989.

55. Henneman E, Clamann HP, Gillies JD, Skinner RD. Rank order of motoneurons within a pool, law of combination. *Journal of Neurophysiology.* 1974; 37: 1338-1349.

56. Henneman E, Somjen G, Carpenter DO. Functional significance of cell size in spinal motoneurons. *Journal of Neurophysiology.* 1965; 28: 560-580.

57. Holcomb WR, Lander JE, Rutland RM, Wilson GD. The effectiveness of a modified plyometric program on power and the vertical jump. *Journal of Strength and Conditioning Research.* 1996; 10(2): 89-92.

58. Hori N, Newton RU, Nosaka K, Stone MH. Weightlifting exercises enhance athletic performance that requires high-load speed strength. *Strength and Conditioning Journal.* 2005; 27(4): 50-55.

59. Hori N, Newton RU, Andrews WA, Kawamori N, McGuigan MR, Nosaka K. Does performance of hang power clean differentiate performance of jumping, sprinting, and changing of direction? *Journal of Strength and Conditioning Research.* 2008; 22(2): 412-418.

60. Jones K, Bishop P, Hunter G, Fleisig G. The effects of varying resistance-training loads on intermediate- and high-velocity-specific adaptations. *Journal of Strength and Conditioning Research.* 2001; 15(3): 349-356.

61. Kanehisa H, Miyashita M. Specificity of velocity in strength training. *European Journal of Applied Physiology and Occupational Physiology.* 1983; 52(1): 104-106.

62. Kaneko M, Fuchimoto T, Toji H, Suei K. Training effect of different loads on the force-velocity relationship and mechanical power output in human muscle. *Scandinavian Journal of Medicine and Science in Sports.* 1983; 5(2): 50-55.

63. Kawamori N, Haff GG. The optimal training load for the development of muscular power. *Journal of Strength and Conditioning Research.* 2004; 18(3): 675-684.

64. Kawamori N, Crum AJ, Blumert PA, et al. Influence of different relative intensities on power output during the hang power clean: Identification of the optimal load. *Journal of Strength and Conditioning Research.* 2005; 19(3): 698-708.

65. Knuttgen HG, Kraemer WJ. Terminology and measurement in exercise performance. *Journal of Applied Sport Science Research.* 1987; 1: 1-10.

66. Komi PV. The stretch-shortening cycle and human power output. In: Jones NL, McCartney N, McComas AJ, eds. *Human Muscle Power.* Champaign, IL: Human Kinetics; 1986: 27-40.

67. Komi PV, Häkkinen K. Strength and power. In: Dirix A, Knuttgen HG, Tittel K, eds. *The Olympic Book of Sports Medicine.* Boston, MA: Blackwell Scientific; 1988.

68. Kraemer WJ. Involvement of eccentric muscle action may optimize adaptations to resistance training. In: *Sports Science Exchange.* Chicago, IL: Gatorade Sports Science Institute; 1992.

69. Kraemer WJ, Newton RU. Training for muscular power. *Physical Medicine and Rehabilitation Clinics of North America.* 2000; 11(2): 341-368.

70. Kyröläinen H, Avela J, McBride JM, et al. Effects of power training on muscle structure and neuromuscular performance. *Scandinavian Journal of Medicine and Science in Sports.* 2005; 15(1): 58-64.

71. Lamas L, Aoki MS, Ugrinowitsch C, et al. Expression of genes related to muscle plasticity after strength and power training regimens. *Scandinavian Journal of Medicine and Science in Sports.* [ePub] 2009.

72. Lesmes G. Muscle strength and power changes during maximal isokinetic training. *Medicine and Science in Sports and Exercise.* 1978; 10: 266-269.

73. Lyttle AD, Wilson G, Ostrowski KJ. Enhancing performance: Maximal power versus combined weights and plyometrics training. *Journal of Strength and Conditioning Research.* 1996; 10(3): 173-179.

74. Malisoux L, Francaux M, Nielens H, Theisen D. Stretch-shortening cycle exercises: An effective training paradigm to enhance power output of human single muscle fibers. *Journal of Applied Physiology.* 2006; 100(3): 771-779.

75. Matavulj D, Kukolj M, Ugarkovic D, Tihanyi J, Jaric S. Effects of plyometric training on jumping performance in junior basketball players. *Journal of Sports Medicine and Physical Fitness.* 2001; 41(2): 159-164.

76. McBride JM, Triplett-McBride T, Davie A, Newton RU. The effect of heavy- vs. light-load jump squats on the development of strength, power, and speed. *Journal of Strength and Conditioning Research.* 2002; 16(1): 75-82.

77. Moffroid MT, Whipple RH. Specificity of speed of exercise. *Physical Therapy.* 1970; 50: 1692-1700.

78. Moss BM, Refsnes PE, Abildgaard A, Nicolaysen K, Jensen J. Effects of maximal effort strength training with different loads on dynamic strength, cross-sectional area, load-power and load-velocity relationships. *European Journal of Applied Physiology and Occupational Physiology.* 1997; 75(3): 193-199.

79. Narici MV, Roi GS, Landoni L, Minetti AE, Cerretelli P. Changes in force cross-sectional area and neural activation during strength training and detraining of the human quadriceps. *European Journal of Applied Physiology.* 1989; 59: 310-319.

80. Newton RU, Kraemer WJ. Developing explosive muscular power: Implications for a mixed method training strategy. *Strength and Conditioning Journal.* 1994; 16(5): 20-31.

81. Newton RU, Kraemer WJ, Häkkinen K. Effects of ballistic training on preseason preparation of elite volleyball players. *Medicine and Science in Sports and Exercise.* 1999; 31(2): 323-330.

82. Newton RU, Kraemer WJ, Häkkinen K, Humphries B, Murphy AJ. Kinematics, kinetics, and muscle activation during explosive upper body movements. *Journal of Applied Biomechanics.* 1996; 12: 31-43.

83. Newton RU, Rogers RA, Volek JS, Häkkinen K, Kraemer WJ. Four weeks of optimal load ballistic resistance training at the end of season attenuates declining jump performance of women volleyball players. *Journal of Strength and Conditioning Research.* 2006; 20(4): 955-961.

84. Newton RU, Häkkinen K, Häkkinen A, McCormick M, Volek J, Kraemer WJ. Mixed-methods resistance training increases power and strength of young and older men. *Medicine and Science in Sports and Exercise.* 2002; 34(8): 1367-1375.

85. Newton RU, Murphy AJ, Humphries BJ, Wilson GJ, Kraemer WJ, Häkkinen K. Influence of load and stretch shortening cycle on the kinematics, kinetics and muscle activation that occurs during explosive upper-body movements. *European Journal of Applied Physiology and Occupational Physiology.* 1997; 75(4): 333-342.

86. Roman WJ, Fleckenstein J, Stray-Gundersen J, Alway SE, Peshock R, Gonyea WJ. Adaptations in the elbow flexors of elderly males after heavy-resistance training. *Journal of Applied Physiology.* 1993; 74(2): 750-754.

87. Sale DG. Influence of exercise and training on motor unit activation. *Exercise and Sport Science Review.* 1987; 15: 95-151.

88. Schilling BK, Stone MH, O'Bryant HS, Fry AC, Coglianese RH, Pierce KC. Snatch technique of collegiate national level weightlifters. *Journal of Strength and Conditioning Research.* 2002; 16(4): 551-555.

89. Schmidtbleicher D. Training for power events. In: Komi PV, ed. *Strength and Power in Sport.* Oxford: Blackwell Scientific; 1992: 381-395.

90. Schmidtbleicher D, Buehrle M. Neuronal adaptation and increase of cross-sectional area studying different strength training methods. *Biomechanics.* 1987; X-B: 615-620.

91. Schmidtbleicher D, Gollhofer A, Frick U. Effects of a stretch-shortening typed training on the performance capability and innervation characteristics of leg extensor muscles. In: de Groot G, et al., eds. *Biomechanics XI-A.* Amsterdam: Free University Press; 1988: 185-189.

92. Simenz CJ, Dugan CA, Ebben WP. Strength and conditioning practices of national basketball association strength and conditioning coaches. *Journal of Strength and Conditioning Research.* 2005; 19(3): 495-504.

93. Stone ME, Johnson R, Carter D. A short term comparison of two different methods of resistive training on leg strength and power. *Athletic Training.* 1979; 14: 158-160.

94. Stowers T, McMillian J, Scala D, Davis V, Wilson D, Stone M. The short-term effects of three different strength-power training methods. *NSCA Journal.* 1983; 5(3): 24-27.

95. Toji H, Kaneko M. Effect of multiple-load training on the force-velocity relationship. *Journal of Strength and Conditioning Research.* 2004; 18(4): 792-795.

96. Toji H, Suei K, Kaneko M. Effects of combined training loads on relations among force, velocity, and power development. *Canadian Journal of Applied Physiology.* 1997; 22(4): 328-336.

97. Tricoli V, Lamas L, Carnevale R, Ugrinowitsch C. Short-term effects on lower-body functional power development: Weightlifting vs. vertical jump training programs. *Journal of Strength and Conditioning Research.* 2005; 19(2): 433-437.

98. van Leeuwen JL. Optimum power output and structural design of sarcomeres. *Journal of Theoretical Biology.* 1991; 149: 229-256.

99. Wathen D. Position statement: Explosive/plyometric exercises. *NSCA Journal.* 1993; 15(3): 16-19.

100. Widrick JJ, Stelzer JE, Shoepe TC, Garner DP. Functional properties of human muscle fibers after short-term resistance exercise training. *American Journal of Physiology—Regulatory, Integrative and Comparative Physiology.* 2002; 283(2): R408-R416.

101. Wilson GJ, Murphy AJ, Walshe AD. Performance benefits from weight and plyometric training: Effects of initial strength level. *Coaching Sport Science Journal.* 1997; 2(1): 3-8.

102. Wilson GJ, Newton RU, Murphy AJ, Humphries BJ. The optimal training load for the development of dynamic athletic performance. *Medicine and Science in Sports and Exercise.* 1993; 25(11): 1279-1286.

103. Winchester JB, McBride JM, Maher MA, et al. Eight weeks of ballistic exercise improves power independently of changes in strength and muscle fiber type expression. *Journal of Strength and Conditioning Research.* 2008; 22(6): 1728-1734.

104. Winter DA. *Biomechanics and Motor Control of Human Movement.* New York, NY: Wiley; 1990.

105. Young WB. Training for speed/strength: Heavy versus light loads. *NSCA Journal.* 1993; 15: 34-42.

106. Young WB, Bilby GE. The effect of voluntary effort to influence speed of contraction on strength, muscular power, and hypertrophy development. *Journal of Strength and Conditioning Research.* 1993; 7(3): 172-178.

107. Zatsiorsky VM, Kraemer WJ. *Science and Practice of Strength Training.* 2nd ed. Champaign, IL: Human Kinetics; 2006.

Chapter 6

1. Costill DL, Coyle EF, Fink WJ, Lesmes GR, Witzmann FA. Adaptations in skeletal muscle following strength training. *Journal of Applied Physiology.* 1979; 46: 96-99.

2. Dudley GA, Abraham WM, Terjung RL. Influence of exercise intensity and duration

on biochemical adaptations in skeletal muscle. *Journal of Applied Physiology.* 1982; 53: 844-850.

3. Fitts RH. Substrate supply and energy metabolism during brief high intensity exercise: Importance in limiting performance. In: Lamb DR, Gisolfi CV, eds. *Energy Metabolism in Exercise and Sport.* Madison, WI: Brown & Benchmark; 1992: 53-105.

4. Gjovaag TF, Dahl HA. Effect of training with different intensities and volumes on muscle fibre enzyme activity and cross sectional area in the m. triceps brachii. *European Journal of Applied Physiology.* 2008; 103: 399-409.

5. Hoffman JR. *Physiological Aspects of Sports Training and Performance.* Champaign, IL: Human Kinetics; 2002: 93-108.

6. Houston ME, Wilson DM, Green HJ, Thomson JA, Ranney DA. Physiological and muscle enzyme adaptations to two different intensities of swim training. *European Journal of Applied Physiology.* 1981; 46: 283-291.

7. Howald H, Hoppeler H, Claassen H, Mathieu O, Staub R. Influence of endurance training on the ultrastructural composition of the different muscle fiber types in humans. *Pflugers Archives.* 1985; 403: 369-376.

8. Jacobs I, Esbjornsson M, Sylven C, Holm I, Jansson E. Sprint training effects on muscle myoglobin, enzymes, fiber types, and blood lactate. *Medicine and Science in Sports and Exercise.* 1987; 19: 368-374.

9. Jansson E, Sjodin B, Tesch P. Changes in muscle fibre type distribution in man after physical training. *Acta Physiologica Scandinavica.* 1978; 104: 235-237.

10. Jansson E, Esbjornsson M, Holm I, Jacobs I. Increases in the proportion of fast-twitch muscle fibres in sprint training in males. *Acta Physiologica Scandinavica.* 1990; 140: 359-363.

11. Kraemer WJ, Gotshalk LA. Physiology of American football. In: Garrett WE, Kirkendall DT, eds. *Exercise and Sport Science.* Philadelphia, PA: Lippincott, Williams and Wilkins; 2000: 795-813.

12. Kraemer WJ, Patton JF, Gordon SE, et al. Compatibility of high-intensity strength and endurance training on hormonal and skeletal muscle adaptations. *Journal of Applied Physiology.* 1995; 78: 976-989.

13. Lepretre PM, Vogel T, Brechat PH, et al. Impact of short-term aerobic interval training on maximal exercise in sedentary aged subjects. *International Journal of Clinical Practice.* 2009; 63: 1472-1478.

14. Linossier MT, Dormois D, Perier C, Frey J, Geyssant A, Denis C. Enzyme adaptations of human skeletal muscle during bicycle short-sprint training and detraining. *Acta Physiologica Scandinavica.* 1997; 161: 439-445.

15. MacDougall JD, Ward GR, Sale DG, Sutton JR. Biochemical adaptations of human skeletal muscle to heavy resistance training and immobilization. *Journal of Applied Physiology.* 1977; 43: 700-703.

16. Parra J, Cadefau JA, Rodas G, Amigo N, Cusso R. The distribution of rest periods affects performance and adaptations of energy metabolism induced by high-intensity training in human muscle. *Acta Physiologica Scandinavica.* 2000; 169: 157-165.

17. Sharp RL, Costill DL, Fink WJ, King DS. Effects of eight weeks of bicycle ergometer sprint training on human muscle buffer capacity. *International Journal of Sports Medicine.* 1986; 7: 13-17.

18. Simoneau JA, Lortie G, Boulay MR, Marchotte M, Thibault MC, Bouchard C. Human skeletal muscle fiber type alteration with high intensity intermittent training. *European Journal of Applied Physiology.* 1985; 54: 240-253.

19. Staron RS, Milicky ES, Leonardi MJ, Falkel JE, Hagerman FC, Dudley GA. Muscle hypertrophy and fast fiber type conversions in heavy resistance trained women. *European Journal of Applied Physiology.* 1989; 60: 71-79.

20. Staron RS, Karapondo DL, Kraemer WJ, et al. Skeletal muscle adaptations during early phase of heavy resistance training in men and women. *Journal of Applied Physiology.* 1994; 76(3): 1247-1255.

21. Staron RS, Leonardi MJ, Karapondo DL, et al. Strength and skeletal muscle adaptations in heavy resistance trained women after detraining and retraining. *Journal of Applied Physiology.* 1991; 70(2): 631-640.

22. Tanisho K, Harikawa K. Training effects on endurance capacity in maximal intermittent exercise: Comparison between continuous and interval training. *Journal of Strength and Conditioning Research.* 2009; 23: 2405-2410.

23. Troup JP, Metzger JM, Fitts RH. Effect of high-intensity exercise on functional capacity of limb skeletal muscle. *Journal of Applied Physiology.* 1986; 60: 1743-1751.

24. Walter AA, Smith AE, Kendall KL, Stout JR, Cramer JT. Six weeks of high-intensity interval training with and without beta-alanine supplementation for improving cardiovascular fitness in women. *Journal of Strength and Conditioning Research.* 2010; 24: 1199-1207.

Chapter 7

1. Baechle TR, Earle RW, NSCA (US). *Essentials of Strength Training and Conditioning.* 3rd ed. Champaign, IL: Human Kinetics; 2008.

2. Bompa TO. *Periodization: Theory and Methodology of Training.* 4th ed. Champaign, IL: Human Kinetics; 1999.

3. Borg G. Perceived exertion as an indicator of somatic stress. *Scandanavian Journal of Rehabilitation Medicine.* 1970; 2: 92-98.

4. Boulay MR, Simoneau JA, Lortie G, Bouchard C. Monitoring high-intensity endurance exercise with heart rate and thresholds. *Medicine and Science in Sports and Exercise.* 1997; 29: 125-132.

5. Budgett R. Overtraining syndrome. *British Journal of Sports Medicine.* 1990; 24: 231-236.

6. Cavanagh PR, Williams KR. The effect of stride length variation on oxygen uptake during distance running. *Medicine and Science in Sports and Exercise.* 1982; 14: 30-35.

7. Coyle EF, Coggan AR, Hopper MK, Walters TJ. Determinants of endurance in well-trained cyclists. *Journal of Applied Physiology.* 1988; 64: 2622-2630.

8. Cureton KJ, Sparling PB, Evans BW, Johnson SM, Kong UD, Purvis JW. Effect of experimental alterations in excess weight on aerobic capacity and distance running performance. *Medicine and Science in Sports.* 1978; 10: 194-199.

9. Daniels J. Training distance runners—A primer. *Gatorade Sports Science Exchange.* 1989; 1-5.

10. Edge J, Bishop D, Goodman C, Dawson B. Effects of high- and moderate-intensity training on metabolism and repeated sprints. *Medicine and Science in Sports and Exercise.* 2005; 37: 1975-1982.

11. Evans M. *Endurance Athlete's Edge.* Champaign, IL: Human Kinetics; 1997: 229.

12. Fry RW, Morton AR, Garcia-Webb P, Crawford GP, Keast D. Biological responses to overload training in endurance sports. *European Journal of Applied Physiology and Occupational Physiology.* 1992; 64: 335-344.

13. Fry RW, Morton AR, Keast D. Overtraining in athletes. An update. *Sports Medicine.* 1991; 12: 32-65.

14. Gastin PB. Energy system interaction and relative contribution during maximal exercise. *Sports Medicine.* 2001; 31: 725-741.

15. Gibala MJ. High-intensity interval training: A time-efficient strategy for health promotion? *Current Sports Medicine Reports.* 2007; 6: 211-213.

16. Helgerud J, Hoydal K, Wang E, et al. Aerobic high-intensity intervals improve $\dot{V}O_2$max more than moderate training. *Medicine and Science in Sports and Exercise.* 2007; 39: 665-671.

17. Hoffman JR. The relationship between aerobic fitness and recovery from high-intensity exercise in infantry soldiers. *Military Medicine.* 1997; 162: 484-488.

18. Holloszy JO, Coyle, EF. Adaptations of skeletal muscle to endurance exercise and their metabolic consequences. *Journal of Applied Physiology.* 1984; 56: 831-838.

19. Howarth KR, Moreau NA, Phillips SM, Gibala MJ. Coingestion of protein with carbohydrate during recovery from endurance exercise stimulates skeletal muscle protein synthesis in humans. *Journal of Applied Physiology.* 2009; 106: 1394-1402.

20. Kerksick C, Harvey T, Stout J, et al. International Society of Sports Nutrition's position stand: Nutrient timing. *Journal of the International Society of Sports Nutrition.* 2008; 5: 17.

21. Koutedakis Y, Budgett R, Faulmann L. Rest in underperforming elite competitors. *British Journal of Sports Medicine.* 1990; 24: 248-252.

22. Kraemer WJ, Ratamess NA. Fundamentals of resistance training: Progression and exercise prescription. *Medicine and Science in Sports and Exercise.* 2004; 36: 674-688.

23. Kyle CR, Caiozzo VJ. The effect of athletic clothing aerodynamics upon running speed. *Medicine and Science in Sports and Exercise.* 1986; 18: 509-515.

24. Matvyev L. *Fundamentals of Sports Training.* [English translation of the revised Russian edition.] Moscow: Progress; 1981

25. McArdle WD, Katch FI, Katch VL. *Exercise Physiology: Energy, Nutrition, & Human Performance.* 6th ed. Baltimore, MD: Lippincott Williams & Wilkins; 2007.

26. Morgan DW, Craib M. Physiological aspects of running economy. *Medicine and Science in Sports and Exercise.* 1993; 24: 456-461.

27. Morgan WP, Pollock ML. Psychological characterization of the elite distance runner. *Annals of the NY Academy of Sciences.* 1977; 301: 382-403.

28. Paavolainen L, Hakkinen K, Hamalainen I, Nummela A, Rusko H. Explosive-strength training improves 5 km running time by improving running economy and muscle power. *Journal of Applied Physiology.* 1999; 86: 1527-1533.

29. Pate RR, Branch JD. Training for endurance sport. *Medicine and Science in Sports and Exercise.* 1992; 24: S340-343.

30. Pollock ML, Gaesser GA, Butcher JD, et al. The recommended quantity and quality of exercise for developing and maintaining cardiorespiratory and muscular fitness and flexibility in healthy adults. *Medicine and Science in Sports and Exercise.* 1998; 30.

31. Powers, SK, Howley ET, eds. *Exercise Physiology: Theory and Application to Fitness and Performance.* Dubuque, IA: Brown & Benchmark; 1997.

32. Raglin JS. The psychology of the marathoner: Of one mind and many. *Sports Medicine.* 2007; 37: 404-407.

33. Shepley B, MacDougall JD, Cipriano N, Sutton JR, Tarnopolsky MA, Coates G. Physiological effects of tapering in highly trained athletes. *Journal of Applied Physiology.* 1992; 72: 706-711.

34. Smith AE, Moon JR, Kendall KL, et al. The effects of beta-alanine supplementation and high-intensity interval training on neuromuscular fatigue and muscle function. *European Journal of Applied Physiology.* 2009; 105: 357-363.

35. Smith DJ. A framework for understanding the training process leading to elite performance. *Sports Medicine*. 2003; 33: 1103-1126.

36. Stevinson CD, Biddle SJ. Cognitive orientations in marathon running and "hitting the wall." *British Journal of Sports Medicine*. 1998; 32: 229-234.

37. Tabata I, Nishimura K, Kouzaki M, et al. Effects of moderate-intensity endurance and high-intensity intermittent training on anaerobic capacity and $\dot{V}O_2$max. *Medicine and Science in Sports and Exercise*. 1996; 28: 1327-1330.

38. Zupan MF, Petosa PS. Aerobic and resistance cross-training for peak triathlon performance. *Strength and Conditioning Journal*. 1995; 17: 7-12.

Chapter 8

1. Brown TD, Vescovi JD. Efficient arms for efficient agility. *Strength and Conditioning Journal*. 2003; 25(4): 7-11.

2. Brughelli M, Cronin J, Levin G, Chaouachi A. Understanding change of direction ability in sport: A review of resistance training studies. *Sports Medicine*. 2008; 38(12): 1045-1063.

3. Christou M, Smilios I, Sotiropoulos K, Volaklis K, Pilianidis T, Tokmakidis SP. Effects of resistance training on the physical capacities of adolescent soccer players. *Journal of Strength and Conditioning Research*. 2006; 20(4): 783-791.

4. Cressey EM, West CA, Tiberio DP, Kraemer WJ, Maresh CM. The effects of ten weeks of lower-body unstable surface training on markers of athletic performance. *Journal of Strength and Conditioning Research*. 2007; 21(2): 561-567.

5. Di Michele RD, Di Renzo AM, Ammazzalorso S, Merni F. Comparison of physiological responses to an incremental running test on treadmill, natural grass, and synthetic turf in young soccer players. *Journal of Strength and Conditioning Research*. 2009; 23(3): 939-945.

6. Fry AC, Kraemer WJ, Weseman CA, et al. The effects of an off-season strength and conditioning program on starters and non-starters in women's intercollegiate volleyball. *Journal of Applied Sport Science Research*. 1991; 5(4): 174-181.

7. Gabbett T. Performance changes following a field conditioning program in junior and senior rugby league players. *Journal of Strength and Conditioning Research*. 2006; 20(1): 215-221.

8. Gabbett T, Georgieff B, Anderson S, Cotton B, Savovic D, Nicholson L. Changes in skill and physical fitness following training in talent-identified volleyball players. *Journal of Strength and Conditioning Research*. 2006; 20(1): 29-35.

9. Graham J, Ferrigno V. Agility and balance training. In: Brown, LE, Ferrigno, VA, eds. *Training for Speed, Agility, and Quickness*. 2nd ed. Champaign, IL: Human Kinetics; 2005.

10. Hoffman, JR. *Norms for Fitness, Performance, and Health*. 1st ed. Champaign, IL: Human Kinetics; 2006.

11. Hoffman JR, Cooper J, Wendell M, Kang J. Comparison of Olympic vs. traditional power lifting training programs in football players. *Journal of Strength and Conditioning Research*. 2004; 18(1): 129-135.

12. Hoffman JR, Ratamess NA, Cooper JJ, Kang J, Chilakos A, Faigenbaum AD. Comparison of loaded and unloaded jump squat training on strength/power performance in college football players. *Journal of Strength and Conditioning Research*. 2005; 19(4): 810-815.

13. Kraemer WJ, Hakkinen K, Triplett-Mcbride NT, et al. Physiological changes with periodized resistance training in women tennis players. *Medicine and Science in Sports and Exercise*. 2003; (35)1: 157-168.

14. Markovic G, Jukic I, Milanovic D, Metikos D. Effects of sprint and plyometric training on muscle function and athletic performance. *Journal of Strength and Conditioning Research.* 2007; 21(2): 543-549.

15. McBride JM, Triplett-McBride T, Davie A, Newton RU. The effect of heavy- vs. light-load jump squats on the development of strength, power, and speed. *Journal of Strength and Conditioning Research.* 2002; 16(1): 75-82.

16. Miller MG, Herniman JJ, Ricard MD, Cheatham CC, Michael TJ. The effects of a 6-week plyometric training program on agility. *Journal of Sports Science and Medicine.* 2006; 5: 459-465.

17. Murias JM, Lanatta D, Arcuri CR, Laino FA. Metabolic and functional responses playing tennis on different surfaces. *Journal of Strength and Conditioning Research.* 2007; 21(1): 112-117.

18. Polman R, Walsh D, Bloomfield J, Nesti M. Effective conditioning of female soccer players. *Journal of Sport Science.* 2004; 22: 191-203.

19. Roozen M. Illinois agility test. *NSCA's Performance Training Journal.* 2004; 3(5): 5-6.

20. Sheppard JM, Young WB. Agility literature review: Classifications, training and testing. *Journal of Sports Science.* 2006; 24(9): 919-932.

21. Tricoli V, Lamas L, Carnevale R, Ugrinowitsch C. Short-term effects on lower-body functional power development: Weightlifting vs. vertical jump training programs. *Journal of Strength and Conditioning Research.* 2005; 19(2): 433-437.

22. Young WB, McDowell MH, Scarlett BJ. Specificity and sprint and agility training methods. *Journal of Strength and Conditioning Research.* 2001; 15(3): 315-319.

Chapter 9

1. Abe T, Kumagai K, Brechue WF. Fascicle length of leg muscles is greater in sprinters than distance runners. *Medicine and Science in Sports and Exercise.* 2000; 32(6): 1125-1129.

2. Arthur M, Bailey B. *Complete Conditioning for Football.* Champaign, IL: Human Kinetics; 1998.

3. Balyi I. Long-term athlete development: Trainability in childhood and adolescence. *Olympic Coach.* 2004; 16(1): 4-9.

4. Berg K, Latin RW, Baechle T. Physical and performance characteristics of NCAA division I football players. *Research Quarterly for Exercise and Sport.* 1990; 61: 395-401.

5. Black W, Roundy E. Comparisons of size, strength, speed, and power in NCAA division I-A football players. *Journal of Strength and Conditioning Research.* 1994; 8: 80-85.

6. Bosco C, Vittori C. Biomechanical characteristics of sprint running during maximal and supramaximal speed. *New Studies in Athletics.* 1986; 1(1): 39-45.

7. Cissik J. Means and methods of speed training, part I. *National Strength and Conditioning Association Journal.* 2004; 26 (4): 24-29.

8. Cissik J. Means and methods of speed training, part II. *National Strength and Conditioning Association Journal.* 2005; 27 (1): 18-25.

9. Delecluse C. Influence of strength training on sprint running performance: Current findings and implications for training. *Sports Medicine.* 1997; 24(3): 147-156.

10. Dintiman G, Ward B. *Sports Speed.* 3rd ed. Champaign, IL: Human Kinetics; 2003.

11. Enoka RM. *Neuromechanical Basis of Kinesiology.* 3rd ed. Champaign, IL: Human Kinetics; 2000.

12. Faccioni A. Assisted and resisted methods for speed development (part I). *Modern Athlete and Coach.* 1994; 32(2): 3-6.

13. Faccioni A. Assisted and resisted methods for speed development (part II). *Modern Athlete and Coach.* 1994; 32(3): 8-11.

14. Ferrigno V, Brown L, Murray D. Designing sport-specific programs. In: Brown LE, Ferrigno VA. *Training for Speed, Agility and Quickness.* 2nd ed. Champaign, IL: Human Kinetics; 2005: 71-136.

15. Fry AC, Kraemer WJ. Physical performance characteristics of American collegiate football players. *Journal of Applied Sport Science Research.* 1991; 5: 126-138.

16. Harland MJ, Steele JR. Biomechanics of the sprint start. *Sports Medicine.* 1997; 23(1): 11-20.

17. Harman E. Biomechanics of resistance exercise. In: Baechle TR, Earle RW, eds. *Essentials of Strength Training and Conditioning.* 3rd ed. Champaign, IL: Human Kinetics; 2008.

18. Hoffman JR. *Physiological Aspects of Sport Training and Performance.* Champaign, IL: Human Kinetics; 2002.

19. Komi PV. Stretch-shortening cycle. In: Komi PV, ed. *The Encyclopedia of Sports Medicine: Strength and Power in Sport.* 2nd ed. Oxford: Blackwell Science; 2003: 184-202.

20. Kumagai K, Abe T, Bruechue WF, Ryushi T, Takano S, Mizuno M. Sprint performance is related to muscle fascicle length in male 100 m sprinters. *Journal of Applied Physiology.* 2000; 88: 811-816.

21. Lentz D, Hardyk A. Speed training. In: Brown LE, Ferrigno VA, eds. *Training for Speed, Agility and Quickness.* 2nd ed. Champaign, IL: Human Kinetics; 2005: 17-76.

22. Little T, Williams AG. Specificity of acceleration, maximum speed, and agility in professional soccer players. *Journal of Strength and Conditioning Research.* 2005; 19(1): 76-78.

23. Mero A, Komi PV, Gregor RJ. Biomechanics of sprint running. *Sports Medicine.* 1992; 13(6): 376-392.

24. Plisk S. Speed, agility, and speed endurance development. In: Baechle TR, Earle RW, NSCA, eds. *Essentials of Strength Training and Conditioning.* 3rd ed. Champaign, IL: Human Kinetics; 2008: 471-491.

25. Verkhoshansky YV. Principles for a rational organization of the training process aimed at speed development. *New Studies in Athletics.* 1996; 11(2-3): 155-160.

26. Verkhoshansky YV. Quickness and velocity in sports movements. *New Studies in Athletics.* 1996; 11(2-3): 29-37.

27. Verkhoshansky YV. Speed training for high level athletes. *New Studies in Athletics.* 1996; 11(2-3): 39-49.

28. Verkhoshansky YV, Lazarev VV. Principles of planning speed and strength/speed endurance training in sports. *National Strength and Conditioning Association Journal.* 1989; 11(2): 58-61.

29. Young WB, McDowell MH, Scarlett BJ. Specificity of sprint and agility training methods. *Journal of Strength and Conditioning Research.* 2001; 15(3): 315-319.

Chapter 10

1. Cowley PM, Swensen T, Sforzo GA. Efficacy of instability resistance training. *International Journal of Sports Medicine.* 2007; 28: 829-835.

2. Ebenbichler GR, Oddsson LI, Kollmitzer J, Erim Z. Sensory-motor control of the lower back: Implications for rehabilitation. *Medicine and Science in Sports and Exercise.* 2001; 33: 1889-1898.

3. Goodman CA, Pearce AJ, Nicholes CJ, Gatt BM, Fairweather IH. No difference in 1RM

strength and muscle activation during the barbell chest press on a stable and unstable surface. *Journal of Strength and Conditioning Research.* 2008; 22: 88-94.

4. Kerr ZY, Collins CL, Fields SK, Comstock RD. Epidemiology of player-player contact injuries among US high school athletes, 2005-2009. *Clinical Pediatrics.* December 30, 2010. [Epub ahead of print].

5. Kohler JM, Flanagan SP, Whiting WC. Muscle activation patterns while lifting stable and unstable loads on stable and unstable surfaces. *Journal of Strength and Conditioning Research.* 2010; 24: 313-321.

6. Taube W, Gruber M, Gollhofer A. Spinal and supraspinal adaptations associated with balance training and their functional relevance. *Acta Physiologica Scandanavica.* 2008; 193: 101-16.

7. Uribe BP, Coburn JW, Brown LE, Judelson DA, Khamoui AV, Nguyen D. Muscle activation when performing the chest press and shoulder press on a stable bench vs. a Swiss ball. *Journal of Strength and Conditioning Research.* 2010; 24: 1028-1033.

8. Waterman BR, Owens BD, Davey S, Zacchilli MA, Belmont PJ Jr. The epidemiology of ankle sprains in the United States. *Journal of Bone and Joint Surgery.* 2010; 92: 2279-2284.

Chapter 11

1. Baker D, Wilson G, Carlyon R. Periodization: The effect on strength of manipulating volume and intensity. *Journal of Strength and Conditioning Research.* 1994; 8: 235-242.

2. Behm DG. Periodized training program of the Canadian Olympic curling team. *Strength and Conditioning Journal.* 2007; 28: 24-31.

3. Bompa TO. In training, preparation. [Antrenamentul in perioda, pregatitoare.] *Caiet Pentre Sporturi Nautice.* 1956; 3:22-24.

4. Bompa TO. Criteria pregatirii a unui plan departa ani. *Cultura Fizica si Sport.* 1968; 2:11-19.

5. Bompa TO. *Periodization: Theory and Methodology of Training.* 4th ed. Champaign, IL: Human Kinetics; 1999: 414.

6. Bompa TO, Haff GG. *Periodization: Theory and Methodology of Training.* 5th ed. Champaign, IL: Human Kinetics; 2009.

7. Bondarchuk AP. Periodization of sports training. *Legkaya Atletika.* 1986; 12:8-9.

8. Bondarchuk AP. Constructing a training system. *Track Tech.* 1988; 102: 254-269.

9. Bosquet L, Montpetit J, Arvisais D, Mujika I. Effects of tapering on performance: A meta-analysis. *Medicine and Science in Sports and Exercise.* 2007; 39: 1358-1365.

10. Buse GJ, Santana JC. Conditioning strategies for competitive kickboxing. *Strength and Conditioning Journal.* 2008; 30: 42-49.

11. Chiu LZ, Barnes JL. The fitness-fatigue model revistited: Implications for planning short- and long-term training. *NSCA Journal.* 2003; 25: 42-51.

12. Counsilman JE, Counsilman BE. *The New Science of Swimming.* Englewood Cliffs, NJ: Prentice Hall; 1994: 420.

13. Coutts A, Reaburn P, Piva TJ, Murphy A. Changes in selected biochemical, muscular strength, power, and endurance measures during deliberate overreaching and tapering in rugby league players. *International Journal of Sports Medicine.* 2007; 28: 116-124.

14. Coutts AJ, Reaburn P, Piva TJ, Rowsell GJ. Monitoring for overreaching in rugby league players. *European Journal of Applied Physiology.* 2007; 99: 313-324.

15. Dick FW. Planning the programme. In: *Sports Training Principles*. London: A and C Black; 1997: 253-304.

16. Dick FW. *Sports Training Principles*. 4th ed. London: A and C Black; 2002: 214.

17. Edington DW, Edgerton VR. *The Biology of Physical Activity*. Boston, MA: Houghton Mifflin; 1976.

18. Fleck S, Kraemer WJ. *Designing Resistance Training Programs*. 3rd ed. Champaign, IL: Human Kinetics; 2004: 375.

19. Foster C. Monitoring training in athletes with reference to overtraining syndrome. *Medicine and Science in Sports and Exercise*. 1998; 30: 1164-1168.

20. Fry AC. The role of training intensity in resistance exercise overtraining and overreaching. In: Kreider RB, Fry AC, O'Toole ML, eds. *Overtraining in Sport*. Champaign, IL: Human Kinetics; 1998: 107-127.

21. Fry AC, Kraemer WJ. Resistance exercise overtraining and overreaching. Neuroendocrine responses. *Sports Medicine*. 1997; 23: 106-129.

22. Fry AC, Kraemer WJ, Stone MH, et al. Endocrine responses to overreaching before and after 1 year of weightlifting. *Canadian Journal of Applied Physiology*. 1994; 19: 400-410.

23. Fry AC, Webber JM, Weiss LW, Fry MD, Li Y. Impaired performance with excessive high-intensity free-weight training. *Journal of Strength and Conditioning Research*. 2000; 14: 54-61.

24. Fry RW, Morton AR, Keast D. Overtraining in athletes. An update. *Sports Medicine*. 1991; 12: 32-65.

25. Fry RW, Morton AR, Keast D. Periodisation of training stress—A review. *Canadian Journal of Sport Science*. 1992; 17: 234-240.

26. Gabbett T, King T, Jenkins D. Applied physiology of rugby league. *Sports Medicine*. 2008; 38: 119-138.

27. Garhammer J. Periodization of strength training for athletes. *Track Tech*. 1979; 73: 2398-2399.

28. Garhammer J, Takano B. Training for weightlifting. In: Komi PV, ed. *Strength and Power in Sport*. Oxford, UK: Blackwell Scientific; 2003: 502-515.

29. Goodwin EP, Adams KJ, Shelburne J. A strength and conditioning model for a female collegiate cheerleader. *Strength and Conditioning Journal*. 2004; 26: 16-21.

30. Haff, GG. *Periodization: Let the Science Guide Our Program Design*. United Kingdom Strength and Conditioning Conference, Belfast, Ireland; 2008.

31. Haff GG, Kraemer WJ, O'Bryant HS, Pendlay G, Plisk S, Stone MH. Roundtable discussion: Periodization of training (part 1). *NSCA Journal*. 2004; 26:50-69.

32. Haff GG, Kraemer WJ, O'Bryant HS, Pendlay G, Plisk S,. Stone MH. Roundtable discussion: Periodization of training (part 2). *NSCA Journal*. 2004; 26: 56-70.

33. Häkkinen K. Neuromuscular adaptations during strength training, aging, detraining, and immobilization. *Critical Reviews in Physical and Rehabilitation Medicine*. 1994; 6: 161-198.

34. Häkkinen K, Pakarinen A, Alen M, Kauhanen H, Komi PV. Daily hormonal and neuromuscular responses to intensive strength training in 1 week. *International Journal of Sports Medicine*. 1988; 9: 422-428.

35. Häkkinen K, Pakarinen A, Alen M, Kauhanen H, Komi PV. Neuromuscular and hormonal responses in elite athletes to two successive strength training sessions in one day. *European Journal of Applied Physiology*. 1988; 57: 133-139.

36. Häkkinen K, Kallinen M. Distribution of strength training volume into one or two daily sessions and neuromuscular adaptations in female athletes. *Electromyography and Clinical Neurophysiology.* 1994; 34: 117-124.

37. Halson SL, Bridge MW, Meeusen R, et al. Time course of performance changes and fatigue markers during intensified training in trained cyclists. *Journal of Applied Physiology.* 2002; 93: 947-956.

38. Harre D. *Principles of Sports Training.* Berlin, Germany: Sportverlag; 1982a.

39. Harre D. *Training Doctrine.* [*Trainingslehre*]. Berlin, Germany: Sportverlag; 1982b.

40. Harris GR, Stone MS, O'Bryant HS, Proulx CM, Johnson RL. Short-term performance effects of high power, high force, or combined weight-training methods. *Journal of Strength and Conditioning Research.* 2000; 14: 14-20.

41. Hartmann J, Tünnemann H. *Fitness and Strength Training.* Berlin, Germany: Sportverlag; 1989.

42. Hoffman JR, Ratamess NA, Klatt M, et al. Comparison between different off-season resistance training programs in Division III American college football players. *Journal of Strength and Conditioning Research.* 2009; 23: 11-19.

43. Issurin V. *Block Periodization: Breakthrough in Sports Training.* Yessis M, ed. Michigan: Ultimate Athlete Concepts; 2008a; 213.

44. Issurin V. Block periodization versus traditional training theory: A review. *Journal of Sports Medicine and Physical Fitness.* 2008b; 48: 65-75.

45. Izquierdo M, Ibanez J, Gonzalez-Badillo JJ, et al. Detraining and tapering effects on hormonal responses and strength performance. *Journal of Strength and Conditioning Research.* 2007; 21: 768-775.

46. Jeffreys I. Quadrennial planning for the high school athlete. *Strength and Conditioning Journal.* 2008; 30: 74-83.

47. Kraemer WJ, Fleck SJ. *Optimizing Strength Training: Designing Nonlinear Periodization Workouts.* Champaign, IL: Human Kinetics; 2007: 245.

48. Kraemer WJ, Hatfield DL, Fleck SJ. Types of muscle training. In: Brown LE, ed. *Strength Training.* Champaign, IL: Human Kinetics; 2007: 45-72.

49. Kurz T. *Science of Sports Training.* 2nd ed. Island Pond, VT: Stadion Publishing Company; 2001.

50. Matveyev LP. *Periodization of Sports Training.* Moscow, Russia: Fizkultura i Sport;1965.

51. Matveyev LP. *Periodization of Sports Training.* 2nd ed. [*Periodisterung Des Sportlichen Trainings.*] Moscow, Russia: Fizkultura i Sport;1972.

52. Matveyev LP. *Fundamentals of Sports Training.* Moscow, Russia: Fizkultua i Sport; 1977.

53. Matveyev LP. About the construction of training. *Modern Athlete and Coach.* 1994; 32: 12-16.

54. Medvedev AS. Training content of weightlifters in the preparatory period. *Soviet Sports Review.* 1982; 17: 90-93.

55. Mujika I, Padilla S. Scientific bases for precompetition tapering strategies. *Medicine and Science in Sports and Exercise.* 2003; 35: 1182-1187.

56. Mujika I, Goya A, Padilla S, Grijalba A, Gorostiaga E, Ibanez J. Physiological responses to a 6-d taper in middle-distance runners: Influence of training intensity and volume. *Medicine and Science in Sports and Exercise.* 2000; 32: 511-517.

57. Nádori L. *Training and Competition.* Budapest: Sport; 1962.

58. Nádori L, Granek I. *Theoretical and Methodological Basis of Training Planning With Special Considerations Within a Microcycle.* Lincoln, NE: NSCA;1989.

59. Olbrect J. *The Science of Winning: Planning, Periodizing, and Optimizing Swim Training.* Luton, England: Swimshop; 2000: 282.

60. Ozolin N. *Athlete's Training System for Competition.* [*Sovremennaia systema sportivnoi trenirovky.*] Moscow, Russia: Fizkultura i Sport; 1971.

61. Pistilli EE, Ginther G, Larsen J. Sport-specific strength-training exercises for the sport of lacrosse. *Strength and Conditioning Journal.* 2008; 30: 31-38.

62. Plisk SS. Speed, agility, and speed-endurance development. In: Baechle TR, Earle RW, eds. *Essentials of Strength Training and Conditioning.* Champaign, IL: Human Kinetics; 2008.

63. Plisk SS, Gambetta V. Tactical metabolic training: Part 1. *Strength and Conditioning Journal.* 1997; 19: 44-53.

64. Plisk SS, Stone MH. Periodization strategies. *Strength and Conditioning Journal.* 2003; 25: 19-37. 2003.

65. Rhea MR, Ball SD, Phillips WT, Burkett LN. A comparison of linear and daily undulating periodized programs with equated volume and intensity for strength. *Journal of Strength and Conditioning Research.* 2002; 16: 250-255.

66. Rowbottom DG. Periodization of training. In: Garrett WE, Kirkendall DT, eds. *Exercise and Sport Science.* Philadelphia, PA: Lippicott Williams and Wilkins; 2000: 499-512.

67. Schmolinsky G. *Track and Field: The East German Textbook of Athletics.* Toronto, Canada: Sports Book; 2004.

68. Selye H. *The Stress of Life.* New York, NY: McGraw-Hill; 1956.

69. Siff MC. *Supertraining.* 6th ed. Denver, CO: Supertraining Institute; 2003: 496.

70. Siff, M.C. and Y.U. Verkhoshansky. *Supertraining.* 4th ed. Denver, CO: Supertraining International. 1999.

71. Smith DJ. A framework for understanding the training process leading to elite performance. *Sports Med.* 2003; 33: 1103-1126.

72. Stone MH, Fry AC. Increased training volume in strength/power athletes. In: Kreider RB, Fry AC, O'Toole ML, eds. *Overtraining in Sport.* Champaign, IL: Human Kinetics; 1998: 87-106.

73. Stone, M.H., H.S. O'bryant, and J. Garhammer. A theoretical model of strength training. *NSCA J.* 1982; 3:36-39.

74. Stone MH, O'Bryant HS. *Weight Training: A Scientific Approach.* Edina, MN: Burgess; 1987.

75. Stone MH, Keith R, Kearney JT, Wilson GD, Fleck SJ. Overtraining: A review of the signs and symptoms of overtraining. *Journal of Applied Sport Science Research.* 1991; 5: 35-50.

76. Stone MH, O'Bryant HS, Schilling BK, et al. Periodization: Effects of manipulating volume and intensity (part 1). *Strength and Conditioning Journal.* 1999; 21: 56-62.

77. Stone MH, O'Bryant HS, Schilling BK, et al. Periodization: Effects of manipulating volume and intensity (part 2). *Strength and Conditioning Journal.* 1999; 21: 54-60.

78. Stone MH, Potteiger JA, Pierce KC, et al. Comparison of the effects of three different weight-training programs on the one repetition maximum squat. *Journal of Strength and Conditioning Research.* 2000; 14: 332-337.

79. Stone MH, Plisk S, Collins D. Training principles: Evaluation of modes and methods of resistance training—A coaching perspective. *Sport Biomechanics.* 2002; 1: 79-104.

80. Stone MH, Stone ME, Sands WA. *Principles and Practice of Resistance Training.* Champaign, IL: Human Kinetics; 2007: 376.

81. Verkhoshansky YU. *Fundamentals of Special Strength Training in Sport.* [*Osnovi Spetsialnoi Silovoi Podgotovki i Sporte.*] Moscow, Russia: Fizkultura i Sport; 1977.

82. Verkhoshansky YU. *Programming and Organization of Training.* Moscow: Fizkultura i Sport; 1985.

83. Verkhoshansky YU. *Fundamentals of Special Strength Training in Sport.* Livonia, MI: Sportivy Press; 1986.

84. Verkhoshansky YU. *Special Strength Training: A Practical Manual for Coaches.* Michigan: Ultimate Athlete Concepts; 2006: 137.

85. Verkhoshansky YU. Theory and methodology of sport preparation: Block training system for top-level athletes. *Teoria i Practica Physicheskoj Culturi.* 2007; 4: 2-14.

86. Viru A. *Adaptations in Sports Training.* Boca Raton, FL: CRC Press; 1995.

87. Yakovlev, N.N. *Sports Biochemistry.* Leipzig, Germany: Deutsche Hochschule für Korperkultur (German Institute For Physical Culture), 1967.

88. Zatsiorsky VM. *Science and Practice of Strength Training.* Champaign, IL: Human Kinetics;1995.

Chapter 12

1. Hoffman JR. *Physiological Aspects of Sports Training and Performance.* Champaign, IL: Human Kinetics; 2002: 93-108.

2. Hoffman JR, Kang J. Strength changes during an inseason resistance training program for football. *Journal of Strength and Conditioning Research.* 2003; 17: 109-114.

3. Hoffman JR, Cooper J, Wendell M, Kang J. Comparison of Olympic versus traditional power lifting training programs in football players. *Journal of Strength and Conditioning Research.* 2004; 18: 129-135.

4. Hoffman JR, Maresh CM. Physiology of basketball. In: Garrett WE, Kirkendall DT, eds. *Exercise and Sport Science.* Philadelphia, PA: Lippincott, Williams and Wilkins; 2000: 733-744.

5. Hoffman JR, Maresh CM, Armstrong LE, Kraemer WJ. The effects of off-season and inseason resistance training programs on a collegiate male basketball team. *Journal of Human Muscle Performance.* 1991; 1: 48-55.

6. Hoffman JR, Wendell M, Cooper J, Kang J. Comparison between linear and nonlinear inseason training programs in freshman football players. *Journal of Strength and Conditioning Research.* 2003; 17: 561-565.

7. Hoffman JR, Fry AC, Deschenes M, Kemp M, Kraemer WJ. The effects of self selection for frequency of training in a winter conditioning program for football. *Journal of Applied Sport Science Research.* 1990; 4(3): 76-82.

8. Hoffman JR, Ratamess NA, Klatt M, et al. Comparison between different resistance training programs in Division III American college football players. *Journal of Strength and Conditioning Research.* 2009; 23: 11-19.

9. Kraemer WJ, Fleck SJ. *Optimizing Strength Training—Designing Nonlinear Periodization Workouts.* Human Kinetics: Champaign, IL; 2007.

10. Kraemer WJ, Patton JF, Gordon SE, et al. Compatibility of high-intensity strength and endurance training on hormonal and skeletal muscle adaptations. *Journal of Applied Physiology.* 1995; 78: 976-989.

11. Tremblay A, Simoneau JA, Bouchard C. Impact of exercise intensity on body fatness and skeletal muscle metabolism. *Metabolism.* 1994; 43: 814-818.

12. USA Track and Field. *USA Track & Field Coaching Manual.* Champaign, IL: Human Kinetics; 2000: 35-62.

Index

Note: The italicized *f* and *t* following page numbers refer to figures and tables, respectively.

About the Editor

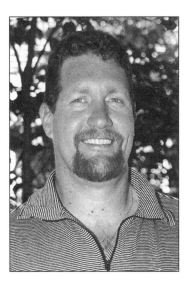

Jay Hoffman, PhD, is a professor of exercise science at the University of Central Florida and coordinator of their sport and exercise science program. Long recognized as an expert in the field of exercise physiology, Hoffman has more than 150 publications to his credit in refereed journals, book chapters, and books, and he has lectured at more than 300 national and international conferences and meetings. He also has more than 17 years of experience coaching at the collegiate and professional levels. This combination of the practical and the theoretical provides him with a unique perspective on writing for both coaches and academic faculty. Hoffman was elected president of the National Strength and Conditioning Association in 2009. He was awarded the 2005 Outstanding Kinesiological Professional Award by the Neag School of Education at the University of Connecticut and the 2007 Outstanding Sport Scientist of the Year by the National Strength and Conditioning Association. He also was awarded the 2000 Outstanding Junior Investigator Award by the NSCA. He is a fellow of the American College of Sports Medicine and serves on the board of directors of the USA Bobsled and Skeleton Federation. He is the author of *Physiological Aspects of Sport Training and Performance* (Human Kinetics, 2002) and *Norms for Fitness, Performance, and Health* (Human Kinetics, 2006).

Contributors

Lee E. Brown, EdD, CSCS*D, FACSM, FNSCA
California State University, Fullerton

James E. Clark, MS
University of Connecticut, Storrs

Brett A. Comstock, MA
University of Connecticut, Storrs

Prue Cormie, PhD
Edith Cowan University, Joondalup, Western Australia

Joel T. Cramer, PhD, CSCS*D, FACSM, FISSN, FNSCA, NSCA-CPT*D
Oklahoma State University, Stillwater

Courtenay Dunn-Lewis, MA
University of Connecticut, Storrs

Avery D. Faigenbaum, EdD, CSCS*D, FNSCA, FACSM
The College of New Jersey, Ewing

John F. Graham, MS, CSCS*D, FNSCA
Lehigh Valley Health Network, Allentown, Pennsylvania

G. Gregory Haff, PhD, ASCC, CSCS*D, FNSCA
Edith Cowan University, Joondalup, Western Australia

Erin E. Haff, MA
Edith Cowan University, Joondalup, Western Australia

Jay R. Hoffman, PhD, CSCS*D, FNSCA
University of Central Florida, Orlando

Andy V. Khamoui, MS, CSCS
The Florida State University, Tallahassee

William J. Kraemer, PhD, CSCS, FNSCA
University of Connecticut, Storrs

Robert U. Newton, PhD, CSCS*D, FNSCA
Edith Cowan University, Joondalup, Western Australia

Nicholas A. Ratamess, PhD, CSCS*D, FNSCA
The College of New Jersey, Ewing

Nejc Sarabon, PhD
University of Ljubljana, Slovenia

Abbie E. Smith, PhD, CSCS*D, CISSN
University of North Carolina, Chapel Hill

Science of Strength and Conditioning Series

The Science of Strength and Conditioning series was developed with the expertise of the National Strength and Conditioning Association (NSCA). This series of texts provides the guidelines for converting scientific research into practical application. The series covers topics such as tests and assessments, program design, and nutrition.

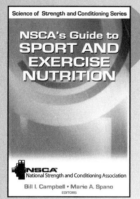

NSCA's Guide to Sport and Exercise Nutrition covers all aspects of food selection, digestion, metabolism, and hydration relevant to sport and exercise performance. This comprehensive resource will help you understand safe and effective ways to improve training and performance through natural nutrition-based ergogenic aids like supplementation and macronutrient intake manipulation. You will also learn guidelines about proper fluid intake to enhance performance and the most important criteria for effectively evaluating the quality of sport drinks and replacement beverages.

NSCA's Guide to Sport and Exercise Nutrition
National Strength and Conditioning Association
Bill I. Campbell, PhD, and Marie A. Spano, MS, Editors
©2011 • Hardback • 320 pp

NSCA's Guide to Program Design moves beyond the simple template presentation of program design to help you grasp the why's and how's of organizing and sequencing training in a sport-specific, appropriate, and safe manner. The text offers 20 tables that are sample workouts or training plans for athletes in a variety of sports, technique photos and instructions for select drills, plus a sample annual training plan that shows how to assemble all the pieces previously presented. Plus, extensive references offer starting points for continued study and professional enrichment.

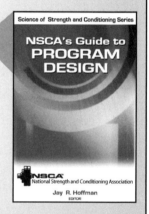

NSCA's Guide to Program Design
National Strength and Conditioning Association
Jay R. Hoffman, PhD, Editor
©2012 • Hardback • 336 pp

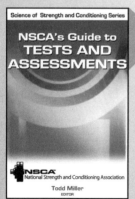

NSCA's Guide to Tests and Assessments presents the latest research from respected scientists and practitioners with expertise in exercise testing and assessment. The text begins with an introduction to testing, data analysis, and formulating conclusions. Then, you'll find a by-chapter presentation of tests and assessments for body composition, heart rate and blood pressure, metabolic rate, aerobic power, lactate threshold, muscular strength, muscular endurance, power, speed and agility, mobility, and balance and stability.

NSCA's Guide to Tests and Assessments
National Strength and Conditioning Association
Todd Miller, PhD, Editor
©2012 • Hardback • 376 pp

For more information, visit our website **www.HumanKinetics.com**.